57792

CLINICAL LABORATORY IMMUNOLOGY

Connie R. Mahon, MS, MT(ASCP)CLS

Adjunct Assistant Professor
Department of Pathology
George Washington University
Washington, DC

Diane Tice, PhD, MT(ASCP)

Associate Professor, Biology
Morrisville State College
Morrisville, New York

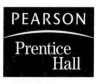

PEARSON

Prentice
Hall

Upper Saddle River, New Jersey 07458

Library of Congress Cataloging-in-Publication Data

Mahon, Connie R.
   Clinical laboratory immunology / Connie R. Mahon, Diane G. Tice.
       p. ; cm. -- (Prentice Hall clinical laboratory science series)
   Includes bibliographical references and index.
   ISBN 0-13-093300-7
   1. Immunodiagnosis.   2. Clinical immunology.
3. Immunology.
   I. Tice, Diane G.   II. Title.   III. Series.
   [DNLM: 1. Immunologic Techniques. 2. Immune System
Diseases--diagnosis.   3. Immune System Diseases--immunol-
ogy.   4. Laboratory Techniques and Procedures.   QW 525
M216c 2006]
   RB46.5.M34 2006
   616.07'9--dc22

                                                        2005013499

Notice:
The authors and the publisher of this volume have taken care that the information and technical recommendations contained herein are based on research and expert consultation, and are accurate and compatible with the standards generally accepted at the time of publication. Nevertheless, as new information becomes available, changes in clinical and technical practices become necessary. The reader is advised to carefully consult manufacturers' instructions and information material for all supplies and equipment before use, and to consult with a health care professional as necessary. This advice is especially important when using new supplies or equipment for clinical purposes. The authors and publisher disclaim all responsibility for any liability, loss, injury, or damage incurred as a consequence, directly or indirectly, of the use and application of any of the contents of this volume.

Publisher: Julie Levin Alexander
Assistant to Publisher: Regina Bruno
Executive Editor: Mark Cohen
Associate Editor: Melissa Kerian
Editorial Assistant: Jaquay Felix
Director of Production and Manufacturing:
   Bruce Johnson
Managing Production Editor: Patrick Walsh
Production Liaison: Julie Li
Production Editor: Jessica Balch, Pine Tree
   Composition

Manufacturing Manager: Ilene Sanford
Manufacturing Buyer: Pat Brown
Design Coordinator: Christopher Weigand
Cover Designer: Joseph DePinho
Director of Marketing: Karen Allman
Channel Marketing Manager: Rachele Strober
Manager of Media Production: Amy Peltier
New Media Project Manager: Stephen Hartner
Composition: Pine Tree Composition, Inc.
Printer/Binder: Courier Westford
Cover Printer: Phoenix Color Corp.

Pearson Prentice Hall™ is a trademark of Pearson Education, Inc.
Pearson® is a registered trademark of Pearson plc.
Prentice Hall® is a registered trademark of Pearson Education, Inc.

Pearson Education Ltd., *London*
Pearson Education Australia Pty. Limited, *Sydney*
Pearson Education Singapore, Pte. Ltd.
Pearson Education North Asia Ltd., *Hong Kong*
Pearson Education Canada, Ltd., *Toronto*

Pearson Educación de Mexico, S.A. de C.V.
Pearson Education—Japan, *Tokyo*
Pearson Education Malaysia, Pte. Ltd.
Pearson Education, Upper Saddle River, New Jersey

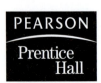

10 9 8 7 6 5 4 3 2 1
ISBN 0-13-093300-7

To my husband Dan,
for his love, support, and understanding;
to my son, Sean Patrick, for his encouragement,
and my daughter Kathleen Elizabeth,
for showing me courage.

—C.M.

To my friends, students, and colleagues
who challenge and stimulate me; to my
family, who support me; to my daughters,
Amanda and Tabitha, who bring me joy;
and to my best friend and husband, Vic,
who sustains me.

—D.T.

CONTENTS

▶ **PART II   Clinical and Laboratory Diagnosis**

FOREWORD

The authors and contributors to *Clinical Laboratory Immunology* present highly detailed technical information and real-life case studies that will help learners envision themselves as members of the health care team, providing the laboratory services specific to immunology that assist in patient care. The mixture of theoretical and practical information relating to immunology provided in this text allows learners to analyze and synthesize this information and, ultimately, to answer questions and solve problems and cases.

Clinical Laboratory Immunology is part of Prentice Hall's Clinical Laboratory Science series of textbooks, which is designed to balance theory and practical applications in a way that is engaging and useful to students. Furthermore, the books in this series are designed to foster various kinds of learning, and some of the titles will be accompanied by computer applications.

We hope that this book, as well as the entire series, proves to be a valuable educational resource.

Elizabeth A. Zeibig, MA, MT(ASCP), CLS(NCA)
CLS Series Editor
Prentice Hall Health

PREFACE

Immunology as a science of study has expanded exponentially during the past several decades. Utilization of immunologic procedures across disciplines in the health sciences has also increased, permeating its applications from detecting agents of infectious diseases and autoimmune disorders to blood abnormalities, genetic disorders, and organ transplantation. Recent developments in technology also include applications of molecular methods in a variety of diagnostic procedures. Students in clinical laboratory sciences therefore must acquire a clear understanding of the principles of immunology and the human immune response to be able to ascertain its applications to laboratory methods and practice.

With this requirement in mind, *Clinical Laboratory Immunology* intends to provide the student with a strong foundation of the basic principles of immunity and the human immune system. To complement the basic concepts, clinical applications are emphasized, demonstrating interdisciplinary relationships in laboratory medicine. We use a building-block type of approach in presenting the concepts, allowing the students to feel comfortable with the background information that they will later apply. Why do we feel that this approach is important in presenting the information to students of immunology?

We find immunology, as a scientific discipline, difficult to introduce to new learners and for new learners to study for several reasons. One is due to the amount of detailed and complicated information available that tends to overwhelm new learners. Trying to assimilate and understand information that constantly evolves as we learn more about human immune diseases and their treatment also tends to be strenuous. Another factor, perhaps just as important, is that the immune system is a complicated network involving several different organ systems interacting with one another, much like athletes on a sports team. New learners find it hard to ascertain the relationships among the "players" in the network, unless a practical approach is used to present the known facts and basic principles. It is, therefore, our intent to provide learners with the basic foundation, concepts, and principles of immunology necessary to understand their applications in clinical laboratory science.

Clinical Laboratory Immunology is divided into three parts. Part I includes chapters that describe the general concepts of immunology, types of immunity, and immune responses. Chapter 1 introduces the learner to the discipline of immunology from a historical perspective. It shows the learner not only how immunology continues to evolve and expand in its clinical applications, but also how concepts interact with one another. An overview of immunity, describing the different immune defenses and the roles they play in defending the human host, is presented in Chapter 2. Chapter 3 presents the structure and functions of immunoglobulins, while Chapter 5 describes the complement system. In Chapter 4, the learner finds an overview of infection and immunity, and a discussion of host-parasite relationships that is unique in an immunology textbook. This chapter provides an impression of how the human host reacts to one of its most common foreign invaders, microorganisms.

Part II presents chapters that discuss principles and procedures involved in the clinical and laboratory diagnosis of infectious diseases (Chapter 7), autoimmune diseases, and other immune disorders. The consequences of "over-reaction" of the immune system expressed as hypersensitivities are presented in Chapter 6; while Chapter 8 covers autoimmune and immune deficiency disorders. We include in Part II chapters in transplantation immunology (Chapter 9), tumor immunology (Chapter 10), and clinical applications of flow cytometry (Chapter 11).

The most outstanding feature of this textbook is the inclusion of molecular diagnostic technology and the multidisciplinary clinical applications of this technology in Part III. We anticipate that within the next several years, clinical laboratory science practitioners will be expected to have had certain, if at least limited, exposure or experience in this technology. Hence, we incorporate chapters that explore the most current applications of molecular methods. Part III begins with a chapter in the principles of hybridization techniques (Chapter 12), followed by a chapter on amplification technology (Chapter 13). Applications of molecular technology in cytogenetics are described in Chapter 14, and in organ transplantation in Chapter 15.

To show the clinical relevance of the content material, each chapter is introduced with a case scenario called Case in Point. This introductory case represents a disease, concept, or principle that is discussed in the chapter text, illustrating the concept or principle through the discussion of the Case in Point. Issues to Consider are points that the learner should be thinking about while reading the chapter, using the Case in Point as place to start. We provide important terms, chapter checklists, points to remember, and learning assessment questions intended help learners understand the key learning elements.

An instructional package is also offered to accompany *Clinical Laboratory Immunology*. The Instructor's Resource Manual contains a wealth of material to help faculty plan and manage the immunology course. It contains chapter outlines, teaching tips, learning objectives, and more for each chapter. The Instructor's Resource CD-ROM provides many resources in an electronic format. First, the CD-ROM contains a complete test bank that allows instructors to create customized exams and quizzes. Second, it includes a lecture package in PowerPoint format. The lectures contain discussion points and embedded images from the textbook to help infuse an extra spark into the classroom experience. Instructors may use this presentation system as it is provided or they may opt to customize it for their specific needs.

Because this textbook is not at all inclusive and is written mainly to provide the learner with a basic but strong foundation of a difficult subject matter, we encourage learners and facilitators to further their experience with additional readings from recommended reference materials. With the attainment of a clear understanding of the basic principles of clinical immunology, we hope that we are able to stimulate the scientific curiosity among learners as much as we, the editors, find this experience rewarding.

Connie R. Mahon
Diane Tice

ACKNOWLEDGMENTS

We are grateful to the contributing authors, especially Kent Weinhold, Steve Mahlen, and Sarah Learmonth, who joined our team at a crucial time of the development process. Special thanks to Linda Smith for taking on an additional chapter and to Bill Nauschuetz for recommending outstanding contributors to this text-book. Many thanks to all others, among them, Beth Zeibig, who made significant suggestions and invaluable comments on ways to improve the outcome of this boc . Thanks to Mark Cohen and Melissa Kerian for their patience and understanding during our most difficult times.

REVIEWERS

Diane Davis, PhD, MT, SC, SLS(ASCP), CLS(NCA)
Associate Professor
Health Sciences Department
Salisbury State University
Salisbury, Maryland

Brandy Greenhill, MS, MT(ASCP)
Education Coordinator
University of Texas—MD Anderson Cancer Center
Houston, Texas

Cecelia W. Landin, MS, MT(ASCP)
Program Director
Clinical Laboratory Science
Affinity Health System
St. Elizabeth's Hospital
Appleton, Wisconsin

Karen Long, MS, CLS(NCA), MT(ASCP)
Associate Professor
Medical Technology Program
West Virginia University
Morgantown, West Virginia

Leslie J. Lovett, MS
Associate Professor
Medical Laboratory Technology
Fairmont State Community and Technical College
Fairmont, West Virginia

Wendy Miller, MS, MT(ASCP)SI
Program Director
Clinical Laboratory Technology
Elgin Community College
Elgin, Illinois

Eileen Patton, MS, MT(ASCP), RM(AAM)
Instructor
Department of Medical and Research Technology
University of Maryland School of Medicine
Baltimore, Maryland

Diane Wyatt, MS, MT(ASCP)
Associate Professor
Program in Medical Technology
University of Tennessee Health Science Center
Memphis, Tennessee

CONTRIBUTORS

Angela Braham-Thompson, BS
Infectious Disease Labs
Walter Reed Army Medical Center
Washington, DC
Chapter 7

Colonel David W. Craft, PhD, D(ABMM)
Chief, Infectious Disease Labs
Walter Reed Army Medical Center
Washington, DC
Chapter 7

Betty Dunn, MS
Cytogenetics Program Director
Department of Clinical Laboratory Sciences
University of Texas Health Science Center
San Antonio, Texas
Chapter 14

Michelle S. Kanuth, PhD, CLS(NCA), MT(ASCP)SBB
Associate Professor
Clinical Laboratory Sciences Department
University of Texas Medical Branch
Galveston, Texas
Chapters 3, 5, & 8

Sarah Learmonth, MS
First Lieutenant, United States Army
Chief, Immunology
Brooke Army Medical Center
Fort Sam Houston, Texas
Chapter 7

Steven Mahlen, PhD
Medical Director, Microbiology
Madigan Army Medical Center
Tacoma, Washington
Chapter 13

Connie Mahon, MS, MT(ASCP)CLS
Adjunct Assistant Professor
Department of Pathology
George Washington University
Washington, DC
Chapters 2 & 4

Linda E. Miller, PhD
Professor, Department of Clinical Laboratory Science
Director, Program in Medical Biotechnology
SUNY Upstate Medical University
Syracuse, New York
Chapter 6

Evan F. Ray, CHS(ABHI), SI(ASCP)
Supervisor, Transplant Immunology
59th Medical Wing/MTLLI
Lackland AFB, Texas
Chapters 9 & 15

LTC Patricia Reilly, PhD
Capability Area Program Officer
Joint Science and Technology Office for Chemical
    and Biological Defense
The Pentagon
Washington, DC
Chapters 9 & 15

John Schmitz, PhD
Director of Histocompatibility/Flow Cytometry
Clinical Microbiology and Immunology
McLendon Clinical Laboratories
UNC Healthcare Systems
Chapel Hill, North Carolina
Chapter 11

Linda A. Smith, PhD, CLS(NCA)
Professor and Graduate Program Director
Deptartment of Clinical Laboratory Sciences
The University of Texas Health Science Center
San Antonio, Texas
Chapters 3, 5, & 8

Diane Tice, PhD, MT(ASCP)
Associate Professor, Biology
Morrisville State College
Morrisville, New York
Chapters 1, 8, & 12

Kent J. Weinhold, PhD
Professor of Surgery and Immunology
Duke University Medical Center
Durham, North Carolina
Chapter 10

Part I • Introduction to Immunology

1

What Is Immunology?

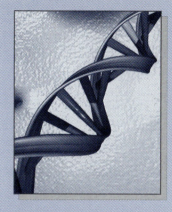

■ CHAPTER CHECKLIST

After reading and studying this chapter, the reader should be able to:

1. Define the immune response in mammals as one that includes an innate response and an adaptive response.
2. Explain the impact of specificity and memory on the adaptive immune response.
3. Discuss the importance of having a functioning immune system using examples from invertebrate and vertebrate species.
4. Speculate as to why the adaptive portion of the immune response has only been found so far in vertebrates, while some form of an innate immune response is present in virtually every multicelled organism.
5. Explain how the field of immunology has progressed over the past century from one driven by clinical needs to one in search of mechanisms and pathways.
6. Describe the sequential nature of research and how experiments build upon each other to advance knowledge of a particular mechanism.

⊚ CASE IN POINT

At a very young age Sophia learned to milk the cows on her family's small farm in turn-of-the century upstate New York. By the time she was six, she was responsible for milking two cows by herself each morning and evening. Winters were bitter, and the cows were warm, so small Sophia leaned her forehead on the cows as she milked. One morning she awoke to find a raised, weeping lesion on her forehead. When the lesion worsened and became encrusted, her worried mother checked with the family doctor. He looked at the lesion and told Sophia and her mother not to worry—the lesion would heal.

ISSUES TO CONSIDER

After reading the patient's case history, consider

⊚ How this story relates to the study of immunology

⊚ How the immune system responds to an invader

⊚ The basis for developing vaccines and the concepts of immunization

⊚ The expected results if Sophia was vaccinated after the lesion healed

IMPORTANT TERMS

Adaptive immunity	Immune response	Memory
Attenuation	Immune system	Recognition phase
Autoimmunity	Innate immunity	Response phase
Cell-mediated immunity	Major histocompatibility	Vaccine
Humoral immunity	complex (MHC)	Variolation

▶ INTRODUCTION

Immunology—the study of the **immune system**—is relatively new. Traditionally immunology was considered an offshoot of microbiology or of blood banking rather than viewed as a separate discipline. Today, immunology is a dynamic field, one that is changing so rapidly that many of the paradigms presented in this text may very well be considered outdated 10 years from now. This chapter introduces the reader to the theories and concepts presented in the following chapters. These principles may be applied in clinical or research science, and not only touch upon humans but also on other mammalian or even nonmammalian species as well. This chapter takes the reader back to early studies that led to the discovery of vaccines and the benefits derived from immunization. The general concepts of the **immune response** and immunology as a scientific discipline that will serve as a foundation for the subsequent chapters are presented.

▶ WHAT IS IMMUNOLOGY?

Immunology as a discipline was originally part of microbiology because the most obvious consequence of the presence or absence of an immune response is either the ablation or continued presence of microorganisms. In the higher phyla, exclusion of pathogens is the most important aspect of the immune system. However, examination of nonmammalian species, or comparative immunology, shows evidence of at least a limited immune response even in nonvertebrate organisms. Therefore, the most primitive aspect of an immune response is the ability to distinguish self from nonself. Even in mammals, the ability to recognize self and not generate an immune response is equally as important as the ability to recognize and mount a response to pathogens.

Although microbiology originally drove the development of clinical reagents such as vaccines and the study of immunologic mechanisms, modern techniques and reagents developed in the immunology laboratory, such as monoclonal antibodies and enzyme-linked immunosorbent assays, are now used throughout all phases of clinical laboratory medicine, research, and industry.

The immune system is amazingly complex. In humans, there is a variety of cells involved in the generation of an immune response. These cells interact with each other, often in a sort of symbiotic relationship where contact of one cell type with another further activates each cell. Chemical "factors" are produced that influence the interaction of the different cell types, the course of the immune response, and, in some cases, memory of the event that triggered the response. The importance of an immune response in an organism is suggested by the redundant pathways for generating an immune response, and confirmed by the consequences to an organism lacking an intact immune system, as discussed in Chapter 8.

If sponges of two different species are disaggregated into separate cells and mixed together, the cells will reaggregate with cells of the same species—self and nonself are distinguished. This is not an immune response per se, but is a demonstration of a primitive ability, generated through cell surface receptors, to recognize self.

A simple form of immunity has been found in every species in every phylum studied. T and B lymphocytes capable of generating **adaptive immunity,** complete with the hallmarks of specificity and memory, have not been found in any invertebrate phyla studied, but these organisms do have mechanisms capable of containing microbes. For example, in *Drosophila melanogaster,* the presence of bacteria or fungi in the body cavity triggers production of antibacterial or antifungal peptides in response. Similar responses are seen in plants invaded by bacteria or fungi. These responses are primitive and are not specific to the particular invader.

Higher plants, invertebrates such as sponges, earthworms, and arthropods; and vertebrates such as cartilaginous fishes, teleost and bony fishes, amphibians, reptiles, birds, and mammals all have some components of the innate immune system. They also produce protective enzymes and enzyme cascades and antimicrobial peptides when invaded by pathogens. In addition, all of these organisms except plants have some type of phagocytic cell. All but plants also have the pattern-recognition receptors important for self–nonself discrimination, and are capable of rejecting grafts from other species. However, as stated previously, only vertebrates have an adaptive immune system, and no T and B cells have been found in any invertebrate species studied to date.

The immune response in any organism is comprised of a **recognition phase** and a **response phase.** The recognition phase might be as simple as a carbohydrate or protein on the surface of the cell which binds to another carbohydrate or protein on the surface of another cell. Recognition may then be of self, in which case the response phase is not begun, or it may be of nonself. If the latter occurs, the response phase of the immune response begins. The innate immune system, which is discussed in detail in Chapter 2, is the more primitive form. In **innate immunity,** recognition is general. It may be a primitive production of antimicrobial or antifungal peptide such as that seen in Drosophila or plants, or, in higher vertebrates, it may be extremely complex, for example, the mannose-binding lectin present on mammalian cells that binds mannose residues present on bacterial cells, which in turn activates the complement system described in Chapter 5.

Higher vertebrates have adaptive immunity in addition to innate immunity. Recognition in the adaptive immune system is highly specific to a small portion of the microorganism or other substance (antigen) which triggered the immune response. The adaptive immune system is also capable of generating **memory** of the antigen trigger, so that should that substance be encountered later, a stronger and more rapid immune response occurs. The ability to generate an almost limitless number of specific recognition molecules from a relatively small portion of the genome is characteristic of the adaptive immune response and is discussed relative to immunoglobulins in Chapter 3. The adaptive immune system of higher vertebrates is geared to eliminate any cells that either do not recognize self, or recognize and respond to self strongly and inappropriately. Should these cells not be eliminated, the consequences may be pathogenic destruction of the organism's own tissues. This abnormal immune response—**autoimmunity**—is described in detail in Chapter 8.

▶ HISTORICAL PERSPECTIVES

EARLY IMMUNOLOGY

Attempts to modify immune responses preceded knowledge of the immune system itself. Early immunology was driven by observations on the effects of pathogenic microorganisms and by the need to modify the immune response to these pathogens—a clinical approach rather than pure research. A brief history of observations in immunology illustrates the progressive nature of the field from early clinical observations on the effects of microorganisms and of the response by the immune system to these organisms to the most recent data collected from molecular biological techniques.

Perhaps the earliest recognition of an innate immune response can be found on documents from ancient Egypt, where inflammation was described. Celsus, a Roman physician in the first century described the four cardinal signs of inflammation: rubor (redness), tumor (swelling), calor (heat), and dolor (pain). Galen, another Roman, added in 200 A.D. function laesa (loss of function). Although the mechanisms leading to these signs would not be determined until almost two centuries later, these cardinal signs are still used in clinical practice today.

Observations on the adaptive immune response, although it was not described as such, were made early in recorded history as well. Thucydides noted in about 430 B.C. in Athens that individuals who became ill with bubonic plague and actually recovered (not a common occurrence) did not contract the disease again. Historical records suggest that not much action was taken based on these observations for several centuries.

A similar set of observations on the epidemiology of smallpox in China and Turkey in the fifteenth century led to the first recorded attempts to intentionally induce an immune response through the use of vaccination with infectious material through cuts in the skin, or variolation. Once again, the Western world did not appear to take note of these observations until Lady Mary Wortley Montagu, wife of the British ambassador to Constantinople, had her children vaccinated in 1718.

COWPOX AND SMALLPOX

Even with the approbation of the British ambassador, vaccination did not readily catch on for another 80 years. **Variolation** for smallpox required that the crusts containing the smallpox virus be inoculated through cuts in the skin or inhaled. Although the virus in these crusts was generally weakened enough to avoid a serious infection, the technique was not perfect, and infection and death from smallpox was always a possibility. Figures 1-1a■ and 1-1b■ show images of smallpox vaccinated sites. Edward Jenner, a British physician, observed that while milkmaids frequently contracted cowpox from infected cows, they did not usually contract smallpox. Cowpox in humans was usually a self-limiting, less serious disease (as illustrated in the case in point at the beginning of this chapter) than was smallpox. In 1798, Jenner inoculated an 8-year-old boy with fluid from a cowpox pustule. In an experiment that would never be condoned by any institutional review board today, he later intentionally infected the boy with smallpox. The child did not become ill, and the utility of vaccination with material containing cowpox virus was quickly accepted in Europe. As in the case of Sophia (see Case in Point), had she been infected with smallpox virus later, her previous exposure to cowpox virus would have offered protection. We know today that vaccination with the cowpox virus led to production by B lymphocytes of antibodies which not only bound specifically to sites on cowpox virus but also cross-reacted with the smallpox virus. **Cell-mediated immunity** generated by T lymphocytes was also induced, along with memory T and B cells. The exposure of the immunized child to smallpox caused the memory cells to become reactivated and to produce specific immunity to the smallpox virus—thus, no clinical disease.

LOUIS PASTEUR AND IMMUNIZATION

Widespread application of the principle of vaccination—immunization with a weaker or related strain of a microorganism in the hope of generating an immune response that would prevent clinical disease upon reexposure to the microorganism—was not applied to other microorganisms for almost another century. Louis Pasteur, who gave his name to the process of pasteurization, might be regarded as the father of vaccination and of immunology. His initial interest was not actually directed toward the immune response but rather to microbiology. In what would be eventually a successful attempt to prove that a culture of a particular bacteria isolated from chickens with fowl cholera could cause the same disease in other chickens, he injected chickens with an old strain of fowl cholera. These chickens developed the disease but recovered—not the usual course of fowl cholera. In an attempt to conserve resources, these same chickens were then reinjected with a fresh strain of the bacteria. The chickens that previously had been injected with the old strain did not show any signs of developing fowl cholera from the fresh strain, but other chickens that had not been previously injected developed the disease and died. Pasteur hypothesized that aging of the bacterial culture had weakened the virulence of the bacteria, rendering them incapable of causing clinical disease. He called the aged strain a **vaccine** and the process **attenuation.**

In 1881, Louis Pasteur attenuated a strain of *Bacillus anthracis* by heating it. He then vaccinated sheep with this strain, and later challenged the vaccinated sheep and unvaccinated control sheep with the virulent strain. As was expected, the vaccinated sheep did not develop the disease whereas the controls did. These results from this intentional experiment combined with those of the serendipitous accident with the fowl cholera led to development of vaccines. In 1885, Pasteur gave the first true vaccine to young Josef Meister, who had been bitten by a rabid dog. The rabies vaccine was a success.

TWENTIETH-CENTURY IMMUNOLOGY

Experiments in immunology in the twentieth century were still driven by clinical needs, but also began to investigate mechanisms, as well as clinical phenomena. A survey of Nobel prizes shows a gradual evolution in immunologic research from "this works" to "this is how this works." For example, in 1890 Emil von Behring and Shibasaburo Kitasato showed that serum from animals immunized to diphtheria could transfer immunity, thus starting to define the mechanisms underlying the success of vaccination. They won Nobel prizes in 1901 for research on these "serum antitoxins" or what we now refer to as immunoglobulins or antibodies. In further experiments by many investigators,

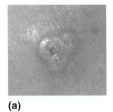
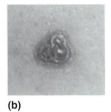

(a)   (b)

■ FIGURE 1-1 (a) Smallpox vaccine inoculation site after 3 days. (b) Same smallpox vaccine inoculation site after 10 days.

serum was shown to have antitoxin properties, to cause precipitation in some instance, and to cause agglutination in others. Elvin Kabat, in 1930, unified these observations by demonstrating that the proteins contained in the gamma globulin portion of serum were responsible for all of these reactions.

Others continued to define the "why" of immunology. Nobel prizes were awarded to Robert Koch in 1905 for his description of cellular immunity to tuberculosis. Jules Bordet was recognized in 1919 for his work on complement-mediated bacteriolysis. Clinical experimentation continued as well. The subdiscipline of serology grew out of Karl Landsteiner's discovery of human blood groups, recognized by the Nobel committee in 1930. An early (1913) recognition of anaphylaxis by Charles Richet was complemented by the development of antihistamines by Daniel Bovet, who was awarded his Nobel Prize in 1957. In yet another recognition of the clinical importance of immunology, Max Theiler was awarded a Nobel medal in 1957 for development of a vaccine to combat yellow fever.

The second half of the twentieth century shows less emphasis on applied immunology combined with greater emphasis on mechanisms. F. Macfarlane Burnet and Peter Medawar were jointly awarded the Nobel Prize in 1960 for their discovery of acquired immunological tolerance—work that laid the foundation for description of the mechanisms of T and B cell tolerance. Porter and Edelman were recognized for defining the chemical structure of antibodies in 1972, the details of which are described in Chapter 3.

Transplantation of solid organs such as kidneys combined basic immunological theory with practical application. There are stories, probably apocryphal, surrounding organ transplants performed in China in 200–300 B.C., as well as stories describing the transplant of one man's leg to another by Saints Cosmos and Damian in the sixth century. Transplants of dog kidneys into humans poisoned by mercury were reported in the mid-1800s. As might be expected with xenografts (organs transplanted from one species to another), these were not successful and were not controlled experiments. Serious experimentation, which included controls, didn't occur until the early twentieth century. In 1908, Alexis Carrel interchanged kidneys in cats. Although the kidneys were ultimately rejected (the reasons for which are discussed in Chapter 9), this study demonstrated that organs function after transplantation. In 1935, a Russian surgeon attempted a human kidney transplant. Unfortunately, this transplant did not survive even for as long as did Alexis Carrel's cat kidneys since there was a blood group mismatch. The

transplant community has since learned that ABO antigens are present on kidney cells, and that naturally occurring anti-A or anti-B antibodies present in virtually all individuals except those of blood group AB attack the mismatched graft immediately, causing hyperacute rejection. The first successful human kidney transplant was performed in 1954 between identical twins, which eliminated the chance of ABO or tissue antigen mismatch and the need for immunosuppression.

Successful organ transplantation was furthered by the description of the **major histocompatibility complex (MHC),** which is discussed in Chapters 9, 11, and 15. George Snell, Jean Dausset, and Baruj Benacerraf were recognized for their seminal work on the MHC in 1980. E. Donnall Thomas and Joseph Murray were awarded a Nobel Prize in medicine for their contributions to transplantation immunology, a growing subfield of immunology, in 1991.

As is both appropriate and important to any emerging field of study, many experiments have led to great controversy among investigators. Elie Metchnikoff, awarded the Nobel Prize in 1908 for his description of the role played by phagocytosis in defense against microorganisms, noted in 1883 that phagocytes could ingest both microorganisms and foreign material, thus contributing to immunity. He also observed motile cells surround rose thorns introduced into starfish larvae and showed that fungal spores could be attacked by the blood cells of Daphnia. He later confirmed this work in mammalian leukocytes, thought today to be polymorphonuclear neutrophils (PMNs) and macrophages. Since the role of "serum antitoxins" in immunity had already been described, a controversy arose between investigators who believed antibodies in the serum to be the prime players in the immune response—**humoral immunity**—and those Metchnikoff and others who believed cell-mediated immunity to be of major importance. While we now know that both cell-mediated and humoral forms of immunity are of equal importance in the adaptive immune response, it is ironic that the cells described by Metchnikoff, which began the controversy, are actually responsible for innate immunity rather than for adaptive immunity and have little to do with the success of a vaccine. Demonstration in chickens in 1964 by Bruce Glick of T lymphocytes (named for their derivation from the thymus) responsible for cell-mediated immunity and B lymphocytes (derived from the bursa of Fabricius) responsible for humoral immunity helped to resolve the dispute.

Because of their importance to the success of vaccination, antibodies (or immunoglobulins) were extensively studied during the twentieth century. In addition to the already mentioned work of von Behring on serum antitoxins and Porter and Edelman on the structure of antibodies, other investigators determined what substances could be recognized by antibodies and demonstrated that an antibody molecule is specific for one particular antigen. In 1900, Jules Bordet showed that antibodies were responsible for specific immunity to the red blood cells of other species. This confirmed the hypothesis that while "serum antitoxins" were originally described as interacting with microorganisms, not all antibodies had to be directed against pathogenic substances. This was further illustrated through work by Karl Landsteiner, who showed that an immune response could be induced to many different organic chemicals.

Observations on the highly specific nature of the adaptive immune response led to more controversy between investigators. Paul Erlich proposed his selective theory in 1900 to explain why some white blood cells could bind to a microorganism. Adapting a mechanism known to be operational in the interaction of enzymes and substrates, he suggested that these cells had "side-chain receptors" which fit structures on the microbe in an interaction analogous to a lock and key. We might speculate today that some of these receptors he proposed were nonspecific pattern recognition receptors on cells of the innate immune system, whereas others may have been the specific recognition structures present on T lymphocytes and B lymphocytes. Erlich also hypothesized that these receptors were formed before the cells were exposed to the infectious agent. Therefore, there must be populations of cells, the "keys" which must be tried out on the microbe to find the right combination.

An alternative to the selection theory hypothesis arose in the 1930s. Proposed by Friedrich Breinl and Felix Haurowitz and supported in the 1940s by Linus Pauling, the instructional theory suggested that there were a limited number of antibody types and that the antigen served as a template around which the antibody would be "instructed" to fit. There was logic underlying this hypothesis. Work by Karl Landsteiner and others had shown that not only were there thousands of natural pathogens to which the immune system must mount a response but also that an immune response could be generated to virtually any organic chemical if presented appropriately. The implication for this was that if the each antibody had a specific binding site formed before an encounter with the appropriate antigen, there would have to be hundreds of thousands of different antibody molecules present in the serum. The chances of having preformed antibod-

ies to substances not normally encountered would either be slight or would imply a tremendously wasteful response by the immune system. Thus, the instructional theory made sense and was popular for a couple of decades.

In the 1950s, the clonal selection theory was championed by Niels Jerne, David Talmadge, and F. Macfarlane Burnet. The underlying hypothesis was similar to that proposed by Erlich five decades earlier—that the specificity of a cell (by now known to be a lymphocyte) was determined before that cell encountered antigen. The clonal selection theory added a proposal that, once a cell encountered antigen, it would be activated and would proliferate to form a clone of cells, all capable of recognizing that antigen. With the advent of molecular biology, the instructional theory was disproven, and the clonal selection theory came to be part of the central dogma of antibody formation and selectivity.

Immunologists continued to investigate the mechanisms used by the immune system. Although the clonal selection theory proposed a mechanism by which cells produced antibodies specific for antigens, it did not explain how the limited amount of genetic information contained in the DNA could code for an almost infinite variety of antibodies. In 1965, Dreyer and Bennett proposed in a theoretical paper the radical idea that two separate genes were responsible for encoding a single immunoglobulin heavy or light chain. This paper challenged the paradigm that one gene coded for one protein or polypeptide chain. Research on other proteins has since shown that immunoglobulins are not unique in this construction. Tonegawa and Hozumi confirmed the theory in 1976 in a paper in *Nature* which provided the first direct evidence that separate genes encode the V and C regions of the immunoglobulin chain and that these genes are rearranged during differentiation. Tonegawa was later awarded the Nobel Prize in 1987 for this work.

The series of experiments and theories described illustrate the sequential nature of immunological research. Most theories do not arise de novo, but are built upon previous observations. The development of monoclonal antibodies by Kohler and Milstein, who were awarded the Nobel Prize for this work in 1987, illustrates this. Previous observations had shown that myelomas were clones of tumor cells that produced a single specificity of antibody and that these clones had an indefinite life span in cell culture. Other research had shown that some viruses caused fusion of cells. Milstein and Kohler used this knowledge to develop hybridomas, a fusion of a myeloma cell with a lymphocyte from an immunized animal. The result of this fusion was a clone of cells that could be maintained indefinitely in the ascites of mice or in cell culture and that produced an antibody of exquisitely defined specificity against one portion or epitope of an antigen—a monoclonal antibody. The development of the hybridoma technique may be second only to the development of vaccines in its impact on the field of immunology. Monoclonal antibodies are now ubiquitous in the clinical laboratory, in research, and in industry. The use of these antibodies are discussed in detail in Chapter 7 and elsewhere throughout the text.

MOVING TOWARD THE TWENTY-FIRST CENTURY

Although B cells and antibodies were the focus of intense investigation during the first three-quarters of the twentieth century, T cells followed in the latter part of the century. The recognition that T cells were also highly specific for antigens suggested that they should have a receptor analogous to immunoglobulin on their surface. This was confirmed when the structure of the T cell receptor was identified. However, T cells do not recognize unprocessed antigen in the same way as do B cells. Zinkernagel and Doherty, awarded a Nobel Prize in 1996, defined the role of the MHC in antigen recognition by T cells. Subsets of T cells re-

sponsible for different functions in the immune response were also defined in the 1990s, as were cytokines produced by T cells.

Although Jerne was awarded a Nobel Prize in 1984 for his work on immune networks and immune regulation, research into the mechanisms responsible for regulation of the immune response, particularly by T lymphocytes, continues.

Molecular techniques have expanded the role of the clinical diagnostic immunology laboratory. These methods are found to be very useful for detection of a wide variety of microorganisms and disease states. Identification of human genes that put individuals at risk for developing certain types of cancer and the move toward a preventive cancer vaccine for tumors may be in the realm of possibility. Histocompatibility (HLA) testing to assess tissue compatibility between a transplant donor and potential recipient prior to transplant to prevent tissue rejection, the development of additional clinical applications of flow cytometry, and new monoclonal antibodies with specificities relevant to particular cells types will serve to continue the expansion of the clinical utility of immunologic analysis.

One area that will become more advanced in the field of molecular immunology is an increase in the level—and reliance—of automation. Amplification methods and applications of gene chip technology will certainly further revolutionize the science of immunology.

SUMMARY

The immune response is an integral function in multicellular organisms. Recognition of nonself underlies the immune response, which is primitive in invertebrates, but becomes increasing complex in vertebrate species, which have not only an innate immune system, but an adaptive immune response capable of exquisite specificity and memory.

Development of vaccines in the latter part of the 19th century fueled investigation into the mechanisms of the immune system and how to manipulate these mechanisms to achieve clinical goals. Research during the twentieth century

produced advances in clinical medicine, such as those seen in organ transplantation, but also provided insight into the cellular and molecular mechanisms of the innate immune response, antibody structure and production, and T lymphocyte function. Although bits of history pertaining to the development of particular concepts or techniques will be presented throughout this text, the brief synopsis provided in this chapter should help to illustrate the importance of the study of immunology.

POINTS TO REMEMBER

▶ The underlying purpose of the immune system is to distinguish self from nonself in order to repel or destroy invaders (usually pathogenic microorganisms) without causing harm to the host. Evidence of at least one component of the innate immune system, which responds to invasion in a nonspecific fashion based on cell surface molecule pattern recognition, has been found in plants, invertebrates, and vertebrates.

▶ The adaptive immune response has only been observed in vertebrates. This portion of the immune response is characterized by specificity and memory. A survey of the history of immunology shows clinical needs, such as the need for vaccines to combat infectious disease, to have been the driving force for research during much of the past century.

LEARNING ASSESSMENT QUESTIONS

1. Rejection of transplanted tissue occurs in:
   a. vertebrates
   b. invertebrates
   c. plants
   d. all of the above

2. Antibodies produced during the course of an adaptive immune response would not be found in:
   a. sharks
   b. chickens
   c. Daphnia
   d. mice

3. Pasteur used heat-treated *Bacillus anthracis* to immunize sheep. These bacteria did not cause anthrax because:
   a. the bacteria were a naturally nonpathogenic strain.
   b. the heat treatment decreased the virulence of the bacteria.
   c. heating bacteria induces antibody formation.
   d. heat treatment increases makes the bacteria more immunogenic.

4. The clonal selection theory proposes that:
   a. the sequence of an antibody is determined after the cell encounters an antigen.
   b. antibodies are folded around the antigen.
   c. side-chain receptors on cells fit into antigen by a lock-and-key mechanism.
   d. surface recognition molecules such as antibodies exist on cells before the cells encounter antigen.

5. _____ proposed that the immune response was primarily cell mediated.
   a. Jenner
   b. Pasteur
   c. Metchnikoff
   d. Pauling

REFERENCES

Burnet, F. M. 1959. *The Clonal Selection Theory of Acquired Immunity.* Cambridge University Press, Cambridge.

Clarke, W. R. 1991. *The Experimental Foundations of Modern Immunology,* 4th ed. John Wiley & Sons, New York.

Dreyer, W. J. and J. C. Bennett. 1965. The molecular basis of antibody formation. *Proc Natl Acad Sci USA* 54:864.

Kimbrell, D. A. and B. Beutler. 2001. The evolution and genetics of innate immunity. *Nature Rev Genet* 2:256.

Paul, W., ed. 1999. *Fundamental Immunology,* 4th ed. Lippincott-Raven, Philadelphia.

Silverstein, A. M. 1989. *A History of Immunology.* Academic Press, San Diego.

Tonegawa, S. 1983. Somatic generation of antibody diversity. *Nature* 302:575.

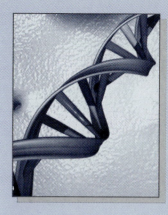

2

Overview of the Immune System

■ CHAPTER CHECKLIST

After reading and studying this chapter, the reader should be able to:

1. Differentiate innate immunity from adaptive or acquired immunity.
2. Describe how physical and chemical barriers can function as effective defense mechanisms of the human body.
3. Identify phagocytic and other cells by their characteristic features and the role of each in innate immunity.
4. Discuss the functions of the phagocytes and other cells involved in the killing of extracellular pathogens.
5. Describe the function of the acute phase proteins involved in the innate immune response.
6. Differentiate between the classical and alternate pathways of complement activation.
7. Explain how complement enhances phagocytosis and the acute inflammatory reaction.
8. List the classical signs of inflammation.
9. Describe how inflammatory mediators drive an inflammatory reaction.
10. Define and differentiate the following terms: antibody, antigen, and immunogen.
11. Describe the function of the lymphoid organs and the process of lymphopoiesis.
12. Compare the humoral immune response with the cell-mediated response.

CASE IN POINT

An unidentified 24-year-old male was transported from the site of a helicopter crash to the burn unit. The patient had multiple injuries, including third-degree burns covering 65 percent of his body. Within 72 hours following admission, the patient experienced fever, chills, and other symptoms of impending septic shock. Exudative bullae formed on his extremities, and *Pseudomonas aeruginosa* was recovered from an infected burn wound.

IMPORTANT TERMS

Adaptive immunity	Hematopoiesis	Natural-killer cell (NK cell)
Antibody	Immunogen	Negative selection
Antigen	Immunoglobulin	Neutrophils
Antigen-presenting cell (APC)	Innate immunity	Opsonins
Apoptosis	Interferon (IFN)	Opsonization
Cluster determinant (CD)	Interleukin (IL)	Phagocytosis
Cytokine	Leukocyte	Phagosomes
Cytotoxic T lymphocyte (CTL)	Lymphocyte	Positive selection
Dendritic cell	Lymphopoiesis	T cell receptor (TCR)
Diapedesis	Macrophages	T helper (T_H) cell
Dohle bodies	Major histocompatibility	Tranferrin
Epitopes	complex (MHC) antigens	Tumor necrosis factor (TNF)

▶ INTRODUCTION

There are two major divisions in the immune system: **innate immunity,** and **adaptive immunity.** The innate immune system, which is sometimes called nonspecific immunity or natural immunity, includes physical, chemical, and other nonspecific mechanical barriers. This form of immunity serves as the first line of defense against microorganisms and other invaders. If the first line of defense is broken and the invading organisms are able to initiate an infection, the adaptive immune system, also called specific or acquired immunity, becomes activated to produce specific re-sponses to the infectious agent. In addition, the adaptive immune system is able to remember the infectious agent and tries to prevent it from causing a similar infection in the future. Table 2-1 © summarizes the differences between innate and adaptive immunity. This chapter introduces the reader to the different components of the immune system. It consists of an overview of the functions each component provides and how the components interact in the defense of the human body. These components and their functions are examined in greater detail throughout the remaining chapters of this book.

✪ TABLE 2-1

Summary of Differences between Innate and Adaptive Immunity		
	Innate	Adaptive
Type of response	Antigen-independent	Antigen-dependent
Timing of response	Immediate-maximal response	Lag time between exposure and maximal reponse
Specificity of response	Not antigen-specific	Antigen-specific
Postexposure results	No immunologic memory	Immunologic memory

► INNATE IMMUNITY

Innate is a nonspecific form of defense inherent to the host. Figure 2-1■ shows the innate immune defenses located at different body sites. As such, it targets any potential pathogen or invader that is presented to the body with stereotyped responses. Nonspecific immunity consists of (1) physical and chemical barriers such as the skin and mucous membranes that line the respiratory tract, gastrointestinal tract, and urogenital tract; (2) secretions such as tears, sweat, saliva, and mucus; (3) plasma proteins such as complement and acute phase proteins that mediate the destruction of microorganisms; (4) cellular components such as polymorphonuclear neutrophils (PMNs), other leukocytes, and **macrophages** that are capable of **phagocytosis.** Innate immunity serves as the first line of defense, and although its ability to defend the host is limited, it does not require previous exposure to the foreign invader in order to quickly mount an effective response.

PHYSICAL AND CHEMICAL BARRIERS

The keratinized layer of intact skin is one of the major effective exterior physical barriers. Tough, waterproof, and equipped with biochemical substances that work against susceptible organisms, the skin prevents microbial invasion and development of infection by forcing most microorganisms to penetrate the skin through a breach in the barrier. The Case in Point at the beginning of this chapter demonstrates the importance of the skin as a barrier. The patient, whose third-degree burns penetrated the skin, had no external barrier to shield him from environmental organisms such as *Pseudomonas aeruginosa.* The patient therefore became susceptible to infection.

Not only did the patient lack the mechanical barrier function provided by the keratinized epidermis of the skin, but also the dermis was destroyed. The dermal layer of the skin contains sebaceous or sweat glands that produce sebum which is comprised in part of lactic and fatty acids. These substances allow the skin to maintain a low pH, which is bactericidal for most microorganisms. In addition, the usual microbial flora present on the skin also serve as an immune defense. The normal microbial flora prevents colonization of potential pathogens by exclusion because the organisms compete for nutrients and space. In patients whose microbial flora has been altered or eliminated by antimicrobial or chemotherapeutic agents, resistant or pathogenic organisms such as *Candida albicans,* a fungal species, may be able to initiate an infection.

The mucous membranes that line the respiratory, gastrointestinal (GI), and urogenital tracts also provide protection. The ciliated epithelial cells of the respiratory tract help by trapping and sweeping away airborne organisms and dust, and the mucus produced by the goblet cells present in all mucous membranes makes a

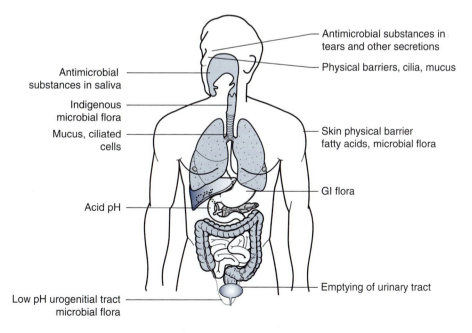

Antimicrobial substances in tears and other secretions

Physical barriers, cilia, mucus

Antimicrobial substances in saliva

Indigenous microbial flora

Mucus, ciliated cells

Skin physical barrier fatty acids, microbial flora

GI flora

Acid pH

Emptying of urinary tract

Low pH urogenitial tract microbial flora

■ FIGURE 2-1 Innate immune defenses located at different body sites

⊘ TABLE 2-2

Physical and Chemical Barriers to Infections

Organ/System	Chemical/Physical Barrier	Mechanism of Action
Skin	Squamous epithelial cells, sweat, sebaceous glands	Desquamation, organic acids, cleansing
Gastrointestinal tract	Columnar cells, mucus lining, mucus, saliva	Peristalsis, low pH, bile acids, flushing
Respiratory tract	Tracheal cilia, mucus	Mucus, surfactants
Eye	Tears	Flushing, lysozyme
Lymphoid organ/circulatory	Phagocytes, natural-killer cells, cytotoxic cells	Phagocytosis, intracellular killing, cytolysis
Plasma/serum	Interferons, TNF-α, lactoferrin, transferrin, fibrinonectin, complement	Antiviral, iron-binding, opsonization, phagocyosis, inflammation

sticky surface. Additionally, such enzymes as lysozome, which is present in tears and saliva, act as chemical barriers that inhibit invasion by microorganisms.

Body secretions such as saliva, fatty acids, and bile acids in the GI tract provide additional chemical barriers. Acute phase proteins, complement, and other substances such as **tumor necrosis factor (TNF) alpha** also provide antimicrobial effects. Transferrin and lactoferrin deprive organisms of iron while lysozyme breaks down the peptidoglycan layer of the bacterial cell wall. **Interferons (IFN)** and TNF inhibit viral replication and activate cellular response. Fibronectin promotes rapid phagocytosis by coating the bacteria **(opsonization)** while the components and products of complement mediate destruction or phagocytosis of microorganisms. Acute phase proteins interact with the complement system. A summary of the physical and chemical barriers to the establishment of infection is shown on Table 2-2⊘.

CELLULAR COMPONENTS

White blood cells (WBCs) or **leukocytes** provide another form of innate immunity. Produced in the bone marrow by **hematopoiesis,** leukocytes differentiate into **neutrophils** or polymorphonuclear cells (PMNs), **lymphocytes,** monocytes/macrophages, eosinophils, and basophils. Of these, neutrophils, monocytes/ macrophages, and lymphocytes play the primary role in host defense, although eosinophils and basophils also contribute. Neutrophils and monocytes/macrophages perform phagocytosis, the process of engulfing, digesting, and destroying foreign invaders such as bacteria. Lymphocytes are responsible for the adaptive immune response. The role of lymphocytes in the immune response is discussed in later chapters.

Neutrophils

Neutrophils are the most abundant of the WBCs and make up about 55–70% of all leukocytes. Morphologically, the mature PMN measures approximately 15 μm, and contains a multilobed nucleus with 2–5 lobes of condensed chromatin connected together by thin strands of chromatin (Figure 2-2a■, peripheral smear, Wright stain and Figure 2-2b■, sputum direct smear, Gram-stained). Immature neutrophils that may occasionally appear in the blood stream are nonsegmented and are called "bands" (Figure 2-3■). The cytoplasm of neutrophils contain three types of granules, the enzymes that function to kill and digest bacteria and fungi: (1) primary or azurophilic granules; (2) secondary or specific granules; and (3) gelatinase-containing granules. Formed during the early stages of maturation, azurophilic granules are nonspecific and are characteristic of immature PMNs. These granules contain lysosomal enzymes, defensins, proteases, lysozyme, and myeloperoxidase. Secondary granules, formed during the myelocyte stage, contain lysozyme, collagenase, transferrin, and B-12

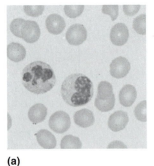 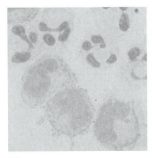

(a)   (b)

■ FIGURE 2-2 (a) Segmented neutrohil, peripheral blood, Wright stain; (b) Segmented neutrophils and macrophages in Gram-stained smear

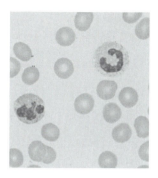

■ FIGURE 2-3 Immature neutrophil or band, peripheral blood, Wright stain

binding factor, but no myeloperoxidase. **Transferrin** is toxic to bacteria and fungi, while collagenase digests connective tissue, allowing the phagocytic cell to reach the affected site. With Wright stain, the primary granules stain purple, and the secondary granules appear light pink. In the metamyelocyte stage, tertiary granules containing plasminogen activator, alkaline phosphatase, and gelatinase are formed.

PMNs remain in the bone marrow for about five days after maturation. Once released into the bloodstream, mature neutrophils may be directed either into marginating pools or circulating pools. About half of the PMNs end up in the marginating pool where cells adhere on the inner surface of the vascular endothelium. If an area of inflammation is encountered, the cells flatten out, squeeze between the endothelial cells, and eventually exit from the blood vessels to enter the tissues in a process called **diapedesis** (Figure 2-4■). They are thought to remain in the tissues for 2–5 days and tend not to return into the

bloodstream but rather die or are destroyed if not involved in an inflammatory response. They are constantly and immediately replaced by the bone marrow with cells in the marrow reserve.

While in circulation, PMNs may become attracted to sites of injury or infection. They immediately adhere to the endothelium of blood vessels in a process called margination after which they squeeze between the endothelial cells to begin phagocytosis of the microorganisms in the affected area. Following phagocytosis, the specific granules coalesce with the membrane-bounded vacuoles, called **phagosomes** (Figure 2-5■), and begin to release their contents. Later, azurophilic granules empty their contents, killing both the invading organism and the PMN.

The major role of PMNs is to remove any infectious or other foreign inflammatory agents that enter the host. Once stimulated, PMNs immediately respond to the site of infection or inflammation. This response to infection and inflammation is reflected by an increase in the relative number of PMNs in the bloodstream, referred to as neutrophilia. Morphologic changes also occur when PMNs are activated. Cytoplasmic alterations include vacuolization, the appearance of toxic granules, and **Dohle bodies** (Figure 2-6■). Toxic granulation can be seen as large clumps of darkly stained granules. Dohle bodies, pale blue aggregated strands of endoplasmic reticulum, may also appear as cytoplasmic inclusions. Highly vacuolated neutrophils also indicate the presence of infection or inflammation. Although these morphologic changes in neutrophils are observed during an inflammatory response, they are considered nonspecific because these features may also be seen in other states such as in pregnancy, drug and toxic reactions, and following severe trauma.

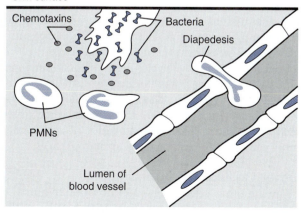

■ FIGURE 2-4 Diapedesis

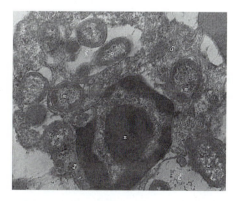

■ FIGURE 2-5 Phagosomes bacterial cells inside a neutrophil (transmission electron microscopy [TEM])

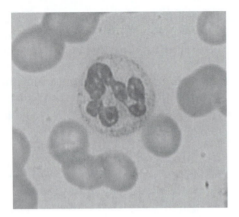

■ **FIGURE 2-6** Neutrophils with Dohle bodies and toxic granulation

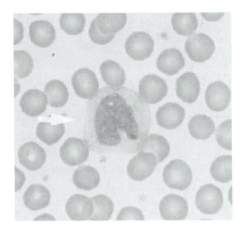

■ **FIGURE 2-7** Monocyte, peripheral blood, Wright stain

Monocytes

Monocytes make up about 2 to 9% of normal WBCs in the peripheral blood and less than 2% of normal bone marrow cells. Monocytes are produced in the bone marrow with monoblasts and promonocytes as precursors before release into the bloodstream. Monocytes remain in the peripheral blood for only about 14 hours after which they move to the tissues to become tissue macrophages.

Monocytes are large cells that measure approximately 15–18 μm (Figure 2-7■). The irregular, dull-grayish blue cytoplasm is large relative to the nucleus and contains small, fine, purplish, evenly distributed granules which give the cytoplasm what is described as "ground-glass" appearance. The cytoplasm may also contain vacuoles, ingested erythrocytes, and other cellular debris. The nuclei of monocytes appear as "brain-like" convolutions and may be kidney shaped. Fine chromatin strands form a lacy network blended with small clumps of chromatin. Although monocytes may be recognized by their characteristic microscopic morphology, monoclonal antibodies against cell surface markers such as CD14 may be used to confirm identification.

Because they enlarge as they mature, it becomes more difficult for monocytes to pass through smaller blood vessels and capillaries. Hence, monocytes move into tissues and transform into the much larger macrophages or histiocytes found in organ systems. Specialized macrophages are found throughout the body tissues. These specialized macrophages are called pulmonary macrophages or dust cells when found in the lung, Kupffer cells in the liver, mesangial phagocytes in the kidneys, microglial cells in the brain, and osteoclasts in the bones. Tissue macrophages typically exist in their chosen environment for approximately 2–4 months. While in the tissues, they acquire several surface receptors for certain complement factors: **immunoglobulins,** other **opsonins,** and chemotactic factors.

Macrophages

Macrophages measure about 25–80 μm and have a round nucleus containing one or two nucleoli (Figure 2-8■). The irregularly sized cytoplasm is vacuolated and contains numerous azurophilic granules. Macrophages seldom reenter the bloodstream but may be found in the circulation during an inflammatory response where they perform numerous functions. In the tissues, macrophages act as scavengers: they engulf, digest, and remove foreign particles and cellular debris. Once digested, foreign proteins (antigens) are processed and displayed on the surface of the macrophage for recognition by antigen-specific T lymphocytes (**CD**+4 and CD+8 cells). Therefore, in addition to serving as phagocytes, they may also participate in the adaptive immune response by functioning as **antigen-presenting cells (APC).** Macrophages also play a vital role in initiating and regulating the immune response and development of inflammatory process by secreting potent substances such as complement factors, lysozyme, and other products that possess antibacterial activity. **Cytokines** and other mediators that enhance the activities of and attract other cell types are also secreted by macrophages.

Other Cellular Components

There are other cells involved in nonspecific immune response. These include **natural-killer (NK) cells,** lymphokine-activated killer cells (LAK cells), and

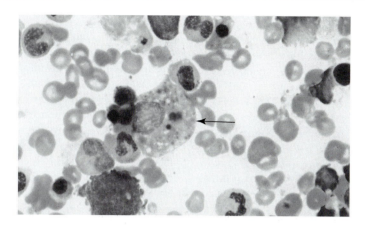

■ **FIGURE 2-8** Macrophage

eosinophils. NK cells resemble large lymphocytes morphologically and are sometimes referred to as large granular lymphocytes. They make up approximately 10–15% of the circulating lymphocytes in the peripheral blood. Although NK cells function in much the same way as do **cytotoxic T lymphocytes (CTL),** NK are neither T nor B lymphocytes since they have neither the immunoglobulin receptors found on B lymphocytes nor the T cell antigen receptor found on T cells. NK cells are capable of destroying tumor and virus-infected cells and discriminate between noninfected cells and malignant or virus-infected cells, but they do lack antigen specificity or prior sensitization.

The cell surface proteins marking NK cells are CD56 and CD16. CD3, a T lymphocyte–specific protein, is absent. The azurophilic granules of the NK cells contain cytolytic proteins such as perforins that participate in cytolysis of the target cells. Upon intimate contact with the target cell, the killer cell binds through glycolipids on the target cell surface. The cytoplasmic granules in the NK cells localize at the contact point and discharge cytotoxic proteins. The lethal burst of chemicals contributes to the lysis and finally death of the tumor or virus-infected cell.

NK cells also contain receptors for cytokines such as **interleukin**-2 (**IL**-2). Interaction with these cytokines can activate NK cells. Once activated, the NK cells become LAK cells. With enhanced cytotoxic capability, these LAK cells broaden their range of target cells. LAK cells have been administered clinically to treat tumors, but the toxic effect of the massive doses of IL-2 required concomitantly has limited the success of this therapeutic regimen. LAK cells also produce IFNγ, TNF α, granulocyte-monocyte colony stimulating factor (GM-CSF), and colony stimulating factor-1 (CSF-1).

Although the ability of NK cells to destroy tumor cells has been well investigated, the primary role of NK cells seems to be protection against infection by intracellular microorganisms such as certain viruses, bacteria, and parasites. Recurrent viral infections, especially with DNA viruses, have been associated with deficiency in NK cells.

ACUTE PHASE PROTEINS, COMPLEMENT, AND INTERFERONS

During the response to infection, the concentration of plasma proteins, referred to as acute phase reactants (APRs) or acute phase proteins, increases 2–100 fold. Predominantly synthesized by hepatocytes in the liver at a constant rate during normal conditions, these proteins play a major role in the defense following invasion of a microorganism. APRs are also produced by other cells such as monocytes, endothelial cells, fibroblasts, and adipocytes. Most APRs such as C-reactive protein (CRP) and complement increase significantly during an inflammatory event, causing these reactants to be referred to as "positive APRs." Other proteins such as albumin and transferrin may be decreased during the acute phase of the reaction, so are termed "negative APRs." This decrease may allow the increased production of the positive APRs by the liver. APRs contribute to the host defense in a variety of ways in the event of or following tissue injury, trauma, or an infection. Activities of APRs include direct neutralization of inflammatory agents, reduction in the amount of damage to the affected tissue, and assistance in tissue repair and restoration.

C-reactive Protein

CRP is one of the classic acute-phase proteins. CRP, first discovered in 1930 by Tillet and Frances, derived its name from the ability of this protein to react with the C-polysaccharide of *Streptococcus pneumoniae*. Inflammatory conditions such as infection, trauma, surgery, burns, and malignant diseases usually lead to as much as an 100–1000 fold increase in CRP. The rapid increase in CRP levels is seen within 4–6 hours following injury or trauma, and reaches peak within 24–72 hours. The level, however, declines just as rapidly after the inflammatory stimuli are removed. Moderate changes in CRP concentrations may be seen after strenuous exercises, heatstroke, and childbirth, while small changes may occur after psychological stress and in severe psychiatric illnesses.

Although an increase in CRP is nonspecific, it reflects the presence and intensity of inflammation. Because this acute phase reactant rises quickly during inflammation, but falls rapidly as well, CRP levels have been useful in assessing and monitoring the severity of inflammation and the success of treatment of an infection. During recent years, investigators have reported the linkage of CRP to coronary heart disease. Because inflammation is believed to play a significant role in the development of cardiovascular events, CRP assays have been considered as a potential marker for detecting people at risk of a heart attack. The action of CRP in the innate immune response is related in part to numerous calcium-dependent binding specificities. It binds to the surface of microorganisms, allowing it to function as an opsonin, assists in the activation of the classical pathway of the complement system, and enhances phagocytic cell function and cell-mediated cytotoxicity. Thus, while nonspecific in its action, CRP is capable of amplifying the immune response.

Alpha1-antitrypsin

Another acute phase reactant, alpha1-antitrypsin, acts against proteases, such as elastase, that are released by neutrophils and that may cause damage to elastin and collagen. For example, alpha1-antitrypsin protects the lung tissue from neutrophil elastase during inflammation. When elastin is degraded, the lungs lose their elasticity, making it difficult to expand and contract. Patients who are deficient in alpha1-antitrypsin may eventually suffer from pulmonary conditions such as emphysema, a condition that makes breathing difficult. These conditions are exacerbated by chemical irritants such as tobacco smoke that, in the process of irritating lung tissue, may initiate white blood cell migration. The increased numbers of neutrophils release elastase into the environment, eventually causing even more lung damage.

Haptoglobin

Haptoglobin is an alpha-2 glycoprotein produced by the liver. Normal values for haptoglobin are 27 to 139 mg/dl. The primary function of haptoglobin is to bind free hemoglobin in the plasma. Free hemoglobin concentrations increase during red blood cell destruction. Once bound, the hemoglobin-haptoglobin complex can be removed from circulation by the cells of the reticuloendothelial system and taken up by the liver. Decreased haptoglobin levels are associated with intravascular hemolysis such as that seen in hemolytic anemias, hemolytic transfusion reactions, and hemoglobinopathies. Haptoglobin may be depressed in liver disease because of decreased synthesis. Because haptoglobin is an APR, increased levels are seen in chronic and acute inflammatory conditions such as rheumatic and neoplastic diseases.

Fibrinogen

Fibrinogen, a glycoprotein, is a main factor in the blood coagulation system. One of the largest and most plentiful of the clotting factors in plasma, fibrinogen is cleaved by thrombin to form a fibrin clot. Fibrinogen is decreased during disseminated intravascular coagulation (DIC), in patients with liver disease, or in hereditary afibrinogenemia. Normal levels range from 110–400 mg/dL. Formation of fibrin clot may or may not benefit the host defense against microorganisms. Formation of a fibrin clot may help contain the spread of infection by trapping microorganisms. On the other hand, organisms contained in fibrin clots are protected from other components of the host's immune defenses.

Alpha-1 Acid Glycoprotein

Alpha-1 acid glycoprotein (AAG) is produced in the liver. The primary function of AAG appears to be inactivation of progesterone and other drugs. As an acute phase reactant, AAG is elevated during inflammation and in autoimmune conditions such as rheumatoid arthritis and systemic lupus erythematosus. Elevated levels are also seen in patients with ulcerative colitis.

Complement

Complement is a collective term used to describe a group of plasma proteins that play a critical role in host defense against infectious agents or during an inflammatory response of any type. The components of the complement system protect the host in a variety of ways: (1) lysis of bacterial cells; (2) opsonization of microorganisms so that invaders such as bacteria, viruses, fungi, and others are primed for phagocytosis; (3) attract phagocytes to the site of invasion or infection (chemotaxis); (4) increase in vascular permeability which allows migration of phagocytic cells to the site of infection or inflammation; and (5) removal of infectious agents.

The complement system consists of more than 25 proteins that may function either as enzymes or as binding proteins, which are present in circulation in an inactive form under normal conditions. When the first component is activated, it sets the system in motion, creating a "ripplelike" effect. As each component is activated, it acts upon the next in specific sequence of regulated events known as the complement cascade.

There are three major pathways of complement activation: classical pathway, alternative pathway, and mannan-binding lectin (MBL) pathway. The activities of the complement system are discussed more fully in a later chapter. Briefly, the classical pathway is activated by antigen-antibody complexes, that is, a foreign particle or an **antigen** bound to an **antibody.** This pathway, therefore, is antibody dependent. The alternative pathway, unlike the classical pathway, is antibody independent. It is activated by invading microorganisms and does not require the presence of antibody for activation. Hence, it plays a major role in host defense against bacterial infections. The most recently described pathway is the MBL pathway. The MBL pathway is triggered by the binding of mannan-binding lectin to carbohydrate structures on microorganisms.

Interferons

Interferons may be produced by macrophages, fibroblasts, NK cells, or T lymphocytes, depending on the type. Type I interferons (IFN-α produced by macrophages; IFN-β produced by fibroblasts) affect all cells by inducing an antiviral state which inhibits viral replication in the affected cells and increases MHC Class I expression. Type I interferons also activate NK cells. Type II interferons, also called immune interferon or IFN-γ, are produced by T lymphocytes and NK cells. Type II interferons are able to activate macrophages (which may then in turn produce more Type I interferon) and can stimulate some antibody responses. Cellular and chemical mediators of innate immunity are summarized on Table 2-3✪.

✪ TABLE 2-3

Cellular and Chemical Mediators of Innate Immunity

Mediator	Function
Phagocytes Macrophages Neutrophils Dendritic cells	Phagocytosis; kill and eliminate pathogens; secrete chemokines and cytokines; function as specialized antigen-presenting cell
Cytotoxic Cells Natural-killer cells Killer cells Lymphokine-activated killer cells	Act on virus-infected cells; recognize altered MHC on infected and cancer cells; activated by IL2 or IFN-γ
Chemokines IL-8 C3a, C5a	Chemoattractants; attract leukocytes to infection site; proinflammatory
Opsonins C3b	Promote phagocytosis; prepare pathogens for phagocytosis by binding phagocyte receptors
Cytokines IL-1 IL-6 TNF-α IFN α/IFN β IL-12	Stimulate release of macrophages, cytotoxic cells, neutrophils Promote release of acute phase reactants Increase body temperature Antiviral action; neutralize viral activity in host cells Promote T-cell proliferation

INFLAMMATION AND PHAGOCYTOSIS

Inflammation

Inflammation is the body's defense response to tissue damage, injury, or foreign particles, including microorganisms. Inflammation helps to localize the infection or injury, to remove or eradicate the foreign body, to repair damaged tissue, and to remove debris from the site of injury.

The classic signs of an inflammatory response are redness, heat, swelling, and pain. This response consists of three major events: (1) increased blood flow to the site of injury (which accounts for the redness and heat seen in inflamed tissue); (2) increase vascular permeability which allows mediators of the immune system to cross the endothelium and reach the site; and (3) migration and accumulation of leukocytes at the site of infection or tissue damage.

There are many factors responsible for the events that occur during an acute inflammatory response. Chemical substances, sometimes referred to as chemical mediators, are released from affected tissues and from leukocytes accumulating in the damaged tissue. Chemical mediators cause increased blood flow, vasodilatation, vascular permeability, emigration of leukocytes, and chemotaxis. These chemical mediators include leukotrienes, histamine, lysosomes, prostaglandins, and serotonin. Although inflammation is an extremely essential and beneficial process in the host's immune defense, the products of an inflammatory response cause the swelling and pain seen during inflammation. Also, altered or enhanced immunological responses such as those seen in hypersensitivity reactions, allergy, or in autoimmune diseases cause inappropriate or excessive reactions that result in tissue damage. Chapter 6 discusses the different types of hypersensitivity reactions; Chapter 8 presents manifestations seen in autoimmunity.

Inflammation may be caused by physical, chemical, or microbial agents. Microbial infection is one of the most common causes of inflammation. Gram-negative bacteria possess endotoxins or lipopolysaccharide (LPS) in their cell walls. These substances stimulate strong inflammatory reactions. Endotoxin, for example, can initiate complement activation that results in vascular dilatation and increased blood vessel permeability. Endotoxins may also activate both the coagulation and fibrinolytic pathways and have been associated with DIC. Certain bacteria may also release specific exotoxins which initiate an inflammatory response. Tissue damage occurring after physical trauma, radiation, burns, or exposure to extremely low temperatures may also cause an inflammatory reaction. Acids, alkali, and other oxidizing agents are corrosive chemical irritants that damage tissues and lead to inflammation.

The acute inflammatory response is initially beneficial to the host. Increased flow of fluids to the site of invasion dilutes toxins that may have been secreted by an infecting organism and makes clearance by lymph vessels possible. In addition, cellular exudates contain inflammatory cells such as neutrophils and macrophages that play major roles in phagocytosis and in clearing away damaged tissues and cell debris. Following an increase in vascular permeability, antibodies are able to enter the extravascular space where they may neutralize toxins, lyse microorganisms in the presence of complement, or mediate phagocytosis by opsonizing microbes. Microorganisms may also be trapped in fibrin clots that inhibit spread of the infection and facilitate phagocytosis. Increased flow of fluid not only brings nutrients essential to inflammatory cells but also allows stimulation of the adaptive immune response when the antigen reaches the lymph nodes.

However, tissue damage may follow as a result of an acute inflammatory response. Lysosomal enzymes such as proteases and collagenases released by inflammatory cells may attack and subsequently destroy normal tissues. The swelling caused by the increased vascular permeability that accompanies inflammation may sometimes be harmful. The acute epiglottitis caused by *Haemophilus influenzae* in children illustrates the deleterious effects of the inflammatory response. Intense swelling of the epiglottis may cause mechanical obstruction of the airway which could be fatal. In the inflammatory responses seen in toxic shock syndrome, chemical mediators released as a response to bacterial endotoxins may result in development of the clinical manifestations of septicemia.

Phagocytosis

Phagocytosis, an essential process in host resistance to infection, involves the ingestion and digestion of extracellular particles. Microorganisms, tissue debris, dead host cells, and other foreign particles are all targets for phagocytosis. Phagocytosis begins with chemotaxis followed by attachment, phagosome formation and ingestion of the particle, digestion, and killing. Figure 2-9■ is a schematic representation of the events that take place in phagocytosis.

Chemotaxis is the directed migration of PMNs into a compromised area (Figure 2-10■). Substances that induce such movement are called chemotactic factors. Chemotactic factors may be produced by complement activation—C5a, a component of complement, is

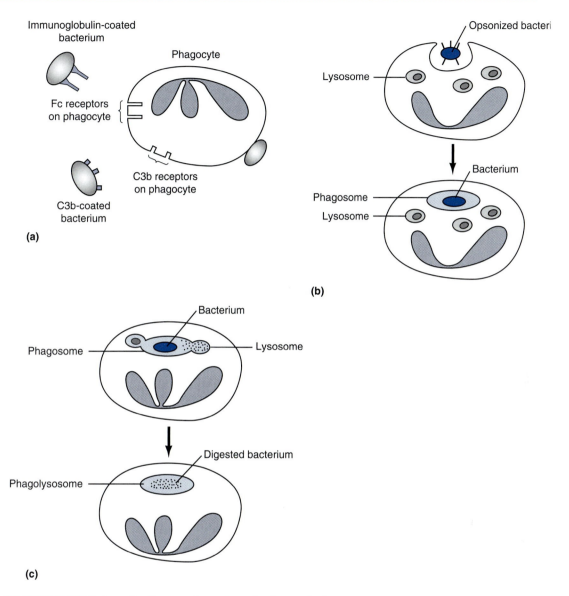

FIGURE 2-9 Schematic diagram of processes in phagocytosis

chemotactic. Other chemotactic factors include bacterial products, products from damaged tissue cells, and mediators produced by other responding inflammatory cells. PMNs and other phagocytic cells constantly patrol the body for foreign particles. When an invader is detected, cells accumulate at the site. PMNs continue to migrate and then squeeze between the endothelial cells lining the blood vessels into the tissues by diapedesis (see Figure 2-4).

Before ingestion can take place, the invading microorganism must first adhere to the PMN membrane. This attachment process is somewhat effective for bacteria but less efficient for proteins or encapsulated organisms. The bacterial capsule is the major structural defense against phagocytosis because it prevents attachment of the bacteria to the PMN membrane. Therefore, encapsulated organisms (Figure 2-11■)— must first be opsonized to facilitate phagocytosis. Opsonization, from the Greek word meaning "prepare for the table," is the process by which microorganisms are altered so that they can be more easily engulfed by phagocytes. Certain host-derived proteins serve as opsonins, substances that may coat particles such as organisms to enhance phagocytosis. Immunoglobulins and complement components are important opsonins. For example, the bacterial cellular structure, lipo-

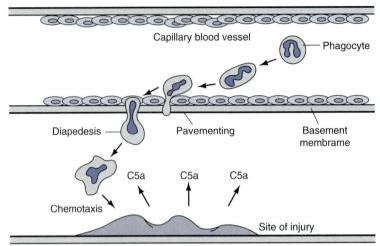

■ **FIGURE 2-10** Chemotaxis. Phagocytes are directed to the site of injury or inflammation. Migration is induced by chemotactic factors such as C5a, a complement component. Other chemoattractants also released by phagocytes adhere to the endothelial cells lining the capillary vessel (pavementing), then squeeze between the cells (diapedesis) to reach the target site.

polysaccharide (LPS), activates complement via the alternative pathway. Activation of the alternative pathway triggers the release of the component C3b, another opsonizing agent. Similarly, immunoglobulins bind to microorganisms by the antigen-binding fragment (Fab), but leave the constant fragment (Fc) component to interact with the Fc surface receptor on PMNs. This then allows the PMNs to attach to the microorganisms. In addition, organisms bound to immunoglobulins can activate the complement via the classical pathway, which then generates C3b. Because phagocytes also express surface receptors for comple-

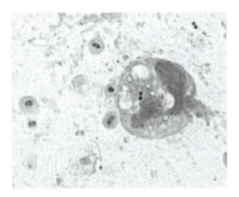

■ **FIGURE 2-11** Encapsulated gram negative bacteria (Gram-stained smear)

ment components, coated particles are targeted for phagocytosis. Figure 2-12■ shows opsonization processes with opsonins C3b and/or immunoglubulin.

Once the phagocyte is attached to the cell surface of the particle to be engulfed, phagocytic pseudopodia extended by the phagocyte engulf the particle, enclosing it in a phagocytic vacuole called a phagosome (See Figure 2-5). The phagosome, bounded by the cell membrane, fuses with lysosomes to form phagolysosome. Lysosomes are membrane-derived vesicles that contain enzymes able to digest and kill microorganisms. Some of these enzymes include proteases, lipases, RNase, DNase, peroxidase, and acid phosphatase. When lysosomes release their potent hydrolytic enzymes into the phagosome, degranulation begins. This degranulation and release of enzymes kills and digests the phagocytized microorganisms. Figure 2-13■ shows remains of degranulation. Granulated cytoplasm is replaced by large cytoplasmic vacuoles.

The metabolic activity of the PMN or macrophage seems to significantly increase upon phagocytosis of a foreign particle. This increase in activity is known as a metabolic or respiratory burst. There is an increase in glycolysis, oxygen use, and production of lactic acid and hydrogen peroxide. The hydrogen peroxide reacts with myeloperoxidase contained in the cytoplasmic granules to produce a bactericidal effect. Additional products of

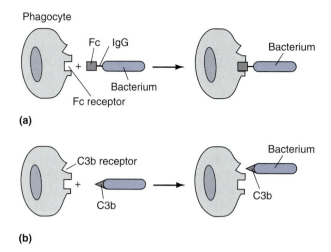

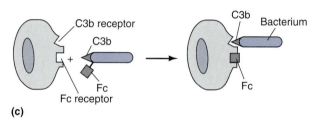

(a)

(b)

(c)

■ FIGURE 2-12 Opsonization process. (a) Antibody-coated bacteria. The antibody attached to the surface of the bacterium minimally binds the Fc phagocyte receptor. (b) Complement-coated bacteria. Complement C3b attached to the surface of the bacterium binds loosely to the phagocyte C3b receptor. (c) Antibody and complement both attached to bacteria. Both antibody and complement C3b are attached to the surface of the bacterium and bound tightly to the phagocyte; allows a greater chance for the phagocyte to engulf the bacterium.

oxygen reduction that contribute to microbial killing include peroxide anions (O_2^-), hydroxyl radicals ($-OH$), and singlet oxygen (1OH). Other enzymes that act on microbes include lactoferrin, lysozyme, and defensins. Lactoferrin chelates iron, which prevents bacterial growth; lysozyme destroys bacterial cells; and defensins increase the permeability of the microbial membranes. The acid pH inside the phagocytic vacuole also contributes to intracellular killing of microorganisms. Therefore, the end result of phagocytosis is the digestion and eventual killing of invading microorganisms.

Certainly, there are microorganisms that are capable of surviving the effects of phagocytosis. These organisms may actually multiply intracellularly. In such cases, other defense mechanisms must be employed. The significance of phagocytosis in immune defense is illustrated in individuals who are deficient in the numbers

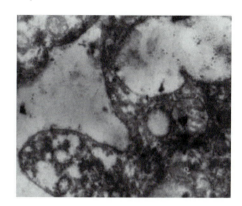

■ FIGURE 2-13 Vacuolated cytoplasm and phagosome (TEM)

or function of phagocytes in their system. These individuals are at risk for a variety of microbial infections.

▶ ADAPTIVE IMMUNITY

Acquired or adaptive immunity enhances and complements innate immunity in protecting the host. However, the ability to respond to a specific foreign substance, or antigen, requires acquired immunity to be much more complex and highly evolved than innate immunity. Adaptive immunity is not only capable of responding to distinct molecules, but also allows development of memory. This immunologic memory engenders a more powerful response to repeated exposures to the same foreign substance. As previously mentioned, adaptive immunity is able to enhance the functions of the innate immune response. Inflammation, a nonspecific innate response that provides signals that activate the adaptive response, is an example of an enhanced innate immune reaction.

ANTIGENS AND ANTIBODIES

Immunogens are substances capable of eliciting an immune response; when they do, they are considered immunogenic. In most cases, the response comes from both humoral and cellular components of the immune system. The immune response comes from clones of B or T lymphocytes whose surface immunoglobulin or **T cell receptor (TCR)** proteins recognize the immunogen. Substances that stimulate antibody production and are capable of binding to the antibody are called **antigens,** hence, they are considered antigenic. Immunogens, therefore, are also antigens. However, not all immunogens are antigenic. Although most immunogens are ubiquitous in the environment and are comprised of a variety of molecules, the immune response is usually directed only against specific molecular components that contain structures recognized as foreign by the immune system. These structures, recognized by the corresponding antibody or TCR, are called antigenic determinants or **epitopes.** In essence, the epitope is the target site to which the immunoglobulin or TCR binds.

The main components of adaptive immunity are immunoglobulins (Ig). Ig, also called antibodies, are proteins that are capable of binding with a specific antigen. The specific antibody matches the antigen that initiated the antibody response, like a lock to a key. Figure 2-14a■ shows a diagram of an immunoglobulin structure and Figure 2-14b, the concept of "lock and key." Although the match is not always precise, the antibody engages with the antigen enough to tag it for destruction. Each antibody has two identical heavy

polypeptide chains and two identical light chains that form the shape of a "Y." The amino acid sequences at the tip of the "Y" arms vary significantly from one antibody to another, and create a pocket ready to enfold a specific antigen. This section is called the variable (V) or Fab region of the immunoglobulin. The stem of the "Y," on the other hand, is called the constant (C) or Fc region and is an area that is identical in all antibodies of the same class. This section of the antibody functions to bind the antibody to other components of the immune defense mechanism such as complement or protein receptors on phagocytes.

There are nine chemically distinct classes of human Ig: IgG (four subclasses), IgM, IgA (two subclasses), IgE, and IgD. Each class of Ig has a specific role in the immune defense strategy. IgG works efficiently in coating microorganisms, preparing them for easy uptake by phagocytes. IgG makes up the major Ig component in

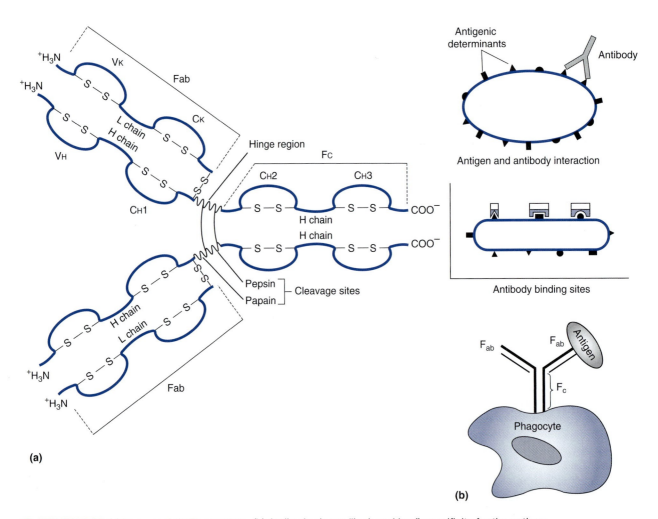

(a)

(b)

■ FIGURE 2-14 (a) Immunoglobulin structure. (b) Antibody shows "lock and key" specificity for the antigen.

the blood although a certain amount may enter the tissues. IgM, concentrated in the bloodstream, is very effective in killing bacteria while IgA is present primarily in body fluids such as tears and sweat, and is secreted by B lymphocytes in the respiratory and gastrointestinal tract mucosa. IgE, usually present in minute amounts, is activated in parasitic infections but is also seen in response to allergic reactions. IgD, embedded exclusively in the membranes of B cells, regulates the activation of these cells. A more detailed discussion of the composition, structure, and functions of antibodies and immunogens is found in Chapter 3.

Lymphoid Organs and Lymphopoiesis

The primary lymphoid organs, thymus and bone marrow, produce and release lymphocytes at a fairly constant rate, regardless of whether the cells are required in the immune response. This production of lymphocytes from uncommitted progenitor or stem cells is termed **lymphopoiesis.** The thymus continues to release T lymphocytes until about the time of puberty at which point this lymphoid organ involutes, becoming much smaller and more acellular than the thymus seen in neonates. Meanwhile, the bone marrow continues to produce B lymphocytes throughout life.

Lymphocytes are white blood cells that play a significant role in the activities of the immune response. Morphologically, a lymphocyte is small, round, and measures approximately 10–12 µm in diameter (Figure 2-15■). It has a spherical nucleus with a dense nuclear chromatin and scanty cytoplasm. Although most may appear morphologically identical, there are several different types of lymphocytes which can be differentiated based on their functions and by the specific protein markers expressed on the cell membrane. In general, there are two distinct types: T, or thymus-derived lymphocytes, and B, or bone-marrow derived, lymphocytes. Common immunologic jargon also refers

to these cells as T cells and B cells. T and B lymphocytes make up about 75% and 10% of all lymphocytes in the peripheral blood, respectively. Natural killer (NK) cells, discussed earlier, account for the remaining 15%.

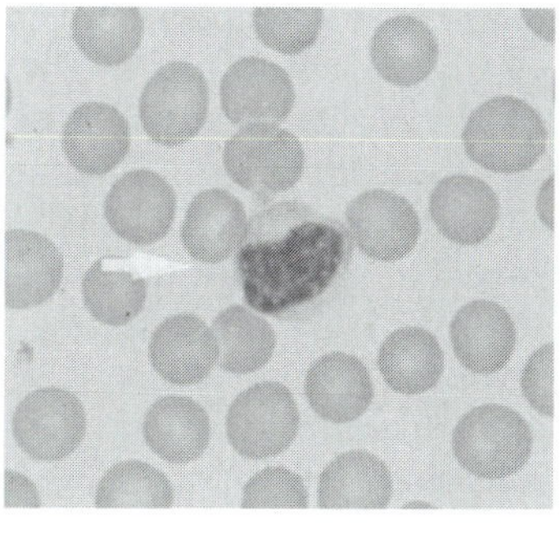

The two major lineages both originate from a common precursor stem cell found in the bone marrow or fetal liver. The progeny of these stem cells follow different pathways to mature into either T or B lymphocytes. While human B lymphocytes develop and mature entirely within the bone marrow, T cells develop from immature precursors in the bone marrow but leave the marrow and move to the thymus where they differentiate into mature T lymphocytes.

When released into the peripheral circulation from the thymus or bone marrow, the mature lymphocytes do not proliferate, although they are capable of undergoing cell division when called upon to perform their immunologic functions. These newly dispersed lymphocytes, sometimes referred to as "naive" lymphocytes, migrate into the secondary lymphoid organs such as the spleen, lymph nodes, tonsils, and Peyers patches (found in the intestinal mucosa), where most immune responses are initiated. Since naive lymphocytes must be activated by an encounter with the antigen for which they are specific, most naive lymphocytes are short-lived and die through **apoptosis** within a few days after they are released from the bone marrow or thymus. The required encounter of naive lymphocyte and antigen in a secondary lymphoid organ is purely serendipitous. Activation of naive lymphocytes takes into effect when cells receive signals that indicate the presence of a foreign material, invader, or pathogen. As soon as activation occurs, naive cells begin their cell division and differentiate into two forms of cells: effector cells that fulfill specific immune functions and memory cells that behave like naive T and B lymphocytes but that may survive for years and are capable of responding promptly of the antigen for which they are specific.

HUMORAL AND CELL-MEDIATED IMMUNE RESPONSES

B lymphocytes

B lymphocytes mature independently of the thymus. Their main function is to secrete antibodies into the body fluids or humors (hence, humoral immunity). Conversely, the only cells in the body capable of secreting antibodies are the B cells or plasma cells (terminally differentiated B lymphocytes) as shown in Figure 2-16■. These Ig interact with the circulating target antigens, such as bacteria and other foreign molecules, but cannot act against microbes sequestered within living cells.

■ FIGURE 2-15 Lymphocyte, peripheral blood, Wright stain

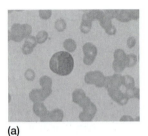 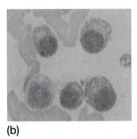

(a)   (b)

■ FIGURE 2-16 (a) Plasma cell (peripheral blood, Wright stain). (b) Plasma cell (bone marrow, Giemsa stain).

T-cells, on the other hand, interact directly with the target cells and can therefore eliminate host cells that have been attacked by viruses. This is referred to as cellular immunity or the cell-mediated immune response.

The major contribution of B cells to is to synthesize Ig. Ig can be expressed on the cell surface of mature naive or memory B cell lymphocyte or can be secreted by effector B cells called plasma cells. While in quiescent state, a B cell may express numerous Ig molecules on its surface. Once activated, B lymphocytes undergo cell division, and whereas some of the progeny become memory B cells, the others differentiate into plasma cells. In addition to the primary function of antibody production, B lymphocytes also possess receptors that when bound to foreign particles send activating signals to T lymphocytes, thus allowing B cells to function as antigen-presenting cells.

Plasma cells are oval in shape with round nuclei eccentrically located in large amounts of cytoplasm (see Figure 2-16). The life span of plasma cells in peripheral circulation is relatively short—only a few days to a week. Antibody levels therefore increase when B cells are activated, but later decline over several days or a few weeks when plasma cells no longer secrete Ig. In order to maintain a source of circulatory antibodies, a certain number of cells committed to becoming plasma cells travel to the bone marrow where they survive for a much longer period of time.

Plasma cells secrete antibodies that recognize and bind to specific antigens. Antibodies that are in circulation account for approximately 25% of total serum protein at a concentration of 7–26 g/L in the adults. Antibodies secreted by plasma cells provide numerous beneficial effects to the host, including opsonization to enhance phagocytosis, agglutination or precipitation of particles, and activation of the complement system leading to lysis of microorganisms.

T Lymphocytes

T lymphocytes make up the major cells involved in adaptive cell-mediated immunity. They arise from multipotential stem cells in the bone marrow which migrate during ontogeny into the thymus. During their tenure in the thymus, the T cell precursors undergo tremendous proliferation induced by IL7 produced by stromal cells in the thymus. Production of mature T cells is a very wasteful process—only about 1% of the T cell precursors produced in the thymus ever reach the periphery.

One of the reasons for this resource-consuming process is the necessity to produce T cells capable of responding to a foreign substance but disinclined to respond aggressively to self. Just as each clone of B cells has a specific receptor for antigen (the immunoglobulin molecule), T cells also possess a specific receptor for antigen. However, unlike B-cells that express Ig, T lymphocytes express surface proteins called T cell receptors which are able to bind to an antigen. These polypeptide receptors, comprised of alpha and beta chains or of gamma and delta chains, are able to bind to specific antigens. As alluded to in Chapter 1, these receptors are the product of multiple gene rearrangements which must be completed successfully before the T cells can leave the thymus.

In an arrangement analogous to that found in B cells (to be explained in detail in Chapter 3), each genetic locus for the different polypeptide chains of the TCR contains multiple variable (V), joining (J), and constant (C) region genes. The locus for the TCR beta gene also contains diversity (D) gene segments. Rearrangement and splicing of the DNA to eliminate all but one of each of the region genes is required before mRNA coding for a receptor chain can be made. These rearrangements are random, and it is pure serendipity that the enormous variation in antigen-binding sites generated interact with the antigens commonly encountered.

If a pro–T cell, which does not express either CD4 or CD8, is to survive, it must express the beta chain of the TCR. If successful, the pro-T cell becomes a pre–T cell. If unsuccessful, the cell dies by apoptosis. Rearrangement of the alpha chain must then take place. Once again, failure to express a complete antigen receptor results in cell death. Successful pre–T cells become immature T cells. These cells are double-positive for both CD4 and CD8 surface proteins.

Immature T cells must then undergo the rigorous processes of **positive selection and negative selection** in the thymus. These processes encourage development of "good" T cells which are capable of recognizing foreign antigens, eliminate the "bad" T cells which react with self-antigen, and further eliminate the "useless" T cells which are not autoreactive but do not have the potential to recognize foreign antigens either. Positive selection preserves immature T cells which weakly recognize either major histocompatibility complex (MHC) Class II and peptide or MHC Class I and peptide. Since, as is explained in more detail later, T cells are only able to recognize short peptides bound to MHC molecules of the same type as the T cells, this is a critical step in assuring that the T cells remaining after the positive selection process are capable of recognizing antigen. The "useless" T cells which do not recognize MHC plus peptide die by apoptosis after positive selection. Negative selection eliminates the "bad" T cells. These are cells that recognize either MHC Class I or MHC Class II plus peptide strongly. These cells have the potential to become autoreactive should they reach the periphery. The implications of this are further discussed in Chapter 8. Cells that survive both positive and negative selection become mature naive T cells. Those that recognized MHC Class I retain CD8 on their surface, while those that recognize MHC Class II retain CD4 (Figure 2-17■).

The naive T cells that leave the thymus do not become activated until they encounter the antigen for which they are specific. Antigen is generally encountered in the peripheral lymphoid tissue, which, as described previously, has the combination of cells necessary to trap and retain antigen and to present antigen to the T cells.

Through the immunoglobulin antigen receptor on their surface, B cells are capable of recognizing many types of antigens, including both large and small peptides, nucleic acids, and polysaccharides. In contrast, T cells can only recognize proteins that have been processed and presented to them in the context of self-MHC either by APC or by infected somatic cells. Antigen recognition is through the TCR complex. This complex is comprised not only of the alpha and beta chains of the TCR, which are responsible for antigen recognition, but also of CD4 or CD8 molecules which bind to MHC Class II or MHC Class I to mediate adhesion and signal transduction. LFA-1 and VLA-4, both cell adhesion molecules, participate in the adhesion of the T cell to its target. However, unlike Ig, these receptors are not secreted by the T cells. Therefore, T cells are not able to attack targets that are at a distance and must depend on direct contact with their targets. These targets may be microbes, or may be the target antigens displayed on the surface of an antigen-presenting cell (Figure 2-18■).

Although just about all types of host cells can present antigens under certain conditions, there are cells that are specifically suited for this function and help keep in check T cell activities. This group of specialized cells, called antigen-presenting cells (APC), includes macrophages, B lymphocytes, and **dendritic cells.** Derived from bone marrow, dendritic cells play a very important role in initiating T cell activity because of their particularly unique structure. Present in almost all tissues, dendritic cells possess numerous cytoplasmic projections, called dendrites that give these cells the characteristic stellate shape. Macrophages, B cells, and dendritic cells are all capable of processing an antigen, digesting it, and presenting a peptide from the antigen in a form recognized by the T cell. Chapter 9 discusses in detail the process of antigen processing and presentation by MHC Class I and Class II antigens. Antigen presentation by APC to CD4+ T cells is also critical for activation of the T cells. APC express on their surface a number of proteins that must bind to an accessory molecule on the T cell in order for the T cell to become activated upon recognition of the antigen. This costimulatory signal for signal transduction occurs when CD28 on the T cells binds to B7-1/B7-2 on the APC surface. Similar binding of CTLA-4 on T cells to the same B7-1/B7-2 receptor acts as a negative regulator. In addition, the binding of T cells to APC is strengthened through binding of the T cell adhesion molecules LFA-1 and VLA-4 to ICAM-1 on APC and endothelial cells, and to VCAM-1 on endothelial cells.

In addition to possessing characteristic T cell morphology, mature T lymphocytes also express surface proteins responsible for specific functions of the T cells. Some of these proteins designated "cluster determinant"

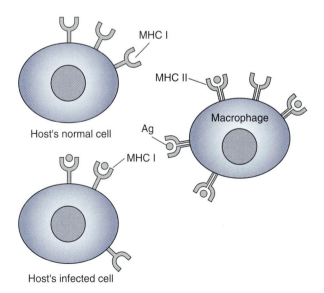

■ FIGURE 2-17 Major histocompatibility complex (MHC) Proteins I and II (MCH I and MCH II)

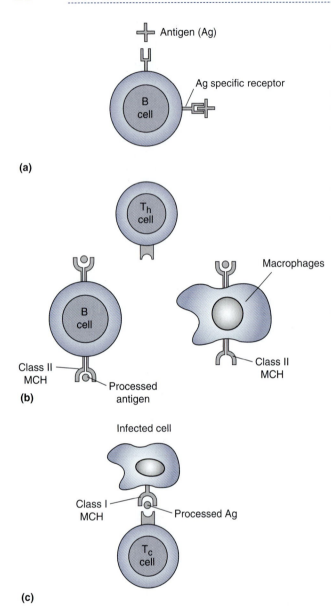

(a)

(b)

(c)

■ **FIGURE 2-18** (a) B cell, anchored in its surface, carry antigen-specific receptors. B cell interacts with the matching antigen ("lock and key") when encountered in blood or other body fluid. (b) B cell and macrophages process antigens encountered, and present processed antigen to T helper cells. B cells, however, can bind only antigens that specifically fit their specific receptor. A helper cell's antigen-specific receptor recognizes antigen presented by APC (Class II MHC). (c) Cytotoxic T cell responds to antigen bound to MHC Class I molecules found on normal or infected body cells.

or CD antigens also serve as markers that aid in the identification of T cells and T cell subset. Among these surface proteins is included the CD3 complex, a group of proteins expressed primarily by T lineage cells, which is used in the laboratory to identify a cell as a T lymphocyte. CD2, which is never found on other cell types, appears at an earlier stage than does CD3. CD2 remains on the surfaces of all T lineage cells, and is therefore a significant marker for identification of all T cells. Because all mature T lymphocytes in the peripheral circulation and in other lymphoid organs express CD2 and CD3 on their surface, they are designated as CD2+CD3+. Within CD2+CD3+ group are T-cell subsets—subpopulations of T lymphocytes that possess their own identifying surface markers and unique immunologic functions.

CD4 and CD8 are the two most significant surface proteins used to designate T cell subsets. Those that express surface marker CD4 are designated as **T helper cells** because they essentially "help" other cells in their proliferation and maturation, as well as in other immunologic activities, by producing cytokines. Although both CD4 and CD8 are expressed on T cells during their maturation in the thymus, the majority of mature T cells in the periphery express either CD4 or CD8. Those that express CD8 proteins are designated as CTL because of their ability to kill cells marked as foreign. CD4 cells (CD4+CD8−) comprise about 70 percent of T cells in peripheral blood and secondary lymphoid tissues; CD8 cells (CD4−CD8+) make up about 25 percent. The remaining T cell populations outside of the thymus are CD4−CD8−, comprising about 4 percent, and those that are CD4+CD8+. The function of this 1 percent of T cells carrying both CD4 and CD8 is not clear. T cells also express CD154 (also known as CD40 ligand), which bind to CD40 on macrophages and B cells. This binding enhances macrophage and B cell activation, which, in turn, either through costimulatory signals from the B cells or production of IL12 by macrophages, enhances T cell activation and effector function.

Although the effector functions of CD4 or CD8 cells were initially associated with helper-inducer (Th) cells and cytotoxic (Tc) cells respectively, these associations are not absolute. For example, although the major function of CD4+ T cells is to produce cytokines which influence the response of many other cells of the immune system, a certain number of CD4 cells may possess cytotoxic activity whereas a few CD8 cells may show helper functions. In addition, Th cells are further divided into Th subsets (i.e., Th1 and Th2 cells) which may stimulate or suppress an immune response. Th1 cells produce IFN-γ which activates macrophages, stimulate production of antibody isotypes which bind to Fc receptors on macrophages, and stimulate expression of MHC class II and B7. Th1 cells therefore promote opsonization and phagocytosis of bacteria, macrophage activation, and indirectly amplify the T cell response through interaction with activated macrophages. Th1 cells also produce IL-2, which is required for T cell proliferation. Th2 cells produce IL4 and IL5, which are required for class switching and for production of the IgE antibodies and activation of eosinophils seen in Type I hypersensitivity reactions (discussed in Chapter 6). Production of IL10 and IL13 inhibit macrophage activation and suppress Th1 cell-mediated immunity.

When activated, T lymphocytes can immediately undergo mitotic division to produce several daughter cells. Daughter cells resemble the parents; CD4+ cells will only produce CD4+ effector cells and memory cells while CD8+ will produce CD8+ effector and memory cells.

MAJOR HISTOCOMPATIBILITY COMPLEX (MHC) ANTIGENS

Before an immune response is launched, the cells of the adaptive immune system must first be activated. The Ig present on the surface of B lymphocytes and the TCR present on T lymphocytes cells allow these cells to recognize bind to target antigens. The Ig on B cells can bind to antigens encountered in the blood and body fluids. These antigens may be protein, carbohydrate, or nucleic acid, and can be soluble or be present on the surface of microorganisms or other cells. T cells, on the other hand, cannot recognize entire proteins or any carbohydrates. Instead, as described previously, T cells are only activated when a very short peptide piece of the antigen is appropriately presented along with protein molecules called **major histocompatibility complex (MHC) antigens** by the APCs.

Originally referred to as human leukocyte antigens (HLA), MHC antigens are proteins on the surfaces of tissue and blood cells that provide identity to a specific individual. These proteins were first identified in individuals who developed antibodies after numerous blood transfusions or multiple pregnancies. These antibodies produced a reaction against membrane proteins on leukocytes from other individuals. It was recognized that T cells from two different individuals react strongly against HLA proteins present on the other leukocytes. MHC proteins have also been associated with rejected transplanted organs. MHC mismatches between organ donor and recipient result in rejection of a transplanted organ or tissue.

There are two types of MHC molecules associated with the presentation of peptides: Class I and Class II. Class I MHC is ubiquitous, found in varying concentrations on most cells in the body. Class II MHC molecules are usually found in quantity only on specialized cells, such as macrophages, dendritic cells, and B cells that can present antigens (see Figure 2-17). MHC molecules therefore serve as a means to indicate the presence of an antigen. For example, in a virus-infected cell, viral proteins are broken up into small peptides, loaded onto MHC I molecules, and transported to the surface of the cell. Cytotoxic T cell lymphocytes (CD8+) can bind specifically to this complex. The MHC Class I proteins loaded with peptide essentially signal the CTL that the cell is infected and should be destroyed. Similarly, macrophages engulf and break up bacterial antigens into small pieces, load these peptides onto class II molecules and display them on their surface to activate helper T cells (CD4+). In sum, cytotoxic T cells (CD8+) recognize MHC Class I and peptide antigens originating from the infected target cells, whereas helper T cells (CD4+) respond to MHC class II and proteins acquired and processed by dendritic cells, macrophages, and B cells. A more detailed discussion of MHC is presented in Chapter 9.

PRIMARY VERSUS SECONDARY ANTIBODY RESPONSE

Primary Response

The first exposure to an antigen requires activation of the B and T cells, proliferation of the activated cells, and generation of the appropriate immune response (production of antibody or a cell-mediated response. Figure 2-19■ shows a schematic diagram of the events that follow an initial exposure to a particular antigen. All of this takes time. This primary immune response is kinetically slow, small in magnitude, and characterized by the appearance of primarily IgM antibodies at first. IgM antibody levels usually peak within one to two weeks following exposure and gradually decline to undetectable levels over the next few weeks or months. At the same time as the IgM antibody levels approach peak, IgG antibodies become detectable and continue to increase for about a month. IgG antibody levels usually remain high for several months and then slowly decline, maintaining a low but detectable level for years.

Secondary Response

A secondary immune response occurs following reexposure to the same antigen. Figure 2-20■ shows the events that occur during a secondary immune

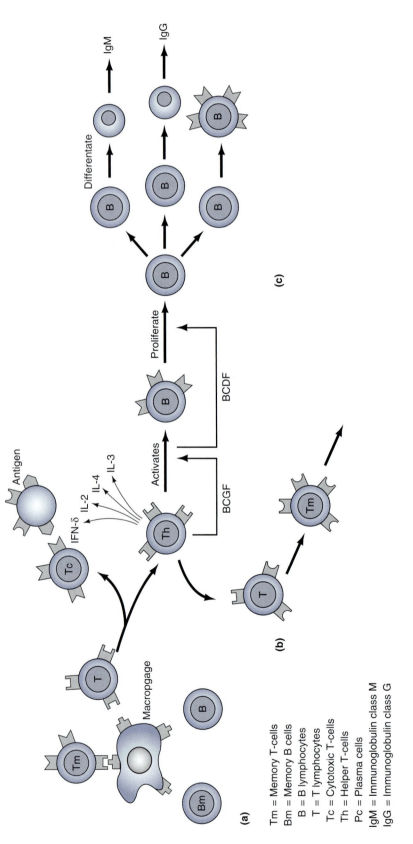

Tm = Memory T-cells
Bm = Memory B cells
B = B lymphocytes
T = T lymphocytes
Tc = Cytotoxic T-cells
Th = Helper T-cells
Pc = Plasma cells
IgM = Immunoglobulin class M
IgG = Immunoglobulin class G

■ **FIGURE 2-19** Primary antibody response—events that follow an initial antigen exposure. (a) APC macrophage presents antigen to T and B lymphocytes and memory cells. No recognition by memory cells. (b) Th and Tc lymphocytes activated. Cytotoxic T cells attack or kill antigen. Th produce lymphocytes and activate B cells. (c) Activated B lymphocytes proliferate, then differentiate into plasma cells to produce IgM first, later IgG. Memory B and T cells are produced.

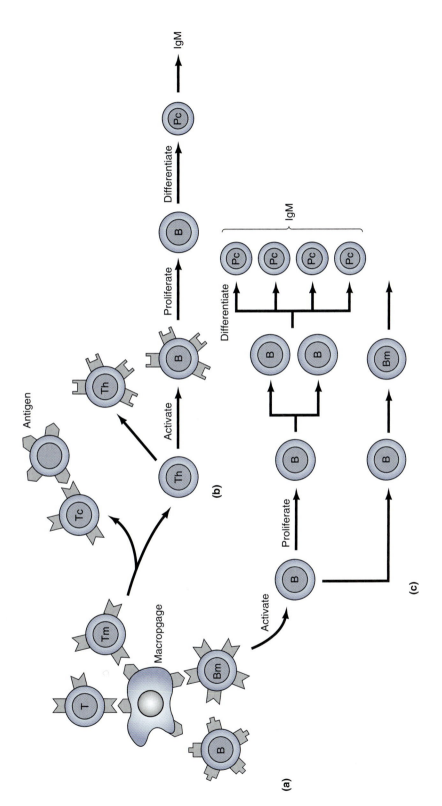

■ **FIGURE 2-20** Secondary antibody, response—events that show the rapid and specific host's immune response to an antigen previously encountered. (a) APC (macrophage) presents antigen to T and B cells and memory cells. T and B memory cells recognize antigen. (b) Memory T cells (1) activate Tc to attack or kill antigen; (2) differentiate to Th; (3) activate B-lymphocytes; (4) produce more memory T cells. (c) Memory B cells differentiate plasma cells to produce imunoglobulins and produce more memory cells.

29

response following a second exposure to the same antigen. In the secondary immune response, larger quantities of Ig G are produced quickly. This increase is more prolonged and shows a more gradual decline than is seen in the primary immune response. Production of IgM antibodies is minor. The difference in responses may be accounted for by the presence and activation of memory cells. A similarly rapid and enhance cell-mediated immune response is also seen upon reexposure to antigen. Figure 2-21■ represents what occurs following the initial reexposure to the same antigen and the corresponding antibody rise and fall following antigen stimulations.

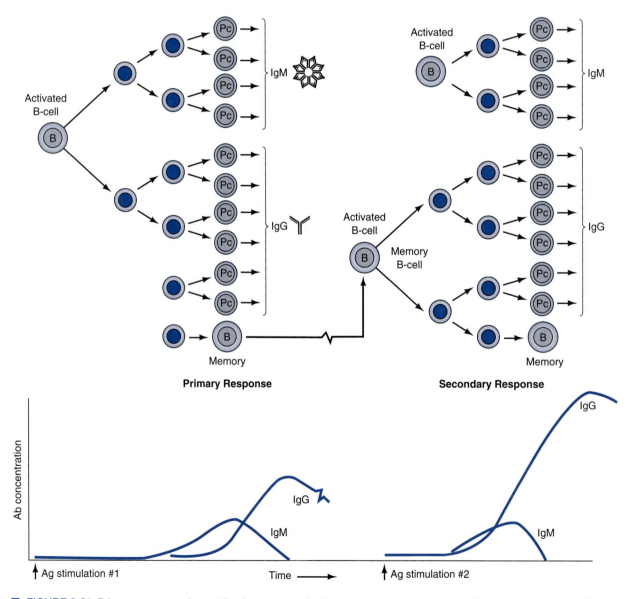

■ FIGURE 2-21 Primary vs. secondary antibody response. Antibody concentration corresponding to the activities of T and B lymphocytes during an initial exposure and subsequent exposure to the same antigen.

SUMMARY

The immune system has evolved with redundancy, as well as checks and balances. The first lines of defense against microbial invasion are chemical and mechanical. As such, these barriers are nonspecific, but can act quickly against most assaults. Should the physical barriers be breached, the cells and chemical factors of the innate immune system function rapidly and nonspecifically. At the same time the innate immune response is containing the potential pathogen, cells and cytokines are initiating the inflammatory response that further contains invaders. The products of the inflammatory response, along with the macrophages and dendritic cells of the innate immune system, then help to activate the B and T cells of the adaptive immune response. After the microbes have been cleared, memory B and T cells remain in a quiescent state, ready to be reactivated should the specific antigens to which they responded reappear. In this way, the immune system has mechanisms by which a quick, nonspecific response can be mounted along with a slower, but exquisitely specific, response. The fine-tuning of these responses insures that the immune system appropriately recognizes threats (pathogens), but does not respond either to its own antigens or to inconsequential antigens. Further chapters in this text discuss the results of a breakdown of this delicate balance.

POINTS TO REMEMBER

▶ Although the immune system is considered to have two divisions, innate immunity and adaptive immunity, these two divisions interact on many levels to produce an immune response to a pathogen.

▶ The first line of defense against pathogens is physical, created by chemical and mechanical barriers. This defense is nonspecific.

▶ The hallmarks of inflammation are the result of chemical factors and cells responding as part of the innate immune response.

▶ Cytokines and antigen-presenting cells from the innate immune response interact with and activate the lymphocytes of the adaptive immune response.

▶ The specificity of the adaptive immune response results from production of antibodies by B cells during the humoral response and activation of particular clones of T cells during the cell-mediated immune response.

▶ B cells bind to a specific antigen through the variable region of surface Ig; T cells recognize antigen through the TCR.

▶ B cells are able to recognize a much more diverse set of antigens than are T cells. T cells must interact with peptides presented by self Class I (if CD8+ cytotoxic T cells) or Class II MHC (if CD4+ helper T cells).

▶ Immunoglobulin serves as both a recognition molecule on B cells and as the effector in the B cell-mediated immune response. T cells utilize the TCR as a recognition structure, but effector functions are generated separately.

LEARNING ASSESSMENT QUESTIONS

1. T lymphocytes recognize antigen by binding to the:
   a. intact antigen.
   b. intact antigen plus MHC.
   c. degraded antigen plus MHC.
   d. degraded antigen presented by APC in the context of MHC.

2. The major contribution of B cells to the immune response is to:
   a. directly cause cytotoxic killing.
   b. produce cytokines.
   c. phagocytize microbes and foreign particles.
   d. produce antibodies.

3. You would expect to see acute response phase proteins secreted:
   a. during an inflammatory response.
   b. following a traumatic injury.
   c. by hepatocytes during normal conditions.
   d. a and b
   e. a, b, and c

4. The major role of PMNs is to:
   a. produce cytokines by which to activate other cells.
   b. ingest and eliminate microorganisms.
   c. make antibodies.
   d. act as antigen-presenting cells for the adaptive immune system.

5. Components of the innate immune system include all of the following EXCEPT:
   a. chemical factors and cytokines.
   b. phagocytes.
   c. lymphocytes.
   d. mechanical barriers.

REFERENCES

Ballou, S. P. and I. Kushner. 1992. C-reactive protein and the acute phase response. *Adv Intern Med* 37:313–36.

Bjorkman, P. J. 1997. MHC restriction in three dimensions: A view of T cell receptor/ligand interactions. *Cell* 89:167.

Ceciliani, F., A. Giordano, and V. Spagnolo. 2002. The systemic reaction during inflammation: The acute-phase proteins. *Protein Peptide Lett* 9:211–23.

Del Prete, G. 1998. The concept of type-1 and type-2 helper T cells and their cytokines in humans. *Int Rev Immunol* 16:427.

Fu Y-X, and D. D. Chaplin. 1999. Development and maturation of secondary lymphoid tissues. *Ann Rev Immunol* 17:399.

Gabay, C. and I. Kushner. 1999. Acute-phase proteins and other systemic response to inflammation. *N Engl J Med* 340:448–54.

Grewal, I. S. and R. A. Flavell. 1998. CD40 and CD154 in cell-mediated immunity. *Ann Rev Immunol* 16:111.

Guermonprez, P., J. Valladeau, J. Zitvogel, C. Thery, and S. Amigorena. 2002. Antigen presentation and T cell stimulation by dendritic cells. *Ann Rev Immunol* 20:621.

Himestra, P. S. and R. Bals. 2004. Series introduction: Innate host defense of the respiratory epithelium. *J Leukoc Biol* 75:3–4.

Johnston, H. L., C. C. Chiou, and C. T. Cho. 1999. Applications of acute phase reactants in infectious diseases. *J Microbiol Immunol Infect* 32:73–82.

Jupe, D. 1996. The acute phase response and laboratory testing. *Aust Fam Physician* 25:324–29.

Kamradt, T. and N. A. Mitchison. 2001. Tolerance and autoimmunity. *N Engl J Med* 344:655–664.

Lanzavecchia, A. and F. Sallusto. 2000. Dynamics of T lymphocyte responses: Intermediates, effectors, and memory cells. *Science* 290:92.

Lipscomb, M. F. and B. J. Masten. 2002. Dendritic cells: Immune regulators in health and disease. *Physiol Rev* 82:97–130.

Mahon, C. R. and G. Manuselis. 2000. *Textbook of Diagnostic Microbiology.* W. B. Saunders, Philadelphia, PA.

McKenzie, SB. 2004. *Clinical Laboratory Hematology.* Prentice-Hall. Upper Saddle River, NJ.

Medzhitov, R. and C. Janeway. 2000. Innate immunity. *N En Jour Med* 343:338–44.

Nemazee, D. 2000. Receptor selection in B and T lymphocytes. *Ann Rev Immunol* 18:19.

Okazaki, T. and T. Nagai. 2002. Usefulness of methemogloin/haptoglonin analysis in the follow-up of severe immune hemolytic anemia. *Chest* 121:1724.

Pichler, W. J. 2003. Delayed drug hypersensitivity reactions. *Ann Intern Med* 139:683–93.

Rock K. L. and A. L. Goldberg. 1999. Degradation of cell proteins and generation of MHC Class I-presented peptides. *Ann Rev Immunol* 17:739.

Sharpe A. H. and G. J. Freeman. 2002. The B7-CD28 superfamily. *Nature Rev Immunol* 2:116.

Starr T. K., S. C. Jameson, and K. A. Hogquist. 2003. Positive and negative selection of T cells. *Ann Rev Immunol* 21:139.

Strieter, R., J. A. Belperio, and M. O. Keane. 2002. Cytokines in innate host defense in the lung. *J Clin Invest* 109:699–705.

Wang, Y., E. Kinzie, F. G. Berger, S. K. Lim, and H. Baumann. 2001. Haptoglobin, an inflammation-inducible plasma protein. *Redox Report* 6:379–85.

Woodhouse, S. 2002. C-reactive protein: From acute phase reactant to cardiovascular disease risk factor. *MLO Med Lab Obs* 34:12–13.

3

Immunoglobulins

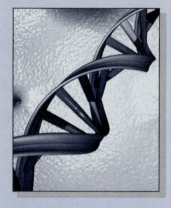

■ CHAPTER CHECKLIST

Upon reading and studying this chapter, the reader will be able to:

1. Describe the processes that occur during B cell maturation.

2. Describe the characteristics of a good immunogen.

3. Illustrate the structure of an immunoglobulin molecule to include heavy chain, light chain, interchain disulfide bonds, intrachain disulfide bonds, and the Fc and Fab (including hypervariable area) regions, and the binding sites for complement, neutrophils, and monocytes.

4. Discuss the rearrangement of the immunoglobulin (Ig) genes and its relationship to production of immunoglobulins.

5. Compare and contrast the function and structure of each of the Ig classes and subclasses.

6. Characterize monoclonal antibodies.

℮ CASE IN POINT

A 25-year-old female presented to her primary care physician in late June with a low-grade fever, anorexia, nausea, vomiting, and severe fatigue. Upon physical examination, the physician noted icteric sclera and hepatomegaly. She ordered a hepatitis panel, liver panel, complete blood count (CBC), and urinalysis. Dark urine was noted when the sample for urinalysis was collected. The serum transaminases were elevated. The hepatitis panel at the time of admission was as follows:

Anti-HAV IgM	positive
Anti-HAV IgG	negative
HBsAg	negative
Anti-HBc IgM	negative
Anti-HBs IgG	positive
Anti-HCV	negative

Upon further questioning, the patient revealed that she had traveled to a coastal area in May and eaten raw oysters. Several of her traveling companions had also begun to have symptoms similar to hers. Her medical history showed that she had been vaccinated for Hepatitis B the previous year. Treatment for symptom relief was ordered, and

CASE IN POINT *(continued)*

she was asked to repeat her laboratory work in four weeks. At that time, the serum transaminases had returned to within reference ranges. The hepatitis panel results four weeks later were as follows:

Anti-HAV IgM	negative
Anti-HAV IgG	positive
HBsAg	negative
Anti-HBc IgM	negative
Anti-HBs IgG	positive
Anti-HCV	negative

ISSUES TO CONSIDER

After reading this patient's case history, consider

● The clinical presentation and laboratory findings presented by this patient

● Which immunoglobulin class shows a positive finding

● The major characteristics and functions of each immunoglobulin class

● Which immunoglobulin class represents an acute, chronic, or convalescent stage of the disease

● How immunoglobulin levels are used as prognostic indicators in certain types of diseases

IMPORTANT TERMS

Adaptive immunity	Epitope	Immunoglobulin
Allotype	Foreignness	Interleukin (IL)
Antibody	Gene rearrangement	Isotype
Antigen dependent	Germline	J chain
Antigenic determinant	Heavy chain	Light chain
Antigen independent	Humoral immunity	Maturation
Antigen presenting cell (APC)	Idiotype	Monoclonal
B cell	IgA	Polyclonal
B cell receptor (BCR)	IgD	Proliferation
Cell surface marker	IgE	Secretory piece
Cytokine	IgG	T helper (T$_H$) cells
Degradability	IgM	Thymus dependent (TD)
Differentiation	Immunogen	Thymus independent (TI)
Domains	Immunogenicity	Variable region

► INTRODUCTION

Although B lymphocytes are only a small proportion of the cells circulating in the peripheral blood, they are arguably one of the most important components of the immune system. In conjunction with **antigen-presenting cells (APCs)** and T lymphocytes, the **B cells** are primarily responsible for the humoral arm of acquired or **adaptive immunity** that protects humans from bacterial and fungal infections through the elaboration of **antibodies.**

The antibody response to invading molecules begins with the "birth" of the B cell. **Maturation, proliferation,** and **differentiation** are all needed to arrive at a cell that actually produces antibodies. This chapter begins with the processes that occur in B cell maturation and how B cells interact with other cells in an immune response. This chapter also characterizes each **immunoglobulin** class, describing the structure and functions. Last, the reader is introduced to the characteristics of monoclonal antibodies and how they are produced.

▶ THE ANTIBODY RESPONSE

B CELL MATURATION

B cell maturation encompasses the initial production of stem cells in the bone marrow through the plasma cell or memory cell. Once the stem cell becomes committed to the B cell line, it becomes a pro-B cell. The pro-B cell in turn matures further into the pre-B cell and then on to the mature B cell. The mature B cell is also called a virgin B cell. The maturation to this point occurs primarily in the bone marrow. During this maturation, the primary activity of the cell is to undergo immunoglobulin **gene rearrangement,** and the stages are recognized by the extent of that process that has occurred (Figure 3-1■).

ANTIGEN INDEPENDENT B CELL MATURATION

Progenitor Cells to Pre-B Cells

B cells are derived from hematopoietic progenitor (stem) cells in the bone marrow, yolk sac, and fetal liver before birth. After birth, the B cells are produced primarily in the bone marrow. There is some production of B cells in the mucosa-associated lymphoid tissue (MALT) in other mammals, but this source has not been proven in humans to date. In the bone marrow, the stem cell commits to the B cell lineage by differentiation into progenitor B cells (pro-B). The pro-B cells are distinguished by the cell membrane expression of CD 45R, a transmembrane tyrosine phosphatase. In the bone marrow, the availability of bone marrow stromal cells (previously called "nurse cells") is necessary for the proliferation and differentiation of the pro-B cells into pre-B cells. The pro-B cells bind to the bone marrow stromal cells through a number of cell adhesion molecules present on the surface of both cell types. The major cell adhesion appears to be through VLA-4 on the pro-B cell binding to VCAM-1 on the bone marrow stromal cell. The pro-B cells then signal the stromal cells to elaborate **interleukin**-7 (**IL**-7) through the binding of a surface molecule called c-Kit, which is a tyrosine kinase, on the pro-B cell to stem cell factor (SCF) on the stromal cells. The IL-7 is a soluble factor that is elaborated into the surrounding medium. This interaction also activates the c-Kit, which signals the transcription of an IL-7 receptor by the pro-B cell and the subsequent expression of this receptor on the surface of the cell. The pro-B cells begin to proliferate while making the IL-7 receptor. Once a number of these pro-B cells are available, they differentiate into pre-B cells that express the IL-7 receptor on the surface. At this point, the pre-B cells no longer require contact with the stromal cells. Figure 3-2■ demonstrates this process.

Immunoglobulin Gene Rearrangement

Germline immunoglobulin DNA is the same in all of our cells, whether or not they become B cells. In order to produce adaptive **humoral immunity** and achieve maximum diversity in the antibodies that can be produced, the DNA in the immunoglobulin gene must be rearranged during the B cell maturation process. The initial process of rearrangement occurs in the pro-B cell stage. The immunoglobulin (antibody) molecule is composed of two types of amino acid chains, a **heavy chain** and a **light chain.** In humans, the genes for the heavy chain of the immunoglobulin molecule are found on chromosome 14, while the genes for the kappa (κ) light chain are on chromosome 2 and those for the lambda (λ) light chain are on chromosome 22.

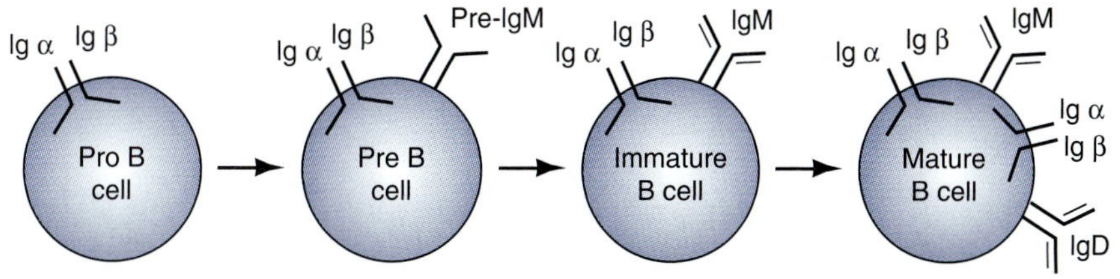

■ FIGURE 3-1 Immunoglobulin expression on B cells during maturation.

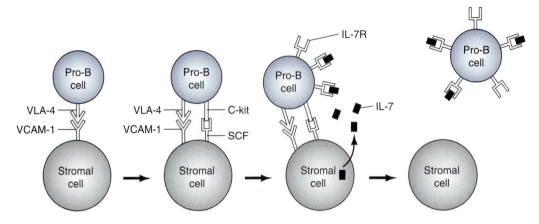

■ FIGURE 3-2 Bone marrow stromal cell involvement in B cell maturation.

The heavy chain is composed of a variable region, which contains the antigen binding site, and a constant region, which determines the isotype (immunoglobulin class) of the molecule. The variable region of the heavy chain is encoded by three separate genes, designated V_H, D_H, and J_H. These V, D, and J regions are rearranged to form the heavy chain half of the antigen binding site (Figure 3-3■). During the pro-B cell stage, the D_H to J_H rearrangement occurs first, followed by the V_H to $D_H J_H$ rearrangement. The heavy chain VDJ rearrangement must produce a configuration that is capable of being transcribed; this is called a productive rearrangement. Since humans have two copies of chromosome 14, the rearrangement is tried using the heavy chain gene from one chromosome first. If the rearrangement is productive, the other chromosome is inactive for this gene. If the rearrangement is not productive, then the second chromosome heavy chain gene is rearranged. A productive rearrangement of the heavy chain gene is essential to the further development of the B cell. The enzyme terminal deoxyribonucleotidyl transferase (TdT) is expressed during this transitional phase. This enzyme catalyzes the insertion of N-nucleotides at the D_H-J_H and V_H-$D_H J_H$ joints. Once this has occurred, the pro-B cell has become a pre-B cell. Note that this process is occurring at the same time as the signaling for the production of IL-7 described earlier.

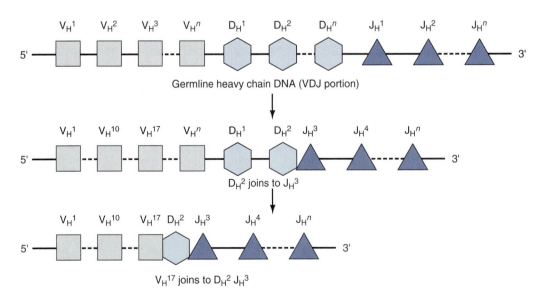

■ FIGURE 3-3 Germline heavy chain DNA is rearranged through DJ joining, then VDJ joining, cutting out intervening sequences. This permanently alters the DNA.

Light chain rearrangement is necessary for further development of the pre-B cell into an immature B cell. Light chains also have variable and constant regions. The genes coding for the variable region in light chains are V and J only. The kappa light chains are the first try to obtain a productive variable region rearrangement. If the V and Jκ rearrange successfully on one chromosome 2, the other chromosome 2 and both chromosomes 22 are inactive for the light chain genes. If no productive rearrangement is obtained, the next try for a light chain is the second chromosome 2. If that is not productive, then the chromosome 22 lambda light chain rearrangement of Vλ and Jλ is tried. Thus, we have four tries (2 κ and 2 λ) to obtain a productive variable light chain rearrangement. This order of rearrangement explains the much larger number of immunoglobulins that are comprised of heavy chains bound to kappa light chains than to lambda light chains.

Completion of successful heavy and light chain rearrangements allow the assembly of the **B cell receptor (BCR),** which is a membrane immunoglobulin molecule (mIg) of the IgM class in association with the Igα-Igβ heterodimer expressed on the surface of the immature B cell (Figure 3-4■). This is the end of the bone marrow stage of B cell development. The immature B cell is not functional at this stage and must undergo a change in the RNA processing of the heavy chain transcript that allows the constant region gene to alternately be spliced into the molecule as the mu (μ) of the IgM isotype or the delta (δ) of IgD. The mature B cell that is released from the bone marrow expresses both membrane IgM and membrane IgD on its surface. These immunoglobulins are the B cell receptor (BCR) that is specific for a single epitope. Each B cell has a unique BCR composed of the variable regions of the heavy and light chains in combination. The VDJ and VJ rearrangements appear to be random in nature to increase diversity or the number of different epitopes that can be recognized by our number of B cells.

Cell Surface Markers

The stage of maturation can be detected by the **cell surface markers** present as illustrated in Figure 3-5■. In the lymphoid stem cell stage, only c-Kit is present. In the pro-B stage, c-Kit is joined by CD45R, CD19, CD24, IL-7R, CD43, and the Igα-Igβ heterodimer. The Igα-Igβ heterodimer, CD45R, CD 19, and CD24 remain for the rest of the B cell sequence. At the pre-B stage, these are joined by CD25 and the mu heavy chain. The immature B cell loses expression of the CD25 and gains the expression of complete IgM. The mature B cell expresses IgD in addition to the markers of the immature B cell. See Table 3-1✪ for the surface markers of each stage of **antigen independent** maturation.

ANTIGEN DEPENDENT B CELL MATURATION

Mature B cells (also called naive B cells by some authors) that are capable of response to antigen, but have not yet encountered antigen, migrate from the bone marrow through the peripheral circulation to the spleen. Once in the splenic follicle, B cells form germinal centers (GCs) upon antigen recognition. Germinal centers are the site of rapid B cell proliferation upon encounters with their specific antigens and with T cells, and are necessary for the formation of memory B cells. Class-switching and plasma cell formation also occur in the GCs, but can also occur elsewhere. GCs also form in other lymphoid tissue, such as the lymph nodes, MALT, appendix, tonsils, and adenoids. The GCs arise from 7 to 10 days after the B cell recognizes its specific epitope that is a **thymus dependent (TD)** antigen.

T CELL AND B CELL INTERACTIONS

B Cell Response to Thymus Dependent Antigens

Thymus dependent antigens require mature B cell contact with **T helper (T$_H$) cells** for a response to occur. TD antigens are primarily soluble proteins. The first signal affecting the B cell is given when antigen is bound to the BCR, cross-linking two BCRs, and then taken into the B cell by receptor-mediated endocytosis. Once inside the B cell, the TD antigen is broken down through the endocytic pathway into small peptides. These peptides are then processed with major histocompatibility complex (MHC) Class II molecules, such that they are situated within the cleft between the α and β chains of the MHC Class II, to allow the T$_H$ cell

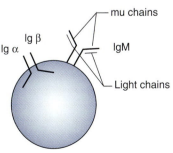

B cell receptor (BCR)

■ **FIGURE 3-4** Structure of the B cell receptor (BCR).

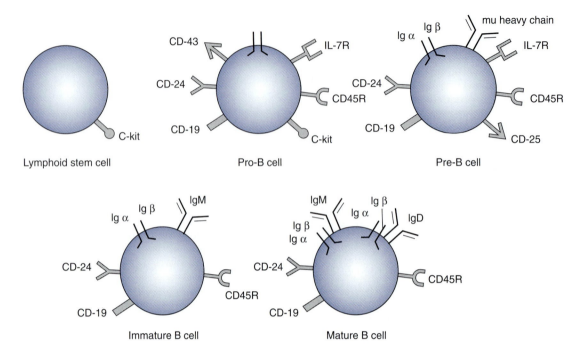

■ FIGURE 3-5 Cell surface markers expressed on B cells during maturation.

to recognize its specific epitope through the T cell receptor (TCR) and the MHC II through the CD4 molecules on the surface of the T_H cell (see Figures 3-6■ and 3-7■). MHC class II molecules are also known as HLA-D antigens and are constitutively produced by B cells; however, their production is up-regulated by the reaction of the antigen with the BCR to enable better antigen presentation by the B cell to the T_H cell.

Once the T_H cell has recognized the antigen presented with MHC II, through the TCR and CD4, the T_H cell is activated, and the B cell up-regulates production and surface expression of CD80/CD86, a costimulatory molecule. This signals the T_H cell to produce and express CD40 ligand (CD40L) on its surface. The CD40L on the T_H cell binds to CD40 expressed on the B cell surface, providing a second B cell signal, while the

✪ TABLE 3-1

Expression of Surface Markers on B Cell Lineage

Cell Stage				
Lymphoid Stem Cell	Pro-B Cell	Pre-B Cell	Immature B Cell	Mature B Cell
c-kit	c-kit			
	CD 45R	CD 45R	CD 45R	CD 45R
	CD 19	CD 19	CD 19	CD 19
	CD 24	CD 24	CD 24	CD 24
	IL-7R	IL-7R		
	CD 43			
		CD 25		
	Igα-Igβ heterodimer	Igα-Igβ heterodimer	Igα-Igβ heterodimer	Igα-Igβ heterodimer
		Mu heavy chain	IgM	IgM and IgD

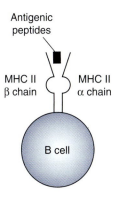

■ FIGURE 3-6 Antigen presentation on the B cell surface in context with MHC class II.

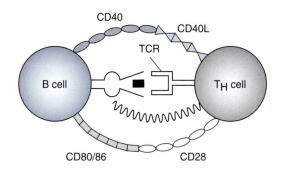

■ FIGURE 3-8 Binding of CD 40 with CD 40L and CD 80/86 with CD 28 enhances cell signaling between the B cell and T_H cell.

CD80/CD86 on the B cell binds to CD28 on the T_H cell, providing costimulation to activate the T_H cell (Figure 3-8■). The CD40-CD40L binding drives the B cell to cycle from G_0, a resting state, to G_1. This second signal is critical to the activation of B cells. At this point, the B cell begins to express **cytokine** receptors for IL-2, IL-4, IL-5, and IL-6. These cytokines, also called interleukins, are produced by the T_H cell and signal the B cells to proliferate when the interleukin binds with its specific receptor on the activated B cell. Cytokine secretion is directed immediately toward the B cell as the T_H cell reorients the Golgi apparatus and secretory organelles toward the T-B interface during T_H activation. IL-5 and IL-6 are also required for induction of B cell differentiation into plasma cells and B memory cells. In addition to activation of B cells, IL-2 produced by T_H cells binds to IL-2 receptors present on the T_H cells. This amplifies the response to the specific epitope by signaling the proliferation of these specific T_H cells, which in turn can activate more specific B cells. Class switching from IgM to IgG, IgA, or IgE responses is characteristic of thymus dependent responses. This class switching is highly dependent on the CD 40 binding to CD 40L, then the presence of cytokines such as IL-4 binding to their receptors on the B cell.

Interleukins and other cytokines are responsible for class switching and affinity maturation of the antibody response (see Table 3-2✪).

B Cell Response to Thymus Independent Antigens

Thymus independent (TI) antigens are able to activate B cells without T cell help. There are two types of these TI antigens. TI type 1 (TI-1) antigens are primarily bacterial cell wall components, such as the lipopolysaccharides (LPS) found in gram negative cell

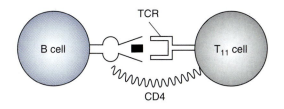

■ FIGURE 3-7 B cell interaction with T helper (T_H) cell through the TCR recognition of antigenic peptides and CD4 recognition of MHC II.

✪ TABLE 3-2

Some of the Cytokines Involved in B Cell Maturation and Differentiation

Cytokine	Action
IL-2	B cell proliferation
	Differentiation to plasma cell
	Initial IgM secretion
IL-4	B cell proliferation
	Differentiation to plasma cell
	Initial IgM secretion
	Class switching to IgG1, IgG4, and IgE
	Possibly class switching to IgG2, IgG3
IL-5	B cell proliferation
	Differentiation to plasma cell
	Initial IgM secretion
IL-6	Differentiation to plasma cell
IFN-γ	Class switching to IgG2 or IgG3
TNF-β	Class switching to IgA

Note: Other cytokines are also involved, and the cytokines listed have other functions in addition to those listed.

walls, and TI type 2 (TI-2) antigens are large molecules with many repetitive sequences.

TI-1 antigens activate B cells in a way that is not well understood at present. When a high concentration of TI-1 antigen is present, all B cells in the vicinity are activated, regardless of the specificity of the BCR. This is known as a polyclonal activation, and the TI-1 antigens capable of this type of B cell activation are called mitogens. However, when present in lower concentrations, the TI-1 antigens can activate only those B cells that have a BCR specific for the antigen.

TI-2 antigens are large molecules with repeating sequences, such as dextran. These antigens activate only the B cells that have BCRs specifically for their epitopes by heavily crosslinking the BCRs. These antigens can activate the B cells without direct T_H contact, but activated T_H cells in the vicinity are required to provide the IL-2, IL-4, and IL-5 cytokines needed for proliferation and differentiation. Antibody produced against TI antigens is primarily of the IgM class.

B Cell Differentiation and Antibody Production

Once the B cell has "seen" its antigen through the BCR and the second signal has been received through either CD40 binding to CD40L or through T independent crosslinking, cytokines are required for proliferation and differentiation. Although several other cytokines may be involved in this process, the primary mediators are IL-4, IL-5, and IL-6. IL-4 promotes vigorous proliferation of the activated B cell, and up-regulates B cell production of MHC Class II molecules. IL-5 stimulates proliferation of activated B cells and differentiation of these cells into plasma cells and memory cells. IL-6 stimulates the differentiation of activated B cells, primarily into plasma cells.

Plasma cells are the end-stage differentiated B cell. They are no longer capable of dividing; all of their cell processes are geared to secrete high levels of antibody molecules. Plasma cells no longer express membrane IgM or IgD. Each plasma cell secretes antibody with a specific variable portion against one specific epitope. Initial antibody production is of the IgM antibody class. Class switching may occur later in the immune response when the response is directed against a thymus-dependent antigen.

Memory B cells are long-lived cells that recirculate through the blood to the bone marrow, lymph nodes, spleen, and other lymphoid tissues. They express high levels of both complement receptors and adhesion molecules, making repeat activation much easier than for a mature B cell.

▶ IMMUNOGENS

Antigens are defined as molecules that stimulate antibody production. The name "antigen" is derived from "*anti*body *gen*erating factor." Although all antigens can elicit an antibody response, some are better at doing so than others. This characteristic is referred to as **immunogenicity.** What factors make an antigen a good **immunogen?** They include complexity, high molecular weight, structural stability, **degradability,** and **foreignness.** In many cases, how immunogenic a molecule is depends also on the dose and route of administration. High doses of a molecule all at once may lead to anergy (immune unresponsivness). One low dose will likely be destroyed too quickly. The best antibody response is obtained when small to medium sized repeated doses of an antigen are introduced into the body.

CHARACTERISTICS OF IMMUNOGENS

The ability of an immunogen to elicit an antibody response is related to both its chemical and physical properties. Characteristics of complexity, high molecular weight, and structural stability are important.

Large, organic molecules make good immunogens. The more complex the molecule, the better the immunogen. Proteins are excellent immunogens because they have a high level of complexity and heterogeneity, are made up of different amino acids, and have a high molecular weight. They are also very stable structures. Lipids are poor immunogens on their own because they are generally less complex and more homogeneous in structure and because they are composed of repeating units. Lipids also break apart more easily. However, lipids combined with proteins can be good immunogens. Glycoproteins and glycolipids are also often good immunogens.

How different the molecule is from the molecules of the host is also important in stimulating an immune response. Foreignness is essential because the individual's B and T cells are "educated" not to respond to host molecules. Many invaders of the body fool the immune system with a structure similar to a host protein, thus stimulating a poor immune response. Lastly, degradability is necessary for an antigen to be a good immunogen. If the molecule is rapidly destroyed in the body prior to being picked up by an APC, it will not go through the antigen presenting process to allow a response. However, it also must be able to be degraded by the APC into appropriately sized pieces for antigen presentation in the cleft of the MHC II molecule.

► IMMUNOGLOBULINS

STRUCTURE OF THE IMMUNOGLOBULIN MOLECULE

Fab and Fc Components

The Fab (fragment antibody) component is the portion of the antibody molecule that contains the antigen-binding site and contains the "variable" region. The Fc (fragment crystallizable) is the portion of the molecule that is "constant." These pieces of the antibody structure were discovered by treating the antibody molecule with enzymes. Papain digestion caused cleavage at the hinge region to reveal two Fab portions and one Fc. The Fab portions were shown to have antibody activity and were about 45 kD each in molecular weight. The Fc portion was inactive when antigen was added and had a molecular weight of about 50 kD. The Fc portion got its name because it crystallized when refrigerated. When a different enzyme, pepsin, is used to digest the antibody molecule, there are two cleavage sites instead on the one site produced with papain. Pepsin cleaves the antibody below the interchain disulfide bonds, to give an F(ab)'2 fragment that contains two binding

sites and degrades the Fc portion of the antibody into very short peptides. Antibody structure, papain cleavage, and pepsin cleavage are illustrated in Figures 3-9■, 3-10■, and 3-11■.

Heavy and Light Chains

The basic structure of the antibody molecule consists of two identical heavy (H) chains and two identical light (L) chains, held together by interchain disulfide bonds at the hinge region. There are five basic types of heavy chains corresponding to the five classes of immunoglobulins: mu (μ) in IgM, delta (δ) in IgD, gamma (γ) in IgG, alpha (α) in IgA, and epsilon (ε) in IgE. There are two types of light chains: kappa (κ) and lambda (λ). Either type of light chain can be used in any class of immunoglobulin, although both L chains are the same in any antibody molecule.

The Variable Region

The N-terminus of the molecule is the antigen-binding site, composed of a region of high variability encoded by the VDJ region of the heavy chain and the VJ region of the light chain. This area is about 110 amino acids in length and is referred to as the **variable region** of the antibody. Each antibody molecule has two N-terminal antigen-binding sites. Within this region are three hypervariable regions called complementary determining regions (CDRs) on each heavy and light chain; each

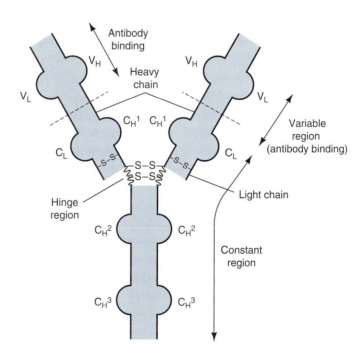

■ FIGURE 3-9 Schematic of antibody structure.

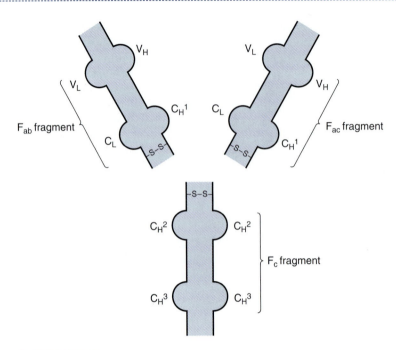

■ **FIGURE 3-10** Schematic representation of papain cleavage of the antibody monomer.

antigen-binding site has six CDRs. The CDRs actually bind the epitope complementary to them, and all six CDRs are involved in the determination of epitope specificity of the antibody molecule. The variable region is organized into one domain, known as V_H in heavy chains and V_L in light chains. The structure is a Y-shape as seen upon electron microscopy. As seen in Figure 3-1, both heavy and light chains have a constant region, as well as a variable region.

The Constant Region

The constant region is identical for all chains of the same type; for example, all κ light chains, all λ light chains, and all heavy chains in an individual have the same constant region structure, regardless of the plasma cell making them. The constant region is encoded in germline DNA and is not rearranged during B cell maturation. The number of amino acids in the constant region varies with the type of chain.

Both the H and L chains are folded into **domains.** Each domain contains around 110 amino acids. The L chains have one constant region domain (C_L). The α, δ, and γ H chains have three constant domains (C_H1, C_H2, C_H3) and a hinge region comprising about 15 amino acids. With the variable region (having a V_H), these heavy chains are 446 amino acids in length. The μ and ε H chains have four constant domains (C_H1, C_H2, C_H3, and C_H4) and no hinge region, although C_H2 in these molecules has "hingelike" function and is where the interchain disulfide bonds are formed. The total length of μ and ε H chains, including the V_H, is about 100 amino acids longer than the other H chains. The domains are held together by intrachain disulfide bonds.

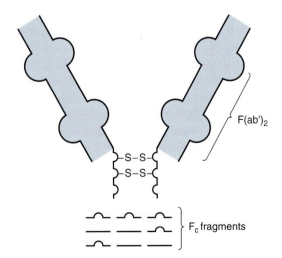

■ **FIGURE 3-11** Schematic representation of pepsin cleavage of the antibody monomer.

✪ TABLE 3-3

Constant Region Domain Functions

Domain	Function	Isotype
C_L	Stabilize VH and VL domains	All
	Extend CDR region	All
C_H1	Stabilize VH and VL domains	All
	Extend CDR region	All
	Molecule flexibility	All
C_H2	Molecule flexibility	All
	Complement binding	IgA, IgD, and IgG
	Macrophage and neutrophil binding	IgA, IgD, and IgG
C_H3	Complement binding	All
	Macrophage and neutrophil binding	All
	Membrane retention	IgD (membrane bound form only)
C_H4	Complement binding	IgM and IgE
	Macrophage and neutrophil binding	IgM and IgE
	Membrane retention	IgM (membrane bound form only)

Table 3-3✪ depicts the functions of each domain in the constant region. The C_H1 and C_L domains help to stabilize the V_H and V_L domains. They also extend the portion of the molecule containing the CDRs to allow greater antigen-antibody interaction. The hinge region is located between the C_H1 and C_H2 domains and is highly flexible, owing to the abundance of prolines in the area. This gives the antibody molecule more possible configurations when bound to antigen. The C-terminal constant region domains (C_H2 and C_H3 for IgA, IgD, and IgG, and C_H3 and C_H4 for IgM and IgE) are important for biologic effects such as complement binding through the C3b component and macrophage and neutrophil activation through Fc receptors on those cells. The receptors for C3b and the ligand for Fc receptors are located in these areas. Also the C_H3 or C_H4 domain on each molecule is important in membrane retention for membrane-bound IgD and IgM, respectively. The structures of this domain are different from those in secreted IgD and IgM, having a transmembrane sequence to anchor the molecule in the B cell membrane.

DIVERSITY OF THE IMMUNOGLOBULIN MOLECULE

Diversity is the key to the adaptive humoral immune response. B cells that recognize and respond to as many different foreign epitopes as possible provide the best chance for human survival. The development of this diversity is essential to the individual's ability to combat diseases caused by bacteria and fungi and is the key to vaccination for bacterial and viral prophylaxis.

As previously discussed, the heavy and light chains that make up antibody molecules are encoded in the germline DNA. However, if all of the B cells used the same DNA to assemble the antigen binding site, only a single epitope would be recognized by all B cells. Therefore, to generate B cells recognizing literally millions of epitopes, the germline DNA for the variable region of both heavy and light chains is subject to rearrangement prior to transcription. If rearrangement that can be successfully transcribed occurs, the B cell can produce a BCR and mature further. If no successful rearrangement occurs, the B cell will undergo apoptosis.

Organization and Recombination of Germline Heavy Chain DNA

The heavy chain germline DNA encodes V_H, D_H, J_H, and C_H gene segments that can be recombined in thousands of different VDJ combinations that then reorient next to the appropriate C_H segment. The C_H segments include C_μ, C_δ, C_γ^1, C_γ^2, C_γ^3, C_γ^4, C_ε, and C_α. The order on the gene from 5' to 3' is V segments, D segments, J segments, then C_μ, C_δ, C_γ^3, C_γ^1, C_α^1, C_γ^2, C_γ^4, C_ε, C_α^2. In humans, there are more than 50 V_H, 27 D_H, and 6 J_H segments, any of which can recombine together. Refer back to Figure 3-3 to visualize this recombination.

In between each V_H, D_H, and J_H segment, there is a recombination signal sequence (RSS). These RSSs are the recognition sequences for the recombinase enzymes that facilitate DNA rearrangement. The first event is the recombination of one D_H segment with one J_H segment. Any of the D_H segments can combine with any of the J_H segments at the RSS. When the recombination has occurred, any intervening DNA between the D_H and J_H segments is deleted to position them as a single $D_H J_H$ gene segment. This occurs at the pro-B cell stage. Subsequent recombination of any one V_H segment to the rearranged $D_H J_H$ gene segment occurs at the RSS, with the intervening DNA deleted. Now there is a ligated $V_H D_H J_H$ gene segment that encodes the entire variable region of the heavy chain to be produced in this B cell.

At this point the germline DNA no longer exists in this cell, as large coding regions have been deleted. This is a permanent deletion; no reversion will occur. Now the heavy chain DNA consists of anything 5' of the V_H segment that was selected to join the $V_H D_H J_H$ gene segment, the $V_H D_H J_H$ gene segment itself, and any DNA 3' of the rearranged gene segment. All of the constant region genes are located 3' of the rearranged $V_H D_H J_H$ gene segment DNA.

When the rearrangement of $V_H D_H J_H$ has been accomplished, RNA polymerase can attach to a promoter 5' of the $V_H D_H J_H$ gene segment and transcribe the entire heavy chain gene through $C\mu$, and $C\delta$ to a stop codon located just 3' of the $C\delta$ gene sequence. The primary transcript is composed of the leader sequence, the $V_H D_H J_H$ gene segment, and the constant region genes for $C\mu$ and $C\delta$. The other constant region gene sequences are located 3' of the stop codon, but remain intact in the DNA of the B cell and can be transcribed later, if the cell undergoes class switching (Figure 3-12■).

Organization and Recombination of Germline Light Chain DNA

Light chain genes are organized in a much similar way to those of heavy chains; however, they are simpler. Kappa (κ) light chain DNA in humans contains about 40 Vκ gene segments, and 5 Jκ gene segments followed by a single Cκ gene segment. The arrangement of the κ germline DNA is similar to that of heavy chain DNA, with the Vκ segments at the 5' end, then the Jκ segments downstream of the Vκ, followed by the Cκ segment at the 3' end. Lambda (λ) light chain DNA contains about 30 Vλ gene segments, 4 Jλ gene segments, and 7 Cλ gene segments that are functional. In humans, any single V segment can combine with any single J segment during VJ recombination of the light chain DNA. The κ light chain tries to recombine first. A successful κ recombination will inactivate both the remaining DNA on the other chromosome 2 and the λ DNA segments on both 22nd chromosomes. Once the $V_L J_L$ recombination event has occurred, the combined segment can be transcribed by RNA polymerase, along with the downstream C_L segment.

Class Switching

As previously mentioned, the order of the constant region DNA is $C\mu$, then $C\delta$, the $C\gamma$ 1, 2, 3, and 4 regions, $C\varepsilon$ and $C\alpha$. Class switching appears to be controlled by interleukins, particularly IL-4. There are special DNA sequences called switch regions, composed of multiple copies of short repeats, which lie about 2 to 3 kilobases (kb) upstream of all of the C_H genes except $C\delta$. According to current theory, enzymes that act as switch recombinases recognize these areas of DNA, bind to them, cut at the repeated sequences and allow recombination of the DNA at the cuts. This "loops out" the intervening DNA containing the C_H genes between the switch regions that have recombined, resulting in a different C_H

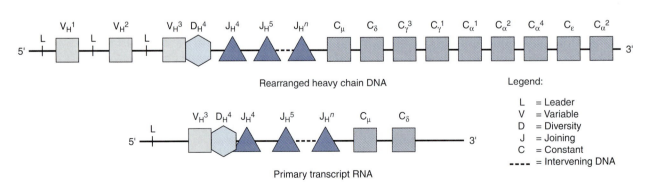

Rearranged heavy chain DNA

Primary transcript RNA

Legend:

L = Leader
V = Variable
D = Diversity
J = Joining
C = Constant
---- = Intervening DNA

■ **FIGURE 3-12** Rearranged heavy chain DNA is transcribed by RNA polymerase to construct the primary heavy chain transcript.

region lying immediately downstream of the rearranged VDJ sequence, as illustrated in Figure 3-13■. The DNA polymerase will now transcribe the $V_HD_HJ_H$ gene segment and the C_H segment closest to it, stopping at the stop codon located after the C_H segment. For example, if class switching has occurred from IgM to IgG1, the switch region upstream from the C_μ segment will recombine with the switch region upstream of the $C_\gamma1$ segment, removing all of the intervening DNA and placing the $C_\gamma1$ segment next to the rearranged $V_HD_HJ_H$ gene segment. The DNA polymerase will now attach to the promoter upstream of the $V_HD_HJ_H$ gene segment, as before, but now will transcribe through the $C\gamma1$ segment and stop, so that this cell will now produce IgG1 antibody rather than IgM. This is shown in Figure 3-14■.

Isotypes, Allotypes and Idiotypes

Immunoglobulins, in addition to being antibodies, can serve as antigens. They have three types of antigenic determinants as part of their structure. An **antigenic determinant** is the structure that elicits an antibody response, and the term has been used interchangeably with the term **epitope.** These structures are composed of chemical and physical elements that can be recognized by the BCR and TCR. The three types of antigenic determinants on immunoglobulins are isotypes, allotypes, and idiotypes. Locations of these structures are demonstrated in Figure 3-15■.

Isotypes are the portions of the heavy chain constant region that differ between imunoglobulin classes (IgG, IgM, IgA, IgD, IgE) and subclasses (IgG1, IgG2, IgG3, etc.). They are also the portions of the light chain constant regions that differ between κ and λ. All individuals possessing a normal immune system have all of the classes and subclasses of immunoglobulins and have antibodies composed of both κ and λ light chains, although all antibody molecules contain only one type of light chain in the individual molecule.

Allotypes are variations of alternative alleles at a single genetic locus. All individuals have only one allotype at the Gm, Am, Mm, and Km locus. Gm, Am, and Mm are located on the C_H region of the immunoglobulin. For example, Gm is an allotype of the IgG immunoglobulin, and all of a person's B cells that produce IgG, regardless of the variable region, will express the same Gm type. Am is a marker on the IgA molecule, Mm is on the IgM molecule, and Km is on the kappa light chain in the C_L region.

Idiotypes are part of the hypervariable (CDR) regions of antibody molecules. Thus, they are unique to the antibodies produced by a single clone of B cells. Antibodies can be made to the idiotypes of any im-

munoglobulin. A person can produce antibodies to idiotype on other antibodies that they are producing. Anti-idiotypes may be part of the regulation of the immune system, by removing antibodies that are no longer needed.

IMMUNOGLOBULIN CLASSES

There are, as previously mentioned, five classes of immunoglobulins: **IgG, IgM, IgA, IgD,** and **IgE.** The major characteristics of each class and some subclasses are summarized in Table 3-3. The constant H chain regions of each class are unique from the others. This structure defines the antibody class. The structures of the five classes are diagrammed in Figure 3-16■.

IgG

Most of the immunoglobulin in human serum, approximately 80 percent, is of this class. The chemical composition of the IgG molecule is two γ H chains and either 2 κ or 2 λ L chains. IgG in humans has been found only in this monomeric form. IgG is the antibody produced in a secondary or anamnestic response and is responsible for long-term immunity to an immunogen. In the case of the patient described at the beginning of this chapter (case in point), the hepatitis panel results at the time of admission showed the presence of anti-HBs IgG, which was a result of previous vaccination. Meanwhile, the patient's posthepatitis profile four weeks later showed a negative anti-HAV IgM negative and anti-HAV IgG positive, indicating convalescence since her immune system has now produced a secondary IgG response to HAV. Other primary functions of IgG include crossing the placenta during pregnancy to provide immunity for the fetus, mediating opsonization by binding to the Fc receptors of macrophages and neutrophils, and activating complement through the classical pathway.

There are four subclasses of IgG, numbered as IgG1, IgG2, IgG3, and IgG4. The subclasses are based on the percentage they contribute to the total serum IgG, with IgG1 having the highest concentration and IgG4 having the lowest. The major differences in structure and function between these subclasses can be found in Table 3-4✪. The differences in the heavy chain structure are minimal, with each subclass being encoded on different germline C region genes. These differences account for only about 5% nonhomology between these genes. The number and position of the disulfide bonds between the two heavy chains of the molecule differ between the subclasses, as do the size of the hinge region. Differences in the biological activities are

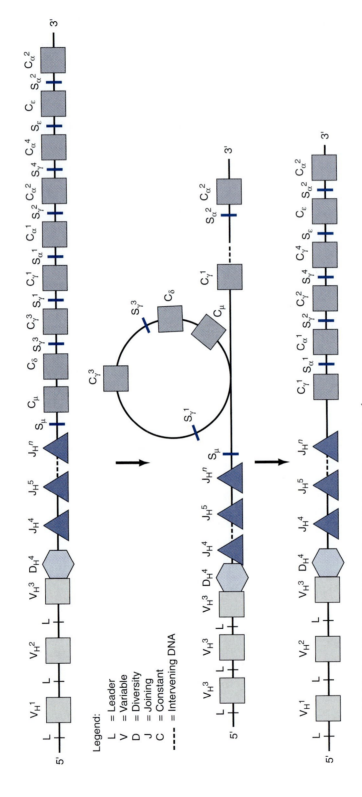

Legend:

L = Leader
V = Variable
D = Diversity
J = Joining
C = Constant
----- = Intervening DNA

■ **FIGURE 3-13** "Looping out" of intervening DNA to produce VDJ-C_γ^1.

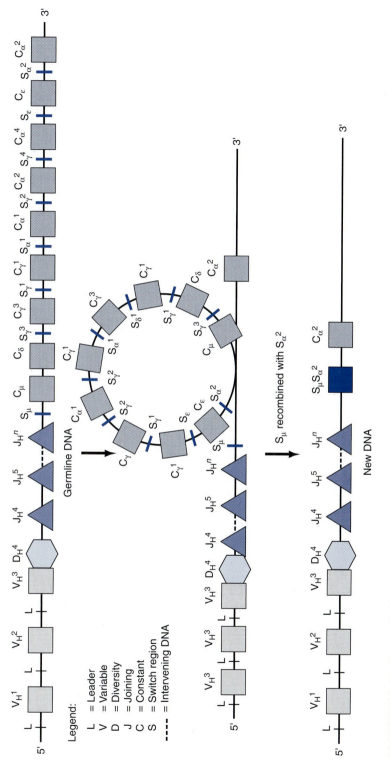

Legend:
L = Leader
V = Variable
D = Diversity
J = Joining
C = Constant
S = Switch region
----- = Intervening DNA

Germline DNA

S_μ recombined with S_α^2

New DNA

■ **FIGURE 3-14** Class switching. In this example, DNA is "looped out" during recombination of switch regions $S\mu$ and $S\alpha$ to obtain DNA with a combined $S_\mu S_\alpha$ and permanent removal of DNA containing the C_μ, C_δ, C_γ, and C_ε genes. This leads to the production of DNA having the same variable VDJ and producing IgA rather than IgM.

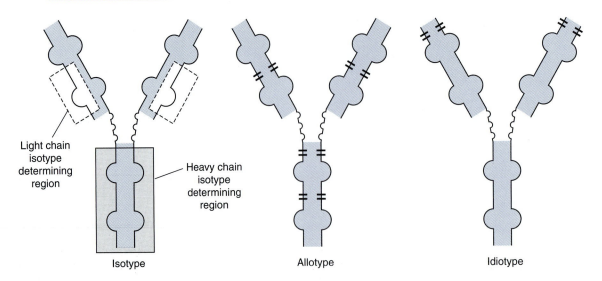

Light chain isotype determining region

Heavy chain isotype determining region

Isotype

Allotype

Idiotype

■ **FIGURE 3-15** Regions of the antibody molecule determining isotypes (a), allotypes (b), and idiotypes (c) are depicted.

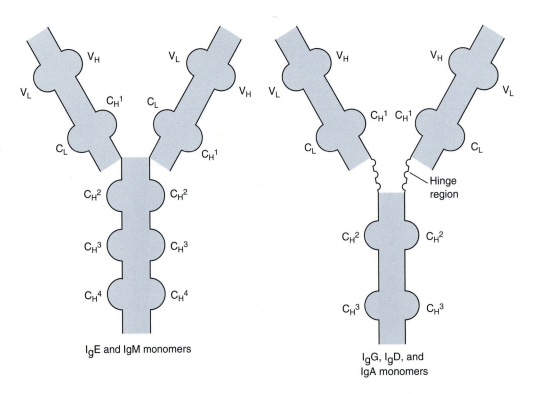

V_H

V_L

V_L

$C_H{}^1$

C_L

C_L

$C_H{}^1$

$C_H{}^2$

$C_H{}^2$

$C_H{}^3$

$C_H{}^3$

$C_H{}^4$

$C_H{}^4$

IgE and IgM monomers

V_H

V_H

V_L

V_L

$C_H{}^1$ $C_H{}^1$

C_L

C_L

Hinge region

$C_H{}^2$

$C_H{}^2$

$C_H{}^3$

$C_H{}^3$

IgG, IgD, and IgA monomers

■ **FIGURE 3-16** Schematic structures of monomeric immunoglobulins. In (a), the monomeric form for IgG, IgD, and IgA is shown. In (b) the monomeric form of IgE and IgM is shown.

✪ TABLE 3-4

Properties of IgG Subclasses

IgG Subclass	# Disulfide Bonds between Heavy Chains	# Gm Allotypes	Crosses Placenta	Activates Complement	Opsonin
IgG1	2	4	Yes	Yes	Yes
IgG2	4	1	Poorly, if at all	Poorly	No
IgG3	11	13	Yes	Yes	Yes
IgG4	4	2	Yes	No	Moderate

also seen in Table 3-4. IgG1 and IgG3 cross the placenta, activate complement well, and mediate opsonization by binding well to Fc receptors. IgG2 crosses the placenta very minimally, does not mediate opsonization, and activates complement rather ineffectively. IgG4 crosses the placenta, mediates opsonization less well than IgG1 and IgG3, and does not activate complement at all.

IgA

IgA is the second most abundant immunoglobulin in human serum, comprising about 10% to 15% of total serum Ig. Serum IgA is most often monomeric, consisting of two α H chains and either two κ L chains or two λ L chains; however, dimmer, trimers, and tetramers are also seen in the serum. IgA is also the predominant Ig in secretions, including the mucus of the nasal, digestive, genital, urinary, and respiratory tracts. It can be found in saliva, breast milk, tears, and most other bodily secretions. Secretory IgA, shown diagrammatically in Figure 3-17■, is either a dimer, composed of two identical monomers, a **J** (joining) **chain** and a **secretory piece** (secretory component), or a tetramer, consisting of four identical monomers, a J chain, and a secretory piece (secretory component). The J chain joins the monomers together through the Fc regions. The secretory component bids to the Fc regions of the monomers and stabilizes the molecule against proteolysis. It is also responsible for the transport of secretory IgA across cell membranes. The primary importance of secretory IgA is in the binding of viral and bacterial surface molecules, preventing attachment of the virus or bacterium to the mucosa and preventing infection. Secretory IgA is also important in breast milk, providing protection against infection for breast-fed newborns, who have little immunity of their own.

There are two subclasses of IgA: IgA1 and IgA2. IgA1 is the more prevalent in serum and differs from IgA2 in the constant region. As with subclasses of IgG, the IgA subclasses are encoded by different constant region genes.

IgM

IgM is third in serum concentration, accounting for between 5% and 10% of total serum Ig. As previously discussed, membrane-bound IgM is found on the cell surface of mature B cells as a monomer, composed of two mu H chains and either two κ L chains or two λ L chains. Serum IgM, illustrated in Figure 3-18■, is a pentamer, consisting of five monomers joined together by a J chain and by interchain disulfide bonds linking their C_H3 and C_H4 domains. The Fc regions of the five monomers are in the center of the molecule, with the 10 Fab portions to the outside of the molecule. The J chain is required for the pentamer to form, but links only two of the mu chains together.

IgM is the first immunoglobulin to be produced, both in a primary response and by infant immune systems. Again, exemplified in the case in point, the patient's anti-HAV IgM showed positive at the time she was seen by the clinician, indicating a primary antibody response against hepatitis A virus and the presence of an acute infection. Four weeks later, her hepatitis panel showed anti-HAV IgM negative and anti-HAV IgG positive, an indication of convalescence. IgM is also found in secretions, although in much lower concentrations than IgA. Having 10 antigen-binding sites allows IgM to be much more efficient in binding highly repetitive epitopes. The proximity of five Fc regions in a single IgM molecule provides greater efficiency in complement activation through the classical pathway than

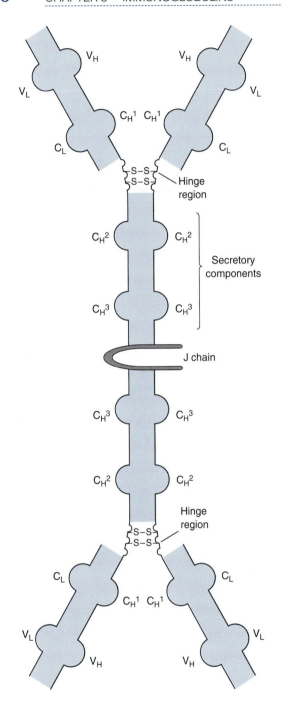

■ **FIGURE 3-17** Secretory IgA is a dimer with a J chain and a secretory component.

IgG, since two Fc in proximity are necessary for this to occur.

Two subclasses of IgM have been postulated and reported in the literature; however, evidence of their existence is scant, and most reliable sources consider IgM not to have subclasses.

IgD

IgD is in very low concentration in the serum, comprising less than 0.2% of total Ig. Only the monomeric form has been seen, composed of two δ H chains and either two κ L chains or two λ L chains. The majority of IgD in humans is membrane-bound to the mature B cell, along with IgM, as the BCR. No other biological function for IgD has been described.

IgE

IgE is also in low concentration in human serum, comprising less than 0.002% of total immunoglobulin. However, IgE is very biologically active. Monomeric IgE is bound to mast cells and basophils through its Fc portion, leaving the Fab to serve as a receptor that binds its epitope and initiates the degranulation of mast cell granules containing histamine and other mediators. This initiates the allergic response, but also provides immune response to parasites. The IgE monomer is composed of two ε H chains and either two κ L chains or two λ L chains.

► MONOCLONAL ANTIBODIES

CHARACTERISTICS OF MONOCLONAL ANTIBODIES

Monoclonal antibodies are identical immunoglobulins with identical variable and constant regions. They are produced by a single clone of B cells. In contrast, a normal immune response to an antigen will be **polyclonal;** that is, it will include responses by many clones of B cells whose BCRs recognize different epitopes on the same antigen. A polyclonal antibody response or reagent will be more likely to detect an antigen than a monoclonal antibody, since a polyclonal antibody will detect most, if not all, epitopes of the antigen. However, polyclonal antibody reagents will also be subject to more false positive reactions due to cross-reaction with similar epitopes on other antigens. Monoclonal antibodies detect only one single epitope of an antigen; thus, they are more specific to the particular antigen being detected. However, monoclonal reagents may be less sensitive in that they may

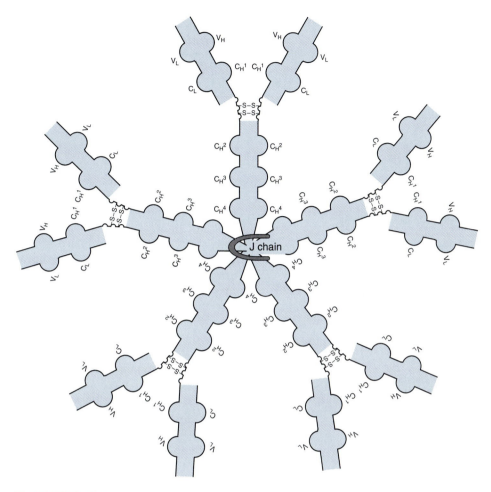

■ FIGURE 3-18 The pentameric form of IgM, diagrammed here, is found in the circulation.

not detect an incomplete antigen or an antigen in which the epitope detected by the monoclonal antibody is hidden due to steric hindrance. For this reason, some commercial monoclonal antibodies are sold as mixed monoclonals. Commercially produced monoclonal antibodies are of high purity and specificity. They can be used for multiple clinical applications, which include, but are not limited to, tumor antigen identification, hormone detection, blood typing, CD identification of leukemia and/or lymphoma cells, bacterial and viral identification, and many more.

PRODUCTION OF MONOCLONAL ANTIBODIES

Monoclonal antibody production begins with the injection of the antigen against which you want an antibody formed into a mouse. The mouse will mount a polyclonal response to the antigen. Then, the mouse's spleen is removed and disrupted to release the B cells. As seen in Figure 3-19■, the mouse spleen cells are then mixed with myeloma cells in the presence of polyethylene glycol (PEG). The PEG allows the cell membranes of the myeloma cells and the mouse spleen cells to fuse, forming hybridomas of myeloma cell fused to spleen cell. Myeloma cells may also fuse to other myeloma cells and spleen cells may fuse to other spleen cells, so the desired hybridomas must be differentiated.

In order to differentiate the desired myeloma-spleen cell hybridomas, the myeloma cells used must have two major criteria: they must be nonantibody producing, and they must be deficient in the enzyme hypoxanthine-guanine phosphoribosyl transferase (HGPRT). The enzyme HGPRT converts hypoxanthine to guanine and allows the cell to use the salvage pathway for

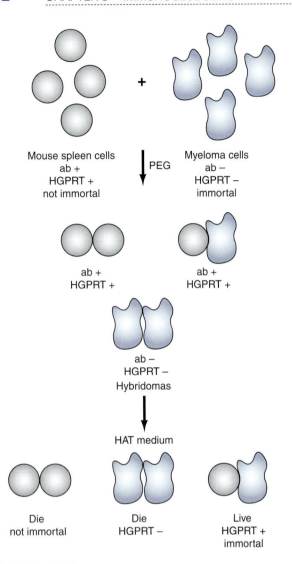

Mouse spleen cells
ab +
HGPRT +
not immortal

PEG

Myeloma cells
ab −
HGPRT −
immortal

ab +
HGPRT +

ab +
HGPRT +

ab −
HGPRT −
Hybridomas

HAT medium

Die
not immortal

Die
HGPRT −

Live
HGPRT +
immortal

■ FIGURE 3-19 The process of making an immortal cell line that generates monoclonal antibodies.

synthesis of the purines and pyrimidines needed to synthesize nucleotides.

Once fusion has occurred, the PEG is removed from the system to stop further hybridization. Then the resulting hybridomas are cultured on HAT medium, containing hypoxanthine, aminopterin, and thymidine. The hypoxanthine and thymidine will allow spleen-spleen cells and spleen-myeloma hybridomas to grow by allowing salvage pathway synthesis of nucleotides. The aminopterin blocks *de novo* synthesis of nucleotides, so myeloma-myeloma fused cells will not grow. The spleen-spleen cells will grow for a short time, since they can use the salvage pathway, but these cells are not immortal and have a finite, short life span. The spleen-myeloma hybridoma cells will grow indefinitely, since they can use the salvage pathway and are immortal. Then, the hydridomas are selected for the desired antibody specificity, and the hybridoma making that antibody is cloned for a theoretical unending source of the monoclonal antibody.

Mouse monoclonals are currently the most common. Mouse-human monoclonals are available for some specificities; these are made using the variable region of the mouse antibody fused to the constant region of a human antibody. Work is underway to produce human monoclonal antibodies using Epstein-Barr infected cells as the immortal cell (myeloma) source.

SUMMARY

B lymphocytes play a major role in immune response. B cells mature, proliferate, and differentiate to antibody-producing cells, the plasma cells. In concert with antigen presenting cells and T lymphocytes, B cells are responsible for the humoral arm of acquired immunity, responsible for protecting human hosts from bacterial and fungal infections by producing antibodies.

Depending on its chemical and physical characteristics, immunogens are able to elicit antibody response when intro-

duced into the body. In general, the more complex the molecule and how different the molecule is from the molecules of the host, the better the immunogen in stimulating an immune response.

There are five classes of immunoglobulins, IgG, IgM, IgA, IgD, and IgE. The constant H chain regions of each class define the antibody class and are unique from the others. Each immunoglobulin class perform specific functions.

POINTS TO REMEMBER

▶ The different processes that take place during B cell maturation

▶ The cell surface markers

▶ T cell and B cell interactions and the role each type of cell play in immune response

▶ Characteristics and functions of each of the immunoglobulin class

▶ Characteristics of monoclonal antibodies and how they are produced

LEARNING ASSESSMENT QUESTIONS

1. The immunoglobulin class that crosses the placenta is
   a. IgA.
   b. IgD.
   c. IgE.
   d. IgG.
   e. IgM.

2. The first rearrangement on the heavy chain immunoglobulin gene is
   a. VDJ.
   b. VJ.
   c. DJ.
   d. VD.

3. CD 40 on the B cell membrane must bind to CD 40L on the T_H cell in order for _____ to occur.
   a. class switching
   b. VDJ rearrangement
   c. antigen recognition
   d. complement binding

4. T independent (TI) antigens activate B cells by
   a. crosslinking BCRs.
   b. elaborating IL-2.
   c. crosslinking MHC II.
   d. activating CD 25 expression.

5. A good immunogen is
   a. a low molecular weight molecule.
   b. highly repetitive.
   c. degradeable.
   d. a protein given in a single, high dose.

6. A pro-B cell expresses on its surface
   a. VCAM-1
   b. CD 45R
   c. IL-7
   d. SCF

7. Delta (δ) heavy chains are seen in
   a. IgA.
   b. IgD.
   c. IgE.
   d. IgG.
   e. IgM.

8. Germinal centers are necessary for the formation of
   a. B memory cells.
   b. switch recombinases.
   c. plasma cells.
   d. TI antigens.

9. Variations of alternative alleles expressed on IgG molecules are called
   a. isotypes.
   b. idiotypes.
   c. allotypes.
   d. C_H1.
   e. C_H3.

10. The IgG subclass that does *not* activate complement at all is
    a. IgG1.
    b. IgG2.
    c. IgG3.
    d. IgG4.

11. Light chain gene rearrangement begins with alignment of
    a. DJ.
    b. VJ.
    c. VD.
    d. VC.

12. J chain is found in the structure of which immunoglobulin class(es)?
    a. IgA and IgD
    b. IgM and IgA
    c. IgM
    d. IgG
    e. IgM and IgE

REFERENCES

Boursier, L., W. Su, and J. Spencer. 2003. Imprint of somatic hypermutation differs in human immunoglobulin heavy and lambda light chain variable gene segments. *Molecular Immunology* 39:1025–34.

Brandtzaeg, P. 2003. Immunology of tonsils and adenoids: Everything the ENT surgeon needs to know. *Int J Pediatr Otorhinolaryngol* 67:S69–76.

Calame, K. L., K-I Lin, and C. Tunyaplin. 2003. Regulatory mechanisms that determine the development and function of plasma cells. *Annu Rev Immunol* 21:205–30.

Cancro, M. P. and S. H. Smith. 2003. Peripheral B cell selection and homeostasis. *Immunol Res* 27:141–48.

Dahl, R. and M. C. Simon. 2003. The importance of PU.1 concentration in hematopoietic lineage commitment and maturation. *Blood Cells, Molecules and Diseases* 31:229–33.

Defrance, T., M. Casamayor-Palleja, and P. H. Krammer. 2002. The life and death of a B cell. *Adv Cancer Res* 86:195–225.

Chung, J., M. Silverman, and J. G. Monroe. 2003. Transitional B cells: Step by step towards immune competence. *TRENDS in Immunol* 24:342–48.

Diaz, M. and P. Casali. 2002. Somatic immunoglobulin hypermutation. *Curr Opin Immunol* 14:235–40.

Do, R. K. G. and S. Chen-Kiang. 2002. Mechanism of BlyS action in B cell immunity. *Cytokine & Growth Factor Reviews* 13:19–25.

Durandy, A. 2003. Activation-induced cytidine deaminase: A dual role in class-switch recombination and somatic hypermutation. *Eur J Immunol* 33:2069–73.

Fleming, H. E. and C. J. Paige. 2002. Cooperation between IL-7 and the pre-B cell receptor: A key to B cell selection. *Seminars in Immunol* 14:423–30.

Gauld, S.B., J. M. Dal Porto, and J. C. Cambier. 2002. B cell antigen receptor signaling: Roles in cell development and disease. *Science* 296:1641–42.

Gorelik, L., K. Gilbride, M. Dobles, et al. 2003. Normal B cell homeostasis requires B cell activation factor production by radiation-resistant cells. *J Exp Med* 198:937–45.

Guzman-Rojas, l., J. C. Sims-Mourtada, R. Rangel, et al. 2002. Life and death within germinal centres: A double-edged sword. *Immunology* 107:167–75.

Iber, D. and P. K. Maini. 2002. A mathematical model for germinal centre kinetics and affinity mazturation. *J Theor Biol* 219:153–75.

Kesmir, C. and R. J. De Boer. 2003. A spatial model of germinal center reactions: Cellular adhesion based sorting of B cells results in efficient affinity maturation. *J Theor Biol* 222:9–22.

Mackay, F. and C. Ambrose. 2003. The TNF family members BAFF and APRIL: The growing complexity. *Cytokine & Growth Factor Review* 14:311–24.

Mackay, F., P. Schneider, P. Rennert, et al. 2003. BAFF and APRIL: A tutorial on B cell survival. *Annu Rev Immunol* 21:231–64.

Magari, M., S. Sawatari, Y. Kawano, et al. 2002. Contribution of light chain rearrangement in peripheral B cells to the generation of high-affinity antibodies. *Eur J Immunol* 32:957–66.

Melchers, F. 2003. Actions of BAFF in B cell maturation and its effects on the development of autoimmune disease. *Ann Rheum Dis* 62:ii25–ii27.

Neuberger, M. 2002. Antibodies: A paradigm for the evolution of molecular recognition. *Biochemical Society Transactions* 30:341–50.

Niiro, H. and E. A. Clark. 2002. Regulation of B-cell fate by antigen-receptor signals. *Nature Reviews/Immunology* 2:945–56.

Parkin, K. G., R. P. Stephan, R-G, Apilado, et al. 2002. Expression of CD 28 by bone marrow stromal cells and its involvement in lymphopoiesis. *J Immunol* 169:2292–302.

Quong, M. W., W. J. Romanow, and C. Murre. 2002. E protein function in lymphocyte development. *Annu Rev Immunol* 20:301–22.

Ratliffe, M. J. H. 2002. B cell development in gut associated lymphoid tissues. *Veterinary Immunol and Immunopasthol* 87:337–40.

Seagal, J. and D. Melamed. 2003. Selection events in directing B cell development. *Histol Histopathol* 18:1–9.

Siegel, R. M. and M. J. Lenardo. 2001. To B or not to B: TNF family signaling in lymphocytes. *Nature Immuno* 2:577–78.

Smith, S. H. and M. P. Cancro. 2003. Cutting edge: B cell receptor signals regulate BLyS receptor levels in mature B cells and their immediate progenitors. *J Immunol* 170:5820–23.

Teitell, M. A. 2003. OCA-B regulation of B-cell development and function. *TRENDS in Immunol* 24:546–53.

VanCompernolle, S. E., S. Levy, and S. C. Todd. 2001. Anti-CD81 activates LFA-1 on T cells and promotes T cell-B cell collaboration. *Eur J Immunol* 31:823–31.

Van Nierop, K. and C. De Groot. 2002. Human follicular dendritic cells: Function, origin and development. *Semin Immunol* 14:251–57.

Vora, K. A., L. C. Wang, S. P. Rao, et al. 2003. Cutting edge: Germinal centers formed in the absence of B cell-activating factor belonging to the TNF family exhibit impaired maturation and function. *J Immunol* 171:547–51.

Wang, L. D. and M. R. Clark. 2003. B-cell antigen-receptor signalling in lymphocyte development. *Immunol* 110:411–20.

4

Infection and Immunity: Host–Parasite Relationships

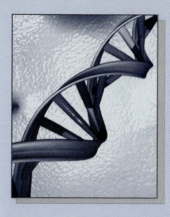

■ **CHAPTER CHECKLIST**

After reading and studying this chapter, the reader should be able to:

1. Differentiate the following terms:
   - usual or indigenous flora
   - resident microbial flora
   - transient microbial flora
   - carrier state

2. Explain how the following factors determine the nature of the microbial flora:
   - amounts and types of nutrients available in the environment
   - pH
   - oxidation-reduction potential
   - resistance to antibacterial substances
   - affinity for specific location or site
   - specific types of epithelial cells to which the usual microbial flora may attach

3. List the predominant flora found in the skin, the respiratory tract, the gastrointestinal tract, and the genitourinary tract of a healthy individual.

4. Explain the role played by the normal microbial flora in the pathogenesis of infectious diseases.

5. Explain the role played by the normal microbial flora in the host defense against infectious diseases.

6. Differentiate the mechanisms leading to infections caused by "true pathogens" from those caused by "opportunists."

7. Give examples of virulence factors that may contribute to the invasiveness of an organism.

8. Explain how organisms apply their virulence structures in evading the host's immune mechanisms.

9. Describe other means by which organisms may resist the host's immune defenses.

CASE IN POINT #1

A 2-year-old boy with acute myelogenous leukemia believed to be in remission, was hospitalized because of fever. Upon admission, his white blood count (WBC) and platelet count were 800 and 67,000, respectively. His temperature was 102°F. Blood cultures were collected and treatment with deftazidime and vancomycin was started immediately. After 4 days of continued febrile episodes, Amphotericin B was added to his regimen of antimicrobial agents. A slender gram negative rod from the blood cultures was detected on the seventh day of incubation.

ISSUES TO CONSIDER

After reading the patient's case history, consider

- The factors that predisposed this patient to his current condition
- The virulence factor(s) utilized by the infectious agent
- The host defense mechanism compromised

CASE IN POINT #2

A 65-year-old woman was admitted to the hospital for hip replacement surgery. After 5 days of uneventful hospitalization, she was released from the hospital with a 10-day regimen of a prophylactic antimicrobial agent. Two weeks after her surgery the patient complained of severe abdominal pain accompanied by diarrhea. She was readmitted to the hospital, and stool examinations were requested.

ISSUES TO CONSIDER

After reading the patient's case history, consider

- Factors that predisposed this patient to her current condition
- Clues that indicate the source of the infection
- Mechanisms microbes use to overcome the host's immune defenses

IMPORTANT TERMS

Carrier state
Chemotaxis
Colonizing (colonized)
Commensalism
Diapedesis
Opportunistic organism

Opportunistic pathogen
Opportunists
Parasitism
Pathogen
Pathogenicity
Resident microbial flora

Symbiosis
Transient microbial flora
True pathogen
Usual (indigenous) microbial
 flora
Virulence

▶ INTRODUCTION

In order to better understand and appreciate how the immune system functions during an infectious process, a clear understanding of the interactions between host and infectious agent in the pathogenesis of disease is necessary. The role of the usual microbial flora in innate immunity was covered in Chapter 2. This chapter expands that presentation and presents the role of the usual microflora at different body sites in the host immune defense and as a source of opportunistic infections. In addition, the chapter discusses the virulence factors that contribute invasion of the host and how microbes are able to evade the host's defenses. Last, this chapter describes factors that may make the host more susceptible to microbial infections.

▶ THE ROLE OF THE USUAL MICROBIAL FLORA

The human body is **colonized** by a wide variety of microbial species. These microorganisms found on or in specific body sites are called **usual (indigenous) microbial flora.** As described in Chapter 2, the usual microbial flora **colonizing** different body sites play a significant role in the host's immune defense. The efficacy of the microbial flora in protecting the human host is indicated by the relatively small number of infections caused by these organisms in immune competent individuals. Nevertheless, these organisms may cause significant, often serious, infections or may exacerbate existing infections in individuals lacking a fully responsive immune system. Table 4-1✪ summarizes the composition of microbial flora at different body sites. Blood, body fluids, and tissues are normally sterile except during a transient bacteremia, such as during heavy chewing or brushing your teeth.

Up until the birth of a child, the environment in which the fetus has existed is sterile. Within a few days after birth, the newborn is exposed to numerous and varied microorganisms encountered in the environment. Microorganisms, upon gaining access onto or into a particular body site of the host, develop a particular relationship with that host. The host-microbe relationship, depending on the circumstance, may be one of **symbiosis, commensalism,** or **parasitism.** Symbiosis is a biological relationship between two or more species with mutual benefits. In commensalism, one species profits and the other remains unharmed, whereas in parasitism, one species gains (parasite) benefits at the expense of the other (host). For example, lactobacilli in the urogenital tract of women provide a symbiotic association, a predictable behavior between host and microorganism. However, while *Proteus mirabilis* is a commensal species in the gastrointestinal tract of humans, it acts as a parasite in the urinary tract and has been known to cause urinary tract infections. There are organisms, however, that are "true" parasites, such as *Neisseria gonorrhoea.* Organisms that parasitize humans exclusively, therefore, are usually not considered part of the usual microbial flora.

Microbial species may colonize a particular body site for a long period of time, such as months, years, or

✪ TABLE 4-1

Microorganisms Usually Encountered at Different Body Sites

Body Site	Microorganisms
Blood	None
Tissue/body fluids	None
Skin/mucous membranes	*Propionibacterium acnes;* Coagulase-negative staphylococci, diphtheroids; streptococci; certain gram negative rods
Mouth	Viridans streptococci; *Neisseria sp.;* occasional *C. albicans* Anaerobes such as *Bacteroides sp.; Fusobacterium sp.; Peptostreptococcus sp.; Actinomyces sp.; Prevotella spp.; Veillonella spp.*
Nasophayrnx	*Staphylococcus aureus; Staphylococcus epidermidis;* Diphtheroids; *Haemophilus parainfluenzae; Haemophilus influenzae; Neisseria meningitidis; Streptococcus pneumoniae; Moraxella catarrhalis*
Esophagus	Same as mouth flora
Stomach	Usually sterile immediately after meals
Small intestine	Few organisms from the colon
Colon	Intestinal anaerobes; Enterobacteriaceae; *Pseudomonas aeruginosa;* yeasts
Vagina/urethra	Skin and mucous membrane flora (depending on the age) Lactobacilli; *Bacteroides* spp.; *S. aureus;* Enterococci; Diphtheroids; *Clostridium* spp.; *Peptostreptococcus* spp.; *C. albicans*

indefinitely. These organisms are called **resident microbial flora.** Organisms that are resident in an area only for a short period of time, perhaps days or weeks, are referred to as **transient microbial flora.** Transient organisms are not able to remain in the area because they are excluded either by the resident microbial flora or by some other form of immune defense mechanism. Certain pathogenic organisms may become established within a host without causing any clinical manifestations; nevertheless, the organisms may be transmitted to and cause infections in susceptible individuals. For example, Group A streptococci may be isolated from individuals who do not experience the clinical disease pharyngitis. Hosts who carry potentially pathogenic organisms but who show no clinical symptoms are called carriers, and their condition is referred to as the **carrier state.** The carrier state may occur as an acute (short-lived) condition or a chronic (long-lasting) condition. For example, a person who becomes infected with *Salmonella typhii* may harbor the organisms long after the clinical disease typhoid fever has resolved. Because *S. typhii* may colonize the gall bladder, the organisms are periodically released with the bile fluids to reinfect the gastrointestinal tract. The carrier state of individuals infected with *Salmonella* lasts for several months, during which time the individual, although no longer ill, becomes a source of infection for other susceptible individuals.

COMPOSITION OF THE MICROBIAL FLORA

Skin Flora

The primary function of normal intact skin is to control the usual microbial flora that are colonizing the skin surface and to protect the underlying tissue from invasion by potential **pathogens.** The number of bacteria present on the skin can be reduced but not completely eliminated by scrubbing and washing. Organisms concentrate most in areas that are moist such as the armpit, groin, and perineum. The apocrine sweat glands in these areas secrete substances metabolized by the skin bacteria, releasing odoriferous amines—the smell that the modern man describes as unpleasant.

The flora on the skin depends on the activity of the sebaceous or sweat glands. The organisms are found on the superficial layers of the skin and the upper portions of the hair follicles. Aerobic diphtheroids are usually found in moist areas such as axillae and toes. *S. epidermidis* and *Propionibacterium* reside in hair follicles and colonize the sebaceous glands because they are resistant to skin lipids and fatty acids, as well as to superficial antiseptic agents commonly used to cleanse the skin. The presence of skin bacteria inhibits the growth of more pathogenic bacterial species, thus providing benefits to the host.

Respiratory Tract Flora

The respiratory tract, commonly divided into upper and lower tracts, is responsible for the exchange of oxygen and carbon dioxide as well as for the delivery of air from the outside of the body to the pulmonary tissues responsible for that exchange. The upper respiratory tract is comprised of the mouth, nasopharynx, oropharynx, larynx; the lower respiratory tract is comprised of the trachea, bronchi, and pulmonary parenchyma. If inhaled particles are to travel through the respiratory tract, they must first penetrate the natural barriers and protective mechanisms that maintain a

sterile environment below the larynx. These barriers include nasal hair, mucosal surfaces equipped with mucociliary cells, and phagocytic inflammatory cells. The physical acts of sneezing, coughing, and swallowing also prevent particles from reaching the alveoli. Any of the defense mechanisms expel organisms that may potentially reach and invade the pulmonary tissue, allowing an extremely efficient clearance of 90% of collect material in one hour. The bronchial secretions also contain antimicrobial substances such as lysozyme that help prevent colonization and establishment of infection in the lower respiratory tract.

Inhaled particles must also survive turbulent flow of humidified air in the upper airway and in the tracheobronchial tree. Turbulence along the air passages causes inhaled particles to collide with and to adhere to mucosal surfaces. The humidified environment causes hydroscopic organisms to increase in size, allowing phagocytosis to occur more easily.

The mouth, nasopharynx, and oropharynx are colonized predominantly with viridans streptococci such as *S. mitis, S. mutans, S. milleri, S. sanguis,* and *Moraxella catarrhalis, Neisseria,* and diphtheroids. Obligate anaerobes reside in the gingival crevices where the anaerobic environment supports these organisms. **Opportunistic pathogens** such as *S. aureus,* which is found in about 30% of healthy individuals, colonize the anterior nares. *Haemophilus influenzae, S. pneumoniae,* and *N. meningitidis,* all potential pathogens, are also found in the nasopharynx of healthy individuals. Individuals who are hospitalized for several days may also become colonized by gram-negative bacteria, particularly members of the enterobacteriaceae, in the upper respiratory tract.

Gastrointestinal Tract Flora

The gastrointestinal tract flora is equipped with numerous defenses and effective antimicrobial factors. Because intestinal pathogens are usually acquired by ingesting organisms contained in contaminated food or drink, host defenses against infections are present throughout the intestinal tract. The stomach is usually sterile, especially after ingestion of a meal causes production of gastric juices, acids, and enzymes which help to protect the stomach from microbial attack. Most organisms, with the exception of spore-forming bacterial species in their spore phase and the cysts of parasites, are susceptible to the acid pH of the stomach. The stomach acidity therefore greatly reduces the number of organisms that reach the small intestine.

The small intestine contains very few, if any, organisms. Organisms that are present are usually from the colon. The constant peristaltic movement in the small bowel provides the major defense of this area, purging the intestinal tract of potential pathogens.

The colon is colonized by a mixture of facultative anaerobes such as members of the enterobacteriaceae and obligate anaerobes. Anaerobes far outnumber aerobes at a ratio of 1000:1. Gram-positive cocci, yeasts, and *Pseudomonas aeruginosa* are also usually present in the large intestine.

Genitourinary Tract Flora

The genitourinary tract is usually sterile although there are a few organisms originating from the perineum that may be found in the distal centimeter of the urethra, particularly in women. The composition of the vaginal flora is consistent with hormonal changes and age. Before puberty and in postmenopausal women, vaginal flora is similar to that of the skin with a few yeasts, gram-negative bacilli, and gram-positive cocci. In contrast, women of child-bearing age have a vaginal pH of about 4–5 as a result of acid produced by lactobacilli. High estrogen levels promote the deposition of glycogen in vaginal epithelial cells. This glycogen is metabolized by lactobacilli to maintain a low pH, creating an environment that is inhibitory to many organisms but that encourages colonization of the vagina with lactobacilli, anaerobic gram-negative bacilli, and gram-positive cocci.

FACTORS THAT DETERMINE THE COMPOSITION OF THE USUAL MICROBIAL FLORA

As previously noted, the composition of the usual microbial flora varies among sites, and to a certain extent, this composition is determined by the environment at that site.

Observations as to the effect of the environment on the composition of the usual microbial flora include

1. Which organisms are present is dictated by nutritional and environmental factors such as the amount and types of nutrients available at the site. For example, more organisms inhabit moist areas than dry areas; these areas are dominated by diphtheroids. Although lipids and fatty acids are bactericidal to most bacteria, *Propionibacterium* colonize the ducts of hair follicles because these bacteria are able to break down the skin lipids to fatty acids. These organisms cannot be removed by washing or scrubbing.

2. pH affects the composition of the female genital tract because most bacteria do not survive at extreme pH ranges. Another example is that the fecal flora found in babies who are breast fed differs from those fed with cow's milk. Human milk, with its high lactose concentration, maintains a pH of 5–5.5 which supports *Bifidobacterium*. Cow's milk, on the other hand, has a greater buffering capacity and therefore is less acidic. Infants fed with cow's milk do not have the high colonization by *Bifidobacterium* found in breast-fed babies, but have instead colon flora similar to that seen in older children and adults.

3. In areas with low oxidation-reduction potential, the environment will support only organisms capable of fermentation, such as seen in the gingival crevices colonized with *Bacteroides* and *Fusobacterium*.

4. The affinity of microorganisms for a specific site depends on the ability of those organisms to resist the antibacterial effects of substances such as bile, lysozyme, or fatty acids, as we have already seen with the usual microbial flora.

ROLE OF THE USUAL MICROBIAL FLORA IN THE PATHOGENESIS OF INFECTIOUS DISEASE

Some organisms that comprise the usual microbial flora are actually parasites that live off the host's nutrients, but in most cases provide some benefit to the host. However, certain members of the usual flora are **opportunists;** they cause disease when there is a disturbance or change in the environment or in the constitution of the host.

In the case of trauma, either accidental or surgical, enough of the usual microbial flora found in the traumatized area may reach other areas in the body where these organisms are not part of the usual microbial flora. For example, leakage following perforation of the colon spills the contents of the colon into the peritoneal cavity, leading to an overwhelming infection by the colon flora. Another example of the potential **pathogenicity** of the usual microbial flora is seen in victims of motor vehicle accidents who become susceptible to infection by environmental organisms, as well as by indigenous microflora.

The immune response may be reduced or altered due to suppression by immunosuppressive drugs, chemotherapy, or radiation. In individuals with lymphoma, leukemia, or other blood disorders where there is a functional defect in phagocytic activity, there is a decrease in the number of functioning cells, or where chemotactic activity is impaired, there may also be a reduced immune response. Case in Point #1 illustrates how opportunistic organisms may initiate a serious infection in individuals who are immunocompromised for some reason. The patient, previously diagnosed with myelogenous leukemia, has a decreased number of white blood cells, therefore becomes very susceptible to infections caused by opportunistic organisms, most of which are members of the indigenous flora.

Members of the usual microbial flora may also initiate an infection or make an infection more serious in patients with chronic illnesses such as diabetes or severe hepatic disease such as cirrhosis. As an example, an amoebic ulcer may become complicated by a secondary bacterial infection.

ROLE OF THE USUAL MICROBIAL FLORA IN THE HOST DEFENSE AGAINST INFECTIOUS DISEASE

Although microorganisms are capable of causing serious infections, these organisms are not necessarily all "bad." The usual microbial flora found at each site serves as a major host immune defense. One of the major functions of the normal flora at each site is to prime the immune system. Consider how a sterile environment might affect a newborn. Antibody production would not be stimulated and the reticuloendothelial system would remain undeveloped. Serum IgG and other antibodies effective against microorganisms would be suppressed, which would make the individual more susceptible to pathogenic species. Without activation by microorganisms and the supporting action of antigen-presenting cells and cytokines, cell-mediated immunity would not develop normally.

The ability of the usual microbial flora to exclude other microorganisms, in particular potential pathogens, is probably the most effective contribution to the host defense system. Organisms compete for nutrients and space. For example, gastroenteritis due to *Salmonella* is generally not treated with antibiotics and is better eliminated by natural exclusion by the colon flora. If the microbial flora has been eliminated, such as is the case in patients receiving antimicrobial therapy or some types of chemotherapy, resistant or more pathogenic species may be able to establish infection. Case in Point #2 illustrates this concept. When present in the gastrointestinal tract, *Clostridium difficile,* an organism associated with antibiotic-associated colitis, may also produce enterocolitis in patients who have recently received antibiotic therapy or chemotherapy.

Candida albicans infection is also common among these patients. *C. albicans* may rapidly multiply and cause diarrhea or infections in the mouth or vaginal tract.

► MICROBIAL FACTORS CONTRIBUTING TO PATHOGENESIS AND VIRULENCE

We have discussed the role of the usual microbial flora in health and in producing disease. Hence, we have begun to recognize that disease does not always occur as the result of every microbial encounter. Certain host defense mechanisms such as the microbial flora will prevent the onset of disease. If every encounter with microbial invaders results in a fatal outcome, what do you think would be the eventual result of the encounter? If you thought of "extinction" of the parasite, then you are right. Microbial invaders, while they parasitize the host, cannot consistently cause the death of the host. If microbes constantly kill their hosts, then they become extinct themselves through lack of an adequate environment for survival. Therefore, we take a look at the host–parasite relationship—how microbes initiate an infectious process and how our body defends itself from the invasion.

PATHOGENICITY AND VIRULENCE

In order to determine the pathogenicity of an organism, that is, the ability of a microbe to produce disease, it must be determined whether the invader is a true pathogen or an opportunistic organism. **True pathogens** are organisms recognized to cause disease in healthy immune competent individuals. *Bacillus anthracis, Yersinia pestis,* and *Francisella tularensis* are examples of a true pathogens. When recovered in clinical samples taken from a body site, there is no doubt that these bacterial species are clinically significant. On the other hand, *Haemophilus influenzae* colonizes the upper respiratory flora of healthy individuals without causing disease, but given the opportunity, may rapidly produce a life-threatening infection. **Opportunistic organisms,** therefore, are those that under usual conditions do not cause disease, and most of these opportunists are members of the microbial flora. However, when the host immune state becomes compromised or suppressed, these organisms are inclined to induce a fulminating infection. *Streptococcus pneumoniae, N. meningitidis,* and *S. aureus* exemplify opportunistic pathogens. Until recent years, the delineation between pathogenic and nonpathogenic organisms is much more simple. With the advent of advances in medicine, that is, the use of prosthetic devices, instrumentation, and organ transplantation, the makeup of the patient population has greatly changed. The use of chemotherapeutic agents and other medical interventions have prolonged lives; however, therapeutic modalities have also caused immunosuppression among these individuals, making them at risk for various types of life-threatening infectious diseases. Under normal conditions, etiologic agents of these diseases do not cause disease. In other words, several years ago, isolation of coagulase-negative staphylococci from clinical sample (i.e., blood cultures) would be interpreted as most likely a contaminant. Today, however, the clinical history, diagnosis, and clinical symptoms are correlated with this result to determine the significance of the isolate. Therefore, microbial species, previously classified as "nonpathogens" are not necessarily harmless anymore.

The **virulence** of the organism, that is, how much harm the organism can cause in the host, depends on those disease-producing factors that are inherent to the organism. For example, *S. aureus* is by nature more virulent than *S. epidermidis,* although both species are known to cause disease. The degree of pathogenicity of an organism is also usually measured by the numbers of microorganisms required to initiate infection in the host. There are organisms that are able to establish infection with as few as 100 organisms, as seen in most *Shigella* infections. Because *Shigella* causes disease with a relatively low infective dose, it is considered more virulent than those that require high numbers to produce an overt infection (i.e., in salmonellosis, 10^6 CFU/mL is necessary to show symptoms). However, certain virulent microbial species may require a relatively high infective dose to produce a fatal outcome.

WHAT DETERMINES MICROBIAL VIRULENCE

The virulence of the organism may therefore depend on certain disease-producing factors inherent to the organism. Factors that determine the pathogenicity and increase the virulence of organisms include their ability to avoid phagocytosis, inherent bacterial structures present, ability to survive intracellularly when phago-

cytosed, and the ability to produce exotoxins and extracellular enzymes.

Ability to Resist Phagocytosis

Phagocytes play a major role in defending the host from microbial invasion. Therefore, one of the microbial factors organisms employ is the ability to resist phagocytosis. There are many ways by which microbial species evade phagocytosis. Certain organisms release potent materials in tissues that kill phagocytes. Streptococci produce hemolysins, which lyze red blood cells but also have toxic effects on white blood cells and macrophages. Pathogenic staphylococci release leucocidins, which induce lysozomal discharge into cell cytoplasm. Staphylococcal leukocidin, called Panton-Valentine, is lethal to leukocytes and contributes to the invasiveness of the organism. Others inhibit **chemotaxis,** and thus, the host is less able to direct PMNs and macrophages into the site of infection.

Bacterial Structures

Bacterial structures such as capsules protect organisms from phagocytosis, increasing their virulence and ability to spread. Encapsulated strains *of S. pneumoniae* and *H. influenzae* are associated with highly invasive infections and are shown to be more virulent than nonencapsulated strains. Fimbrae are cell wall structures used by organisms for adherence and attachment. Fimbrae offer resistance by attachment to target cells, thereby increasing the organism's colonizing ability. Once attached, phagocytosis is less likely to occur. On the fimbrae of Group A streptococci are M proteins, the major virulence factor associated with this organism.

Protein A in the cell wall of *S. aureus* helps the organism avoid phagocytosis by interfering with the inactivation of host's antibodies. Protein A binds to the Fc portion of IgG, thus preventing opsonization and phagocytosis.

Ability to Survive Intracellularly

In most circumstances, when an organism is engulfed by macrophages, lysosomal contents are released in the phagocytic vacuoles, and the organism is killed. In contrast, if the engulfed organism is not exposed to intracellular killing and digestive processes, it is able to survive and multiply inside the macrophage. Bacterial species such as *Chlamydia, Mycobacterium, Brucella,* and *Listeria* are easily engulfed by macrophages and phago-

✪ TABLE 4-2

Examples of Exotoxins Produced by Clinically Significant Organisms

Species	Toxin	Disease
Bacillus anthracis	Edema toxin	Anthrax
Escherichia coli	Shiga toxin	Hemorrhagic colitis
	Heat-labile and heat-stable enterotoxins	Traveler's diarrhea
Clostridium difficile	Enterotoxin(A) Cytotoxin(B)	Antibiotic-associated colitis
Clostridium tetani	Tetanospasmin	Tetanus or "lockjaw"
Corynebacterium diphtheriae	Diphtheria toxin	Diphtheria
Clostridium botulinum	Neurotoxin	Botulism
Staphylococcus aureus	Exfoliative toxin	Scalded skin syndrome
	Enterotoxin	Food poisoning
Streptococcus pyogenes	Erythrogenic	Scarlet fever
Vibrio cholerae	Vibrio enterotoxin	Cholera

cytes; however, these species are not only able to survive inside the macrophages and are protected from other hosts' immune defenses, but also they are able to multiply intracellularly.

Ability to Produce Extracellular Toxins and Enzymes

Another major factor that contributes to the virulence and invasiveness of the organism is the ability of organisms to produce exotoxins and extracellular enzymes. Exotoxins are produced by both gram-negative and gram-positive bacteria and can be secreted or released upon lysis of the organism. Exotoxins are proteins, although others are enzymes, which can cause cell and tissue damage. There are toxins that mediate direct spread of the microorganisms through the matrix of connective tissues. Some organisms produce soluble substances, proteases, and hyluronidases that liquefy the hyaluronic acid of the connective tissue matrix and help spread of bacteria in tissues promoting the dissemination of infection.

Table 4-2✪ shows some examples of specific toxins, such as diphtheria or botulinum, which are potent exotoxins that make these species virulent. Diphtheria toxin inhibits protein synthesis and affects the heart, nerve tissue, and liver. Botulinum toxin is a neurotoxin that blocks nerve impulse transmission, causing flaccid paralysis especially in infants. *S. pyogenes* and *S. aureus* both produce exfoliatins that cause rash and massive skin peeling or exfoliation.

Virulence in microorganisms not only is increased by production of exotoxins, but also can be caused by production of enzymes. Table 4-3✪ shows examples of enzymes that contribute to the pathogenicity of organisms. Collagenase and hyaluronidase, which disintegrate the ground substance of tissues and hydrolyze hyaluronic acid, allow organisms that produce these enzymes to spread and cause tissue necrosis. Coagu-

✪ TABLE 4-3

Examples of Enzymes That Contribute to Microbial Invasiveness

Species	Enzymes	Action
C. perfringens	Collagenase	Disintegrates the ground substance of tissues
S. aureus	Coagulase	Coagulates plasma
	Leukocidin	Kills cells and WBCs
Staphylococci, clostridia, streptococci	Hyaluronidase	Hydrolyzes hyaluronic acid
Many species	Capsule	Resists phagocytosis
Many species	Fimbriae	Attachment to target cells

lase, another enzyme, protects *S. aureus* by forming fibrin walls around the lesions. Leukocidin kills cells and the white blood cells responsible for counteracting a microbial invasion.

THE HOST DEFENSE AGAINST MICROBIAL INVASION

FIRST-LINE DEFENSES

The host's major physical barrier against microbial invaders is the squamous epithelial layer of the skin. The stratified and keratinized epithelium of healthy skin serves as a physical barrier to direct penetration by most microorganisms. Although some microorganisms infect the skin or enter the body via the skin, most of these organisms usually cannot penetrate intact skin. Only a few species (e.g., *F. tularensis, Treponema* spp., and *Leptospira* spp.) are able to enter the body by penetrating unbroken skin. Other organisms require a vector (e.g., an insect or animal bite) or other means by which to facilitate entry and to overcome the mechanical barrier. The antagonism by the microbial skin flora also provides protection, as previously described. The large amount of microbial flora occupies possible attachment sites, competes for nutrients, and helps maintain a low pH. Some accessory organs of the skin, such as the sebaceous glands, may also produce bactericidal substances.

Desquamation of the skin surface, a form of cleansing, disposes of microorganisms colonizing the skin. By continuously shedding the keratinized squamous epithelial layer of the skin, the microbial load on the skin surface is constantly reduced.

The epithelial linings and mucous membranes of the urogenital tract, respiratory tract, paranasal sinuses, and intestinal tract also function as a blockade against pathogens. In addition to serving as a barrier, mucous membranes secrete antimicrobial substances such as lysozyme, lactoferrin, and secretory IgA. The mucous membranes in the respiratory tract are lined with cilia, ready to trap any foreign particles that come in that direction. Nasal hairs, cilia, and mucus secreted by membrane linings trap particles and microorganisms, which are then directed toward the oropharynx, where the particles are either coughed up or swallowed. These mechanisms certainly prevent infectious organisms and other potentially harmful objects from reaching the pulmonary parenchyma. When microorganisms are swallowed, either in food or drink, or as part of the oral secretions containing mouth flora,

most bacteria, except those that are encapsulated, are destroyed by the acidity in the stomach, as previously described. Those that survive encounter mucous secretions, secretory antibody, and phagocytes lining the mucosal surfaces which are prepared to defend the site against potential invaders. The voiding of urine is another form of cleansing: cleansing of the genitourinary tract. Organisms that may have reached the bladder via the urethra, especially in women, are readily eliminated by the flushing action of the bladder.

Antimicrobial substances, produced in the host or secreted by mucous membranes, provide significant contributions to defense against microbial invasion. Lysozyme, for example, hydrolyzes the peptidoglycan layer of bacterial cell walls, killing the organisms. Lysozyme may also act with other substances (e.g., antibody, complement). Antibodies may serve as opsonins to facilitate phagocytosis, or to bind complement and neutralize the infecting organism.

SECOND-LINE DEFENSES

Phagocytosis, chemotaxis, and inflammation are critical components of the host's defense against infectious agents. Phagocytosis by PMNs and macrophages is the primary mechanism by which the host resists extracellular bacterial agents, some viruses, and fungi. As described in Chapter 2, PMNs in the blood are attracted to the site of tissue injury as soon as the cytokines and chemotactic agents of the inflammatory response are released. However, these cells are short-lived, and dead PMNs containing engulfed organisms are taken up by macrophages during most infectious processes.

The body is patrolled by protective cells such as PMNs and other phagocytic cells. Phagocytes circulate through the body, ready to migrate to the site of an infection of penetration of surface barriers by a foreign body. The movement into the tissue of the PMNs through small spaces between the endothelial cells of the blood vessels is called **diapedesis.** This migration of inflammatory cells and phagocytes to an area of injury, or chemotaxis, is an orchestrated event induced by factors serving as chemotactic agents. These factors may be products from the infecting bacteria, damaged tissues, responding inflammatory cells, or components of complement. Although the initial contact of the PMNs with the foreign particle may be random, production of chemotactic factors induced by the invader direct PMNs and other phagocytes to the site of invasion.

The process of inflammation as an immune response has been previously discussed in Chapter 2. Inflammation is one of the body's responses to injury or invading foreign matter. During inflammation, mediators are released by phagocytic cells. These mediators cause increased blood flow to the site of injury, producing erythema. Increased vascular permeability causes edema and the continued accumulation of phagocytes that make up pus. Thus, the hallmarks of inflammation, heat, pain, redness, and swelling occur. The phagocytic cells release enzymes that digest the foreign object, injured tissues, and cell debris. Once the invading particle is removed, the damaged site of invasion repairs and heals.

The adaptive immune response, discussed at length in other chapters of this text, also defends against microorganisms. This response is much slower to develop than are the other defenses, but is also specific to and develops memory for the microorganism. The antibodies produced by the B lymphocyte response combine with the cell-mediated immunity launched by the T cells to eradicate whatever microorganisms have eluded the first- and second-line defenses.

MECHANISMS BY WHICH MICROBES MAY OVERCOME THE HOST DEFENSES

The fact that infectious agents are able to establish disease indicates that the host's immune defense can be overcome by the invader. Organisms employ a variety of antihost mechanisms. These microbial strategies act to counter the host's defenses and include induction of tolerance, immune suppression, absence of the appropriate target for the immune response, and antigenic variation.

Tolerance is the failure of the host's immune system to respond to specific antigens of the infecting microorganisms. However, this failure to respond is not necessarily caused by immune suppression. The reduction in the immune response to microbial antigen may be due to a "feeble antigen": an antigen or antigenic component of an organism that is not able to elicit an immune response from the host. Therefore, the host fails to launch a response or is slow in responding, suggesting tolerance to this antigen. Tolerance to an organism may also develop when the infection occurs during fetal life or in a neonate. For example, it is believed that although the fetus, when infected by the rubella virus, responds and makes its own antibodies, the antibodies are often weak and are unable to contain the infection. Because the T cell response is also poor, the virus is able to persist in the fetus and during the neonatal period. Hence, microor-

ganisms can persist if they are able to survive in the host during prenatal infections without producing an overt form of the disease.

There are certain microorganisms that cause immune suppression in the infected individual. The decreased immune response is often more far-reaching than simply to the antigen of the involved microorganism. Viruses, certain bacteria, and protozoans are examples of microorganisms likely to cause immune suppression in the infected host. These infectious agents multiply in macrophages or in lymphoid tissues. The exact mechanisms of immunosuppression by the infecting organism have not been defined for all organisms. However, individuals infected with viruses such as Epstein-Barr virus and cytomegalovirus show depressed T cell or antibody responses to other unassociated antigens. Reduced immune reactivity caused by an infectious agent is exemplified by that caused by the human immunodeficiency virus (HIV). HIV targets CD4+ T cells. Because the virus destroys the major cells that defend the host against viral, fungal, and protozoan infections, the infected person becomes susceptible to opportunistic infections caused by these organisms.

Certain organisms are able to elude the host immune defenses because of their ability to systematically change their surface antigens during the course of a single infection, even while inside the host. This occurs in relapsing or recurring fever infections with *Borrelia recurrentis*. After an initial incubation period of two to 15 days following transmission of the spirochetes from a tick or louse, high numbers of the organism are found in the blood. The infected individual experiences high fever, rigors, severe headache, muscle pains, and weakness. The febrile period lasts for about three to seven days but ends quickly with the induction of an immune response. However, a similar but less severe course of symptoms recurs several days to weeks later. The relapses are caused by antigen variation by the borreliae. Spirochetemia worsens during febrile periods and diminishes between recurrences.

Another evasion strategy employed by microorganisms is to make themselves unavailable as targets to the host's immune system. Certain organisms such as *Brucella, Listeria,* and *Mycobacteria* evade the host's immune response by surviving inside infected cells. Macrophages that engulfed these microbial species protect them from antibacterial substances and support their growth inside the macrophage. For example, the parasite *Plasmodium* spp., during the exoerythrogenic cycle in liver cells, avoids being a target for the immune response. Malarial parasites can therefore infect red blood cells and cause disease while protected from the host's defense mechanisms.

Hosts also produce antibodies against specific antigenic stimuli as an immune defense. However, if the antibodies produced against an infecting organism are of low avidity, or have a weak antimicrobial effect on the infecting organisms, the ability of the infected host to control the infection is decreased. Therefore, in certain microbial infections, antibodies, although produced, provide little or no protection to the host.

Similarly, interferons play a very significant role in the host defense against foreign invaders. The main function of these cytokines is to stimulate the expression of MHC proteins by T cells. Interferons are also antiviral; IFN-α and IFN-β work against double-stranded RNA viruses while IFN-γ is produced following the activation of T cells. There are instances when viruses escape the effects of interferons, either because they are resistant to the antiviral effects or because the induction of interferon in the host does not take place. For example, vaccinia virus is able to resist the effects of interferons by inactivating IFN-γ. Other viruses may produce persistent infections because these viruses do not induce interferon production.

SUMMARY

In this chapter, we have reviewed the benefits derived by the host from organisms that colonize the skin, the respiratory system, the gastrointestinal tract, and the genitourinary tract—the usual microbial flora. The factors that determine the composition of the usual microbial flora were discussed, as was the role of this flora as opportunists in the pathogenesis of infectious disease. Microbial factors that contribute to the pathogenicity and virulence of microbes were described, including the ability of some microorganisms to resist phagocytosis, the ability to of some to survive intracellularly, and the ability to produce exotoxins and enzymes. Intoxication and adherence were presented as mechanisms capable of causing disease. We also reviewed the host defense against microbial invasion and noted ways by which microbes may evade the host's immune system.

POINTS TO REMEMBER

▶ Humans do not exist in a sterile environment. Colonization of the body by microorganisms begins at birth.

▶ The usual microbial flora benefits the normal host by priming the immune system, out-competing potential pathogens for nutrients and creating a hostile environment for other microbes.

▶ The usual microbial flora present at each site in the body is dictated by nutritional and environmental factors.

▶ Some species of the usual microbial flora may be opportunists, capable of causing disease in an immunocompromised host.

▶ True pathogens cause disease in all individuals.

▶ The host defense system against microorganisms includes physical, mechanical, and chemical barriers; components of the innate immune system such as phagocytes, complement, cytokines, and the products of inflammation; and the components of the adaptive immune response.

▶ Microbes have mechanisms to evade the host defenses, including the ability to evade phagocytosis, the production of enzymes and exotoxins, the ability to induce tolerance in the adaptive immune system or to suppress the adaptive immune system, and the ability to avoid recognition by the adaptive immune system by varying the antigens present on the surface of the microorganism.

LEARNING ASSESSMENT QUESTIONS

1. A long-term resident species of bacteria in the gastrointestinal tract produces vitamin K, which is required for blood clotting in mammals. This is an example of:

a. commensalism.
b. parasitism.
c. symbiosis.
d. opportunism.

2. The usual microbial flora helps to:
   a. prime the host immune system.
   b. produce substances toxic to more pathogenic species.
   c. decrease the numbers of pathogenic organisms by competing for nutrients.
   d. All of the above.

3. "Lockjaw" is the result of:
   a. an inflammatory response to *C. tetanii*.
   b. the action of an exotoxin produced by *C. tetanii*.
   c. overwhelming sepsis caused by *C. tetanii*.
   d. an autoimmune response generated after exposure to *C. tetanii*.

4. "First-line defenses" include:
   a. antibody production.
   b. chemotaxis.
   c. mechanical barriers.
   d. the inflammatory response.

5. Certain microorganisms, such as *Mycobacteria*, evade the host immune response by:
   a. causing immune tolerance.
   b. inducing immunosuppression in the host.
   c. proliferating inside of phagocytic cells.
   d. frequently mutating surface antigens.

REFERENCES

Koneman, E., et al., eds. 1997. *Color Atlas and Textbook of Diagnostic Microbiology.* 5th ed. Lippincott and Wilkins, Philadelphia, PA.

Mandell, G., J. Bennett, and R. Dolin. 2000. *Mandell, Douglas and Bennett's Principles and Practice of Infectious Diseases,* 5th ed. Churchill Livingstone, New York.

McKenzie, S. B. 2004. *Clinical Laboratory Hematology.* Pearson-Prentice-Hall. Upper Saddle River, NJ.

Mims, C., A. Nash, and J. Stephen. 2001. *Mim's Pathogenesis of Infectious Disease,* 5th ed. Academic Press, San Diego, CA.

Sheldon, H. 1992. *Boyd's Introduction to the Study of Disease,* 11th ed. Lea & Febiger, Philadelphia, PA.

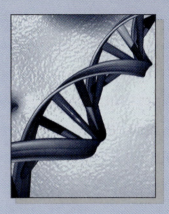

5

The Complement System

■ CHAPTER CHECKLIST

After reading and studying this chapter, the reader should be able to:

1. Describe the nomenclature for the complement components.
2. Explain the classical complement cascade.
3. Describe the alternate complement pathway and the mannose-binding lectin pathway.
4. List each of the complement components and their subunits.
5. Describe the biological activity of each complement component.
6. Determine a differential diagnosis between the various complement disease states based on laboratory findings.

CASE IN POINT

A 6-year-old male was taken to his pediatrician. His mother noted he had been complaining of fever, headache, stiffness of the back and neck. He had Brudzinski's sign and a petechial rash on his lower extremities and abdomen. His medical history revealed that he had experienced many bacterial infections throughout his life with some being extremely severe. The clinician ordered a urinalysis, chemistry profile, CBC, blood culture, and spinal tap, and the results were as follows:

Blood

Hemoglobin	14.5 g/dL	WBC: 13.5×10^9/L	
Differential	Neutrophils: 60%	Lymphocytes: 9%	
	Monocytes: 4%	Bands: 27%	
BUN	Normal	Glucose: 90 mg/dL	
Electrolytes	Normal	Culture: Negative	

CSF

Appearance	Cloudy	WBC: 2800/mm³
Differential	Neutrophils: 98%	Glucose: 30 mg/dL
Protein	150 mg/dL	Gram Stain: Many WBCs
		Gram-negative diplococci
Culture	*Neisseria meningitidis*	

IMPORTANT TERMS

Activation unit	Complement receptor	Membrane attack complex
Alternate pathway	Complement regulatory	(MAC)
Amplification loop	molecules	Opsonin
Anaphylotoxin	Decay accelerating factor	Paroxysmal nocturnal
C1 inhibitor (C1INH)	(DAF)	hemoglobinuria (PNH)
C3 convertase	Factor H	Properdin
C4 binding protein (C4BP)	Factor I	Recognition unit
Chemotactic agent	Hereditary angioedema (HAE)	S protein
Classical pathway	Immune adherence	Total hemolytic complement
Complement	Mannose-binding lectin	(CH_{50}) assay
Complement fixation test	(MBL) pathway	

▶ INTRODUCTION

The complement system is comprised of at least 30 proteins that function to initiate some of the biological processes involved in the immune response. Although **complement** is considered a part of the innate immune system encoded in the germ line cells, it is also a bridge between that system and the adaptive immune system. As such, it works in tandem with an antibody developed against specific antigens as a defense against bacterial infection by aiding in the presentation of antigen to phagocytic cells or by causing lysis of the organism. It also assists in disposing of immune complexes and the products of inflammation or injury. Fragments produced during activation serve as **chemotactic agents, opsonins,** and **anaphylotoxins.** Finally, the complement cascade is also linked to coagulation, fibrinolytic, and kinin systems.

The three complement pathways discussed in this chapter are the **classical pathway** which is antibody-dependent, the **alternate pathway** which is antibody-independent and can be triggered by surface receptors on bacteria, and the **mannose-binding lectin (MBL) pathway** which involves the interaction of specific bacterial carbohydrates with complement components. The first sections of the chapter discuss the activation of each of the pathways; the later sections cover the regulators that help prevent inappropriate activation of complement and the diseases that are associated with complement deficiencies.

The nomenclature of complement components can be problematic when first studied. Components are designated by either a letter or number, depending on the pathway. Some components are common to all three pathways; others function only in one (Figure 5-1■). In the classical pathway the components are numbered (C1, C2, C5, etc.). When certain components are split, the fragments are given the letters a or b. With the exception of C2 fragments, the larger fragment is designated b and is attached to the target cell. The smaller a fragment is released into the plasma. In the MBL pathway the initial components are given letter abbreviations (MBL, MASP). From C2 through the final component, the letters and numbers in the MBL

are the same as in the classical pathway. In the alternate pathway some components, known as factors, are designated by a letter (e.g., Factor B). In the alternate pathway the components that are identical to those in the classical pathway retain their numbers (C3, and C5 through C9). Regulatory proteins have names derived from their function or are identified by the cluster differentiation system (e.g., CD21).

The complement molecules interact in a cascade-like fashion similar to that seen in coagulation. Some of the complement proteins initiate the cascade, and others serve as regulators to block the cascade. There are approximately 20 proteins that act in the plasma phase and 10 that serve as either regulators or cell membrane receptors. The majority of the components are manufactured in the liver. C1 is made by the epithelial cells of the intestine and, in some situations, by activated macrophages. Factor D, which is involved in the alternate pathway, is made in adipose tissue. C3 is the most abundant of the components with an average concentration of approximately 1200–1600 µg/ml. C4, a β_1 globulin, is the next most abundant with a concentration of 600 µg/ml (0.6 mg/ml) (Table 5-1✪). The components are heat labile,

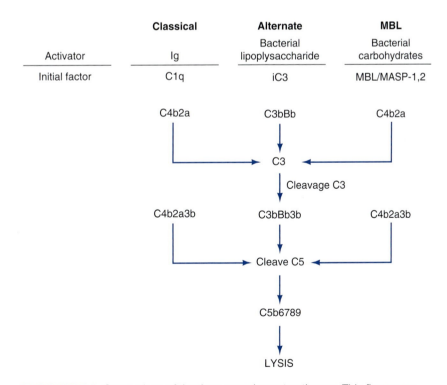

■ FIGURE 5-1 Comparison of the three complement pathways. This figure compares the three pathways of complement activation. Note that although each pathway has a different mechanism for activation and different C3 convertases, they all share the C5-9 membrane attack complex.

✪ TABLE 5-1

Serum Concentration of Complement Components

Factor	Approximate Serum Concentration (µg/ml)
Classical	
C1q	70–100
C1r	30–34
C1s	30–31
C2*	25–30
C3**	1200–1600
C4*	430–600
Lectin	
MBL	0.05–20
MASP1	1–10
Alternate	
B	200–240
D	1–2.5
Properdin	22–25
Membrane attack complex (MAC)—all pathways	
C5	70–80
C6	60–65
C7	50–55
C8	55–80
C9	60–160
Control proteins	
C1INH	150–200

*Also part of the lectin pathway.

**Also part of the alternate and lectin pathway.

and heating serum at 56°C for 30 minutes can destroy their activity.

Although these proenzyme molecules (zymogens) circulate in the plasma, they are inactive until a specific event initiates the pathways. Once initiated, the inactive molecules are cleaved to expose an active site. Some fragments are cleaved, with the larger fraction capable of enzymatically cleaving the next molecule in the cascade, whereas the smaller fragment has an inflammatory effect. The pathway may continue to completion or may be inhibited by innate regulators.

The **complement regulatory molecules** serve to balance the reaction between activation by foreign antigens and inhibition of complement interactions with normal cells. Although the end stage of complement activation is usually thought of as lysis of the cell under attack, fragments of the complement molecules are involved in other activities, including opsonization, chemotaxis, initiation of mast cell degranulation,

immune adherence, clearing of immune complexes, and enhancement of the inflammatory process. Therefore, deficiencies in complement may predispose an individual to recurrent bacterial infections or increased risk for certain autoimmune diseases. The young patient described in the case study had a history of recurrent bacterial infections, presumably due to some abnormality in his complement system.

Complement may be used by organisms to increase virulence. Some viruses may use cell-bound **complement receptors** or regulatory proteins to gain entry into a cell. For example, Epstein-Barr virus (EBV) uses CD21 (complement receptor type 2) to enter B lymphocytes. Other organisms such as mycobacteria use a coating of C3b to bind to a cell's complement C3 receptor.

Complement is required for proper processing and clearance of self-antigens. Normally apoptotic cells are opsonized with complement fragments to enhance phagocytosis that is mediated by complement receptors on phagocytic cells. When these self-antigens are not cleared properly, there is increased risk of developing autoimmune disease. The autoantigens are taken up by immature dendritic cells in the presence of cytokines such as TNF-α and IL-1. These cytokines induce the maturation of these dendritic cells into mature antigen presenting cells capable of presenting these antigens to T cells and able to initiate an immune reaction with autoreactive B cells.

Complement possesses some anti-inflammatory functions stemming from its ability to clear immune complexes from the circulation and tissues. Soluble immune complexes in the circulation are coated by complement fragments (usually C3b) to prevent tissue deposition and to increase **immune adherence.** The complexes react with CR1 receptors on erythrocytes. In the liver and spleen, tissue macrophages remove the complexes without destruction of the erythrocyte. If the immune complexes are allowed to precipitate in the vasculature, then inflammation will develop.

▶ THE COMPLEMENT PATHWAYS

CLASSICAL PATHWAY

The classical pathway has nine numbered proteins in the cascade, but C1 is made up of three separate proteins (C1q, C1r, C1s), bringing the total number of proteins to 11. There are three units in the classical pathway—the recognition unit made up of C1q, C1r, and C1s; the activation unit made up of C4, C2, and

✪ TABLE 5-2

Components of the Complement Pathways

	Classical	Alternate	Lectin
Recognition and initiation	Immunoglobulin (IgM or 2 IgG) molecule reacts with C1qrs	Bacterial antigen	Bacterial carbohydrate with mannose binding protein and MASP1 and MASP2
Activation	C4b2a	Ticking over of C3 Interaction with Factor B, D, properdin	C4b2a
C3 Convertase	C4b2a	C3bBb	C4b2a
C5 Convertase	C4b2a3b	C3bBb3b	C4b2a3b
MAC	C5b6789	C5b6789	C5b6789

C3; and the membrane attack complex (MAC) which is composed of C5b-C9 (Table 5-2✪).

Immunoglobulins bound to antigen are required to activate the classical pathway. This can be a single IgM molecule or two IgG molecules no further apart than 30–40 nm on the cell or in a circulating complex. As mentioned in chapter 3, C1q binds to a receptor in the C_H3 domain of IgM and the C_H2 domain of IgG. IgM, which is produced early during the course of an infection, is the most efficient antibody in fixing complement because of its pentameric structure. When attached to a target antigen, there are multiple domains available for complement binding. Of the four subclasses of IgG, only IgG_1, IgG_2, and IgG_3 can bind complement with IgG_3 being the most efficient and IgG_2 the least. Because of the distance constraint for C1q binding, at least 1000 molecules of IgG must be present on a cell surface to get two molecules close enough for complement to bind.

Recognition Unit

The **recognition unit** involves only one complement component C1, which is composed of three proteins—C1q, C1r, and C1s (Figure 5-2■). C1q resembles a bouquet of six flowers with the six globular heads serving as the attachment sites and triple stranded polypeptide chains (stalks) extending from the heads. Prior to activation the unit is linear, but after activation C1r and C1s loop around the stalks of C1q in a loose figure eight. Calcium ions (Ca^{++}) are required to stabilize the molecule. Once two of these C1q heads bind to the appropriate domains on the Ig molecule, C1r is activated, acquires serine protease activity, and proteolytically cleaves C1s. Once C1s is cleaved, it too acquires serine protease activity. This activated molecule is now capable of cleaving C4 and C2.

Activation Unit

The cleaving of C4, C2, and C3 are the phases involved in the **activation unit** of the classic pathway. C4, a molecule with three polypeptide chains known as α, β, and γ, is the first molecule cleaved. C4a, the smaller fragment is released into the plasma. C4b binds to the cell surface near the C1 molecule. C4b must bind to the cell membrane within a few seconds or it is inactivated. Once C2 is cleaved by C1s, C2a binds to C4b on the membrane, and C2b is released into the plasma. Mg^{++} is required to stabilize the molecule. This molecule C4b2a—known as **C3 convertase**—is highly active and can split up to 200 C3 molecules into active fragments. C3 is initially split into C3a, a small anaphylactic molecule released into the plasma, and C3b, which covalently binds to proteins on the cell surface. If the C3b molecule is deposited on the cell membrane within a distance of approximately 40 mm of the C4b2a complex, then it is capable of interacting with these fragments to form C4b2a3b (C5 convertase). C3b fragments that are deposited at distances greater than this do not combine but remain on the cell membrane and serve as opsonins (Figure 5-3■). If the entire process is terminated at the C3b stage, the fragments already deposited can also serve as opsonins.

Membrane Attack Complex

Once the activated C4b2a3b molecule begins cleavage of C5, this initiates the final stage of complement activity leading to lysis. This stage, known as the **membrane attack complex (MAC),** involves components C5–9. C5 is first cleaved into a small C5a fragment that is a potent anaphylatoxin released into the plasma, and C5b, which is deposited on the membrane, serves as a binding molecule for C6–9. C6 and C7 are deposited, and lysis is initiated with the addition of C8. At the deposition of C8, a small channel

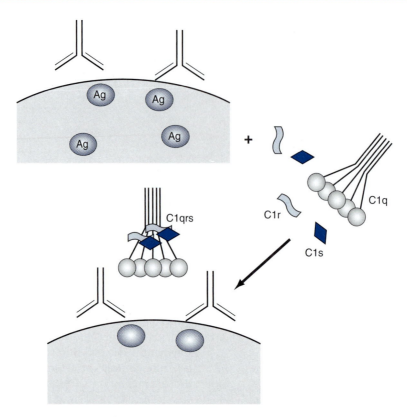

■ **FIGURE 5-2** Formation of C1q. This figure shows the mechanism by which the C1qrs molecule is assembled.

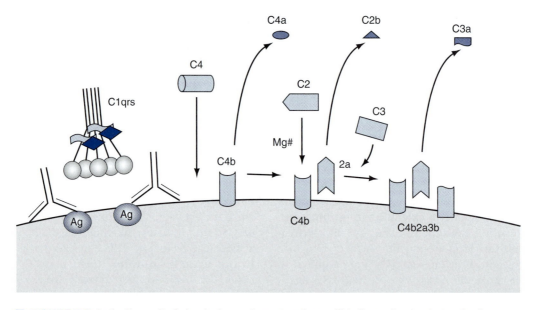

■ **FIGURE 5-3** Activation unit of classical complement pathway. This figure demonstrates the formation of C3 convertase, the final molecule in the activation phase. Fragments of the activated C4, C2, and C3 are given off into the plasma where they function in other immune response activities.

(about 10 A) is formed in the cell membrane that allows the leakage of intracellular potassium and other cellular components. Each C8 molecule can bind up to 10–14 C9 molecules, which complete the formation of the transmembrane channel. At this stage the channel, which can reach a diameter of 1000 A, allows the influx of sodium ions, calcium ions, and water resulting in cell lysis (Figure 5-4■).

ALTERNATE PATHWAY

The alternate pathway is considered to be antibody-independent, meaning that activators are not immunoglobulins, but rather components of the cell walls of bacteria, fungi, viruses, and some parasites. For example, lipopolysaccharides from gram-negative bacteria and teichoic acid from the cell walls of gram-positive bacteria are two compounds known to activate this pathway.

Some of the proteins involved in the alternate pathway differ from those found in the classical pathway in name but parallel the action. These include factor D, which is similar in function to C1qrs and Factor B, which is similar to C2. **Properdin** acts as a stabilizing molecule in this pathway (see Table 5-2).

The initial stages of the pathway differ from that of the classical pathway, but once C3 has been cleaved, the process for formation of the MAC is identical. The activating stage is referred to as "ticking over." The unstable C3 in the plasma is slowly and spontaneously activated by water molecules to iC3. This is converted to a hydrolyzed C3b-like molecule referred to as iC3b when an internal thioester bond reacts with an exposed $-OH$ or $-NH2$ group. This molecule, in the presence of Factor D and magnesium ions, can then combine with factor B to form iC3bBb, the fluid phase C3 convertase. If the molecule is deposited on autologous cells, it usually binds to sialic acid or inhibitor proteins and is inactivated. If it is deposited on nonhuman cells such as bacteria, the pathway will continue because there are no regulatory proteins present. Properdin, the only positive complement regulator protein, stabilizes this molecule and increases the half-life from about five minutes to 30 minutes.

At this point, iC3bBb can split additional C3 in a positive feedback or **amplification loop** (Figure 5-5■). The C3b produced has two fates. One outcome is that as the C3 convertase cleaves C3 and deposits multiple molecules of C3b over the surface of the cell, leading to increased opsonization by neutrophils or macrophages with C3 receptors. The other is that the C3b will combine with C3bBb to form C3bBb3b or C5 convertase. This molecule, which cleaves C5, will drive the reaction through the MAC and cell lysis.

LECTIN PATHWAY

The lectin pathway, also known as the mannose-binding lectin (MBL) pathway, is considered part of the innate immune system and is the second type of path-

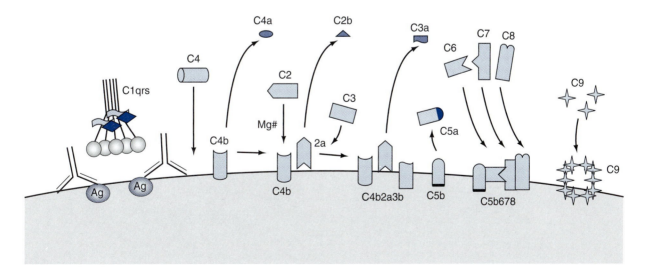

■ **FIGURE 5-4** Formation of the membrane attack complex (MAC). This figure demonstrates the formation of the C5b-9 or membrane attack complex (MAC). The addition of C8 and C9 are responsible for the pore formation and lysis of the cell membrane.

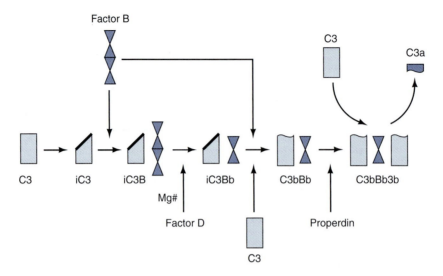

■ **FIGURE 5-5** Tick-over of C3 in the alternate complement pathway. This figure demonstrates the normal tick-over of C3 in the serum and the formation of C3 convertase in the alternate pathway. Note that properdin, Factor B and Factor D play a role in the formation of the molecule.

way involving reactions of complement with carbohydrates located on the cell membrane of fungi, bacteria, yeast, viruses, and parasites. The pathway functions during the early part of a bacterial infection and is thought to be of particular importance in children during the period between decrease of passive maternal antibody and full development of the adaptive immune system (between 6–18 months of age).

Carbohydrates that can bind to MBL include mannose, N-acetylglucosamine, fucose, and glucose. Along with the MBL there are mannose associated serine proteases (MASP) that noncovalently bind to MBL and serve as initiators of the pathway. These are MASP-1 and MASP-2, with MASP-2 being the most important in complement activation. MBL is structurally related to C1q, and the MASPs are similar to C1r and C1s. The MBL binds to carbohydrates on the cell wall and recruits MASP-2. MASP-2 initiates the sequential cleaving of C4 and C2. As with the classic pathway, calcium is required to stabilize the molecule. The sequence now proceeds in a manner identical to that seen in the classic complement activation pathway (Figure 5-6■).

BIOLOGICAL ACTIVITIES OF COMPLEMENT

The lytic activity of the MAC is well known, but complement activation also results in production of biologically active fragments that function in the general immune response by promoting opsonization, phago-

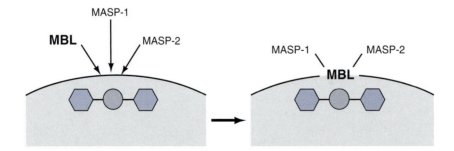

■ **FIGURE 5-6** Formation of initial unit in the lectin pathway. This figure shows the initial step in the mannose lectin pathway. Notice the similarity of this to the formation of C1qrs in the classical pathway. From this point on the steps in the lectin pathway are identical to those in the classical pathway.

cytosis, chemotaxis, and anaphylaxis. In addition there is evidence that certain fragments facilitate activation of B cells, especially memory cells. These activities are most often dependent on the presence of specific receptors on cells that allow the complement fragments to bind to the cell. The major complement fragments involved in these activities are C3a, C4a, C5a, C3b, iC3b, and C3d (Table 5-3✪).

The MAC formed by any of the three complement pathways is capable of lysing a variety of cell types, including microbial organisms. Gram negative and gram positive bacteria differ in their susceptibility to complement mediated lysis. Gram positive organisms have thick peptidoglycan cells wall components that inhibit or prevent penetration of C8-C9 complex.

C3b, iC3b, and C4b are opsonins. These fragments coat the cell membrane of an organism and enhance phagocytosis of the organism. Macrophages and neutrophils possess complement receptor 1 (CR1) that binds to these fragments so that C3b or C4b coated cells are engulfed and phagocytized more effectively than noncoated organisms. CR3 and CR4 bind C4b and iC3b, respectively. C3b also binds to soluble immune complexes which in turn react with CR1 receptors on erythrocytes. These complexes are carried to the liver and spleen where the immune complex is removed from the erythrocyte and phagocytized (Figure 5-7■).

C3a, C4a, and C5a are low molecular-weight peptides referred to as anaphylotoxins, with C5a being the most active and C4a the least. The effects of anaphylotoxins begin when fragments attach to specific recep-

tors on cells such as mast cells or basophils. In these cells, the complement fragments stimulate the release of histamine from intracellular granules. Histamine stimulates smooth muscle contraction, increases capillary permeability, causes release of lysosomal enzymes, and induces the respiratory burst. The resulting influx of plasma promotes movement of phagocytic cells and antibody to the area.

C5a, the most potent, also possesses chemotactic activity that activates neutrophils and macrophages and causes migration to the source of antigen and inflammation. It increases vascular adherence by myeloid cells. C5a also plays a role in upgrading the number of CR1 receptors on activated phagocytic cells and will stimulate segmented neutrophils to release enzymes and chemokines that amplify the inflammatory response. In addition it serves an immune adherence molecule for nonphagocytic cells such as erythrocytes, B lymphocytes, and endothelial cells. In this process complement and antibody work together to bind a bacterium, virus, or immune complex to the erythrocyte surface using complement receptors. This allows the erythrocyte to transport the molecule to phagocytic cells.

Another function of complement involves viral infectivity. In some cases complement will cause direct lysis of the viral particle. In other cases it coats the viral particle and therefore blocks the ability of the virus to attach to host cells. In essence it neutralizes infectivity. Presence of C3b on the virus will also increase phagocytosis by those cells with CR1 receptors. The in-

---

✪ TABLE 5-3

Biological Function of Selected Complement Fragments

Function	Fragment Involved				
	C3a	C4a	C5a	C3b	C4b
Anaphylotoxis	x	x	**x**		
Degranulation of mast cells/basophils					
Increased vascular permeability					
Smooth muscle contraction					
Chemotaxis			x		
Release of neutrophilic granules	x		x		
Increased CR1 receptor expression			x		
Opsonization				**x**	x
Immune complex clearance				x	

Note: Bold face type indicate this fragment is the major fragment involved in the function.

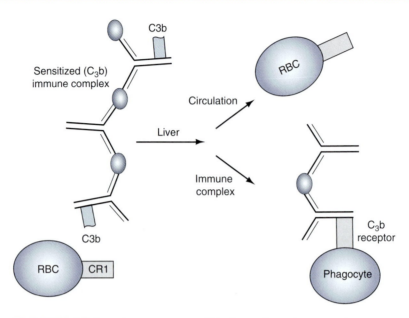

■ **FIGURE 5-7** Complement receptor. This figure shows how complement receptor 1 (CR1) functions in helping to clear immune complexes from the blood. Notice that while the immune complex with C3b is removed from the cell in the liver by phagocytes with C3b receptors, the erythrocyte is not affected.

teraction of C2b with plasmin creates kininlike activity, including smooth muscle contraction and increased mucus secretion.

COMPLEMENT REGULATORY PROTEINS

Much of the regulation of the complement cascade occurs passively simply because the components are inherently unstable and, if not activated rapidly, have a short half-life. In other words, a molecule is inactivated quickly if the next component does not interact and the cascade stops. For example, in the alternate pathway when C3 is normally "ticked over" into C3b, that molecule has approximately 60 microseconds to bind to an amino or hydroxyl group on the cell surface, or it will become inactivated.

There are, in addition, molecules that function as regulators. These molecules actively inhibit or prevent inappropriate complement activation in plasma or on human cells. Most of these molecules are coded on Chromosome 1 within a closely linked gene cluster. The regulator proteins act at three major points: blocking initiation of the cascade, preventing formation of the C3/C5 convertase, or inhibiting the formation of MAC (Table 5-4✪).

C1 inhibitor (C1INH) and **Factor I** act to prevent initial activation. **Decay accelerating factor (DAF),** complement receptor 1 (CR1), membrane control protein (MCP), **C4 binding protein (C4BP),** and **Factor H** inhibit convertase formation by either preventing binding of the necessary complement protein or causing dissociation or degradation of molecules. CD59 and **S protein** block the MAC.

Some regulatory proteins are found as soluble plasma molecules. These include C1INH and C4BP in the classical pathway, factor H in the alternative pathway, Factor I, and complement S-protein in the MAC of all pathways. Others, which are part of the cell membrane, include complement receptor types 1 through 4 (CR1, CR2, CR3, CR4), DAF, MCP and CD59.

Regulatory Proteins in the Classic Pathway

C1INH is a serine protease and the only molecule that acts on C1. It combines irreversibly with activated C1r and C1s to cause dissociation from C1q. Although C1q remains bound to immunoglobulin, this dissociation prevents formation of C3 convertase and, in turn, inhibits cleavage of C3 into C3b. Factors such as kallekrein, plasmin, and activated factor XII (Hageman factor) may also be inhibited by C1INH. Factor I can act in both the alternate and the classical pathway to

⊘ TABLE 5-4

Complement Regulator Proteins

Soluble Proteins (Serum)	Function	Pathway
C1 inhibitor (C1INH)	Dissociation of C1r and C1s from C1q	C*
C4 binding protein	Binds C4b and increases decay of C4b2a; prevents C3 convertase	C, L
Factor I	Cleaves C3b and C4b	C, L, A
Factor H	Binds C3b/blocks C3 convertase formation	A
Properdin	Stabilizes C3bBb	A
S-Protein	Binds C5b67 complex; stops insertion in cell membrane	
Cell membrane proteins	**Function**	**Pathway**
Complement receptor 1 (CR1)	Binds C4b and prevents C3 convertase formation	C, L, A
Membrane cofactor protein (MCP)	Binds C4b and prevents C3 convertase formation	C, L, A
Decay accelerating factor (DAF)	Promotes decay of C3 convertase	C, L, A
C8 binding protein (C8bp)	Prevention of MAC formation	C, L, A
CD59	Prevention of MAC formation by blocking insertion of complex and C9 polymerization	C, L, A

*C—classical pathway; A—alternate pathway; L—lectin pathway.

cleave the cell bound C3b molecule in several places. Two membrane-bound inactive molecules, C3c and C3dg, are the result of this cleavage. Formation of C3dg stops the complement cascade. However, C3d is not a highly efficient opsonin because macrophages lack receptors for the molecule.

C4 binding protein (C4BP) acts as a cofactor to Factor I and inhibits the classic pathway formation of C3 convertase by displacing C2a from the molecule or by inactivating C4b, causing degradation to C4c and C4d.

DAF, also known by its cluster designation CD 55, and CR1 are membrane molecules responsible for preventing the binding of C2 to C4b for dissociation of C3bBb or C2a from the C3/C5 convertase molecules (Figure 5-8■). MCP (CD46) is instrumental in the catabolism of C4b. DAF is present on peripheral blood cells, especially erythrocytes, and vascular endothelial cells. This molecule protects the individual's own erythrocytes from complement-induced lysis by increasing Factor I degradation activity on C3b. Thus it prevents opsonization, lysis, the release of anaphylotoxins, and decreases the inflammatory reaction.

Regulatory Proteins in the Alternate Pathway

Properdin is the only molecule that acts to prolong the life of a complement fragment or activated molecule. It increases the half-life of the C3bBb molecule so that conversion of additional C3b can occur. Factor I competes for the same binding site as factor B in the alternate pathway. Therefore, if Factor I binds, no C3bBb can form.

Factor H, a soluble factor that is an analogue to C4BP, affects the alternate pathway by preventing formation of C3 convertase. It inhibits binding of Factor B to membrane-bound C3b, thus preventing cleavage of B to Bb. It competes with factor B to bind to C3b

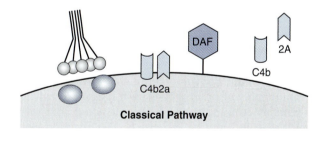

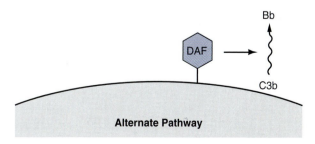

■ **FIGURE 5-8** Action of selected complement regulators. This figure shows how decay accelerating factor (DAF) can act to dissociate or to hinder attachment of molecules.

and causes dissociation into separate C3b and Bb molecules. The end result of this dissociation is that no C3 convertase is formed. Factor H can also serve as a cofactor for Factor I to catabolize C3b.

Regulation of MAC in All Pathways

CD59 is a membrane bound molecule found on all blood cells, as well as endothelial and epithelial cells. It inhibits lysis by binding to the C5b-8 complex and inhibits insertion of the complex into the cell membrane. It also prevents C9 attachment to complete the MAC molecule.

S protein is a serum protein produced in the liver. Its primary function is to prevent incorporation of early stages of the MAC complex (C5b-8) into the cell membrane and subsequent polymerization of C9. In addition, it may perform some scavenger functions that increase clearance of molecular complexes.

Homologous restriction factor (HRF), which occurs on homologous cells only, is a membrane protein of erythrocytes and platelets, and white cells that inhibits channel formation. Membrane cofactor protein (MCP, CD46), also a glycoprotein, is present on epithelial and endothelial cells and on all hematopoietic cells except erythrocytes. This molecule binds to C3b and C4b so that they are susceptible to inactivation by Factor I.

COMPLEMENT RECEPTORS

Complement receptors are molecules that specifically react with fragments of the complement molecule. Three opsonization fragments C3b, iC3b, and C3dg and four complement receptors (CR1, CR2, CR3, and CR4) are involved in this process (Table 5-5✪).

CR1 (CD35), a glycoprotein, is the only one of the receptors present on erythrocytes. It is also present on a number of cells in the body, including follicular dendritic cells, neutrophils, monocytes, macrophages, B lymphocytes, and some T lymphocytes. It serves as a receptor for C3b and acts as a cofactor to Factor I in the process of cleaving C3b to C3c and C3dg. It possesses some decay accelerating factor-like activity with both C3 and C5 convertases. It has an additional role on erythrocytes—it will bind complement-bearing immune complexes to transport them to the phagocytic cells in the liver or spleen. A deficiency of CR1 receptor may be a predisposing factor in the development of systemic lupus erythematosus. This molecule has also become a target for complement regulation therapy for certain inflammatory conditions. In its soluble recombinant form, it has been used to decrease tissue damage in burns and shock syndromes.

CR2 (CD21) is found on B lymphocytes and follicular dendritic cells. It primarily reacts with iC3b and C3dg. On dendritic cells it serves a role in B cell stimulation. As previously mentioned it also serves as a receptor for entry of the Epstein-Barr virus (EBV) into B lymphocytes. CR3 is present on myeloid cells and mediates phagocytosis of cells coated with iC3b. CR4 plays a minor role in calcium-dependent iC3b binding to tissue macrophages and myeloid cells.

▶ DISORDERS OF COMPLEMENT FUNCTION

COMPLEMENT AND MICROBIAL ORGANISMS

Microbial organisms, including viruses, bacteria, and parasites, can evade complement-mediated lysis or can use complement receptors to invade host cells and therefore promote their pathogenicity. Some gram-negative organisms have lipopolysaccharide layers that direct complement away from their membranes so that opsonization or lysis does not occur. Other organisms such as *Neisseria* species may have a capsule with in-

✪ TABLE 5-5

Complement Receptors

Receptor	Cells Involved	Complement Fragment Bound
CR1 (CD35)	Erythrocytes, neutrophils, B and T lymphocytes, monocytes and macrophages, follicular dendritic cells	C3b, C4b, iC3b
CR2 (CD21)	B lymphocytes, follicular dendritic cells	C3d, C3dg
CR3	Neutrophils, monocytes, macrophages, NK cells	iC3b
CR4	Neutrophils, monocytes, macrophages, NK cells	iC3b
C1q	B lymphocytes, macrophages, monocytes, platelets	C1q with immune complex

creased amounts of sialic acid that causes C3b to bind to Factor H, not Factor B. In this case, C3 convertase is not formed, and the amplification loop of the alternate pathway does not occur. Parasites such as the trypomastigotes and the schistosomes have regulatory molecules similar to those on human cells that protect from complement binding or affect the stability of the C3 convertase. For example, the trypanosomes have decay accelerating factor (DAF) and CD59-like molecules whereas schistosomes actually absorb soluble DAF from the host. Both these molecules promote dissociation of the C3b convertase of the alternate pathway.

In other cases organisms use the membrane-bound molecules as receptors that facilitate entry into the cell. EBV is the classic example of this mechanism in that it uses the CR2 receptor on B lymphocytes as the point of attachment and entry into the cell. The measles virus has been found to use MCP, and there is evidence that West Nile virus may use C3 to help gain entry into cells.

DISEASES LINKED TO COMPLEMENT DEFICIENCIES

There are over 80 primary immunodeficiency conditions and of these approximately 1 to 3% involve complement deficiencies. Most are inherited as autosomal recessive conditions except properdin deficiency, a deficiency that is X-linked. Deficiencies in one or more complement components or in regulators of complement result in a variety of conditions usually charac-

terized by decreased lytic activity or decreased opsonization. If the deficiencies are in the MAC components, then defects are in lytic activity, and the individual may be prone to recurrent *Neisseria meningitidis* infections. The patient in the case study may have had a deficiency in a component of the MAC. Further testing would identify a defect in lytic activity rather than a simple complement deficiency. Deficiency of early components in the classical pathway predisposes the individual to immune complex disorders such as systemic lupus erythematosus (SLE). If the defect is in other complement components, notably C3, then the individual is often prone to recurrent infections with organisms such as staphylococci and streptococci, primarily as the result of ineffective opsonization (Table 5-6✪). Unlike autoimmune diseases where women are affected more frequently, complement deficiencies affect both sexes about equally and are inherited in an autosomal recessive pattern.

Links to Autoimmune Disorders
Complement deficiency has been linked to a number of diseases, the most prominent of which is SLE. Individuals with deficiencies in the early components of the cascade (C1q, C2, or C4) show a strong predisposition to the development of immune complex diseases such as SLE, but there has been no strong association between SLE and deficiencies of the MAC components. This association is thought to be related to the ineffective clearance of apoptotic material, allowing self-antigens to initiate an immune response. Comple-

✪ TABLE 5-6

Complement Deficiencies and Associated Conditions or Diseases

Component—Classical Pathway	Condition/Disease
C1q, r, s	Collagen vascular disease (lupuslike syndrome)
C2	SLE, discoid lupus, glomerulonephritis; recurrent bacterial infection
C3	Increased susceptibility to bacterial infections, glomerulonephritis
C4	Collagen vascular disease (lupuslike syndrome)
C5, 6, 7, 8	Recurrent *Neisseria* infections
C9	None
Component—Alternative Pathway	**Condition/Disease**
Properdin	*Neisseria* infection (sepsis)
Factor H or Factor I	Recurrent pyogenic infections
Regulators	**Condition/Disease**
Decay accelerating factor (DAF)	Paroxysmal nocturnal hemoglobinuria (PNH)
CR3	Bacterial skin infections
C1 inhibitor (C1INH)	Hereditary angioedema (HAE)

ment is not only important in defense against microorganisms, but also is a key player in the scavenging of necrotic and apoptotic cells and in handling immune complexes. Complement deficiency may promote nuclear antigen presentation and trigger autoantibody formation.

Since C1q enhances phagocytosis of apoptotic cells by macrophages, a deficiency leads to accumulation of cells. When these antigens are not deleted, dendritic cells encounter these exposed nuclear antigens on blebs from the cells, leading to stimulation of autoantibody formation by activation of self-reactive B cells. Patients with C1q deficiency often present with symptoms involving renal and skin presentations before age 20.

Deficiencies in C2 and C4 lead to insufficient production of C3 convertase. This results in inadequate C3b and C4b deposits on membranes. The lack of these opsonins inhibits removal of immune complexes, a mediator of inflammation in the host.

Prevalence of SLE disease in homozygous C1q deficiency may be as high as 90% but is lower with C4 or C2 deficiencies.

In C1q deficiency most patients are under 20 years of age and show skin and renal manifestations. Autoantibodies are directed against extractable nuclear antigens (ENA). In homozygous C4 deficiency cutaneous lesions are seen, and anti-SSA (anti-Ro) and anti-SSB (anti-La) are frequently encountered.

Because the MBL pathway is a first line of defense in preventing bacterial infection, deficiency in MBL has been associated with increased susceptibility to bacterial infections, including those causing acute pneumonia or urinary tact infections in children.

Links between deficiencies in regulator proteins and development of autoimmune diseases such as myasthenia gravis are also being investigated.

Acquired complement deficiencies, on the other hand, occur in diseases in which immune complexes activate the pathway. Several of these conditions include SLE or other collagen vascular diseases and disseminated intravascular coagulation (DIC). In DIC, the decrease occurs because C3 is consumed by enzymes that are active in fibrinolysis. In SLE, the reaction of autoantibody with nuclear antigens and the deposition of immune complexes in the vasculature activate the classic pathway and increase consumption. Fragments such as C3a, C3b, and C5a mediate inflammatory response and lead to additional tissue damage.

C1INH is the only plasma protease inhibitor that inactivates C1r and C1s and therefore is the primary regulator of the classic pathway. There is also some evidence that it may regulate the MBL pathway. The lack of C1INH has also been linked to development of autoimmune diseases. In this case, inadequate regulation of complement activity results in decreased levels of C2 and C4. C1INH regulates production of bradykinin by inactivation of kallikrein and Factor XIIa and regulates intrinsic coagulation pathway by inactivation of Xla and Xlla. Although it is able to inactivate plasmin, it does not usually play a role in fibrinolysis. An acquired angioedema also exists that is due to development of an autoantibody to C1INH.

Hereditary Angioedema

The most well-recognized link between a specific disease and a deficiency of a complement component is that of C1 inhibitor (C1INH) deficiency and **hereditary angioedema (HEA),** a disease characterized by recurrent, nonpainful, localized edema of the skin or mucosa of the larynx or gastrointestinal tract. The condition is linked to a heterozygous deficiency of plasma C1INH due to either deletions or missense mutations in the controlling gene.

In this condition, the low level of C1INH leads to activation of the complement system. There are decreases in C2 and C4 and an increase in bradykinin. Edema in the gastrointestinal tract may lead to colicky pain, nausea, and vomiting. There is no fever nor is there an increase in white blood cells which help to distinguish it from acute intestinal disorders. Attacks last 48–72 hours and spontaneously resolve. The edema occurs with a loss of endothelial barrier function, resulting in excessive vascular permeability without the presence of inflammation, and does not respond to steroids.

Paroxysmal Nocturnal Hemoglobinuria

Although the clinical signs of **paroxysmal nocturnal hemoglobinuria (PNH)** have been known since the 1880s, the actual cause was not identified until 100 years later. This acquired hemolytic disorder occurs as a result of a somatic mutation in hematopoietic cell precursors. The result is an altered enzyme responsible for stabilizing two of the regulatory proteins on cell membranes—decay accelerating factor (CD55) and protectin (CD59). The resulting mutation in phosphatidylinositol glycan Class A (or a GPI anchored protein) leads to increased susceptibility to complement-mediated lysis.

The PNH syndrome is characterized by increased susceptibility to complement activation leading to intravascular hemolysis, hemoglobinuria, hemosiderinuria, and a predisposition to thrombosis. The lack of the molecule on platelets causes release of granules and increased prothrombin activity, which increases the risk of thrombosis. Older diagnostic tests for PNH included the sucrose hemolysis test for screening and Ham's acid hemolysis test for confirmation. Newer techniques include the use of flow cytometic analysis for CD55 and CD59.

Other Conditions Related to Complement Deficiency

Two deficiencies of regulatory factors have been identified as causes of atypical (nondiarrheal, nonverocytotoxin) hemolytic uremic syndrome (HUS). The first is a mutation in Factor H and can often be seen in families. This mutation decreases the binding of Factor H to C3b and predisposes the individual to excess complement activation. Normal Factor H has decay accelerating factorlike activity. Conversely, the altered molecule allows for increased stability of C3 convertase (C3bBb). The second molecule deficiency associated with atypical HUS is membrane cofactor protein, a surface-bound regulator. This molecule, which is part of the host tissue membrane, normally inhibits complement activation by regulating C3b deposition. When there is a mutation, complement activation is increased.

Deficiency in the components of the MAC leads almost exclusively to *Neisseria meningitidis* infections because these intracellular organisms are not killed once inside the cell. When the MAC components are deficient, *N. meningitidis* is not able to be killed in plasma. The young patient present in the case study most likely had either a deficiency of a MAC component or an abnormal protein unable to function in the MAC.

Treatment

In most cases of diseases that result from complement deficiencies, treatment has been focused on resolving the infections that occur or limit the damage that develops in autoimmune disorders. There have been, however, numerous attempts to develop agents that can serve to regulate the complement pathway in persons who may have deficiencies. One of the first, albeit unsuccessful, was use of cobra venom. This bound to Factor B and consumed C3 so that there was none available for functional activities. There have been attempts at developing monoclonal antibodies to serve as inhibitors by blocking cleavage mechanisms. Excessive C5a will deactivate oxidative burst (H_2O_2). Monoclonal anti-C5a has been tried in cases of bacterial sepsis. This molecule deactivates some of the C5a and helps preserve the oxidative burst (H_2O_2) in segmented neutrophils. Other

therapeutics that have been considered include the use of soluble recombinant forms of membrane complement regulator molecules. Recombinant soluble CR1, which inhibits C3/C5 convertase, has been tried with some success to limit the damage due to complement activation in cases of acute myocardial infarction and respiratory distress syndrome.

▶ DETECTION OF COMPLEMENT

ASSESSING IMMUNE DEFICIENCIES

Patients with suspected functional defects in the immune system are given a battery of tests to determine the type of immune deficiency present. Tests might include quantitative IgG, IgA, and IgM levels; complete blood count and enumeration of T lymphocytes; and measurement of serum complement levels and/or assessment of complement functional activity. In addition to determining the total amount and function of the complement proteins, there may be testing to determine whether the deficiency is due to inherited or acquired conditions. Although inherited conditions most often result in decreased amounts or function of complement proteins, acquired conditions can result in increased consumption or decreased production.

Complement comprises about 15% of the total globulin fraction, and when the overall percentage of globulins is significantly decreased, there may be a decrease in complement. Because complement is heat labile, once the serum has been separated from the clot it should be placed at 4°C and tested immediately (within 1–2 hours) or stored at −70°C.

The classic screening test for determining the function of the entire classical pathway is the **total hemolytic complement (CH$_{50}$) assay;** for the alternative pathway it is the AH$_{50}$. The Ch$_{50}$ assay is based on the ability of complement in the patient's serum to lyse a standardized aliquot of antibody-coated sheep red blood cells (SRBC). If there are any factor deficiencies, the CH$_{50}$ value will be decreased. If there is a total lack of complement, then the value is zero. In the test patient serum is serially diluted, and an aliquot of antibody-sensitized SRBC is added to each tube. After incubation the mixture is quantitatively assayed for free hemoglobin. The endpoint is the dilution that lyses 50% of the cells.

The AH$_{50}$ test is a modification of the CH$_{50}$ and is often used along with that test as part of a complement deficiency screen. Rabbit red blood cells, which can activate the alternate pathway, are used instead of SRBC to evaluate the sequence of factors D, B, P, and C5-9.

The amount of hemolysis observed is due to alternate pathway activation. If both assays are abnormal, then the defect must be in a common component (C3-C9). If only the CH_{50} is abnormal, then the defect must be in one of the early components (C1, C4, or C2).

The concentration of individual complement components such as C3 or C4 is most frequently performed by radial immunodiffusion (RID) or nephelometry. These tests require antibody directed against the specific complement component. In RID the antibody is incorporated into a gel matrix. Patient serum is added into a well and allowed to diffuse into the surrounding medium. A line of precipitation will form at the zone of equivalence between antigen and antibody. The diameter of this circle is measured and compared with values plotted on a standard curve.

DIAGNOSTIC TESTING THAT RELIES ON COMPLEMENT

Complement fixation tests are a group of tests used to detect the presence of antibodies to organisms such as viruses, rickettsia, and fungi. The native complement in the patient's serum is destroyed by heating at 56°C for 30 minutes. This serum is mixed with soluble antigen and an external standardized source of complement. After incubation, antibody-coated SRBCs are added. If there is lysis of the SRBC, then the patient lacks antibodies to the specific organism (negative test). If there is no lysis, then complement was tied up by the patient's antibody bound to the soluble antigen and was not available to lyse the antibody coated SRBC (positive test) (Figure 5-9■).

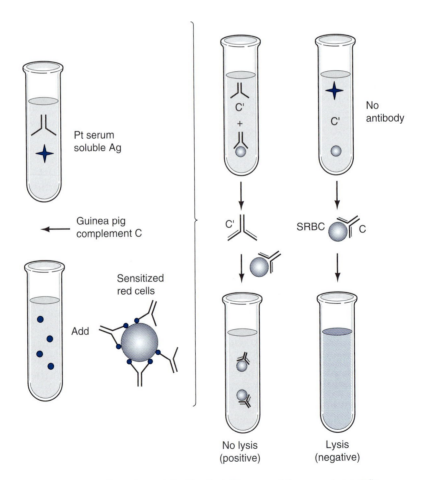

■ **FIGURE 5-9** Complement fixation test. The use of the complement fixation test in demonstrating presence of antibody in a patient's serum is shown in the figure.

SUMMARY

In summary, the complement proteins of each of the three pathways and their associated regulatory proteins serve as a key part of the immune response. These molecules can lyse cells, serve as opsonins to enhance phagocytosis of foreign antigens, or help process and remove immune complexes. In turn, some organisms use the complement pathway and reg- ulator proteins as a mechanism of pathogenesis. Deficiencies of the complement proteins or the lack of functional components may results in disease states such as systemic lupus erythematosus, paroxysmal nocturnal hemoglobinuria, or hereditary angioedema.

POINTS TO REMEMBER

▶ The complement system is a key part of both the innate and adaptive immune responses, and is involved in clearance of self- and foreign antigens.

▶ The system contains over 30 molecules that either activate or regulate the cascade.

▶ There are three separate pathways for activation, all of which act in a cascadelike fashion: classical, alternate, and mannose-binding lectin (MBL).

▶ Activation may result in cell lysis if the entire cascade is completed or in the deposition of immunologically active fragments on cells if the cascade is inactivated during the process.

▶ The classical pathway is activated by immunoglobulins bound to antigen.

▶ The alternate pathway is antibody independent, and is activated by components of the cell wall of bacteria or fungi, or by viruses.

▶ The MBL pathway involves reaction of complement component with carbohydrates on cell membranes of organisms.

▶ The biological activities of complement and its fragments include lysis, stimulation of smooth muscle contraction, increasing capillary permeability, promotion of chemotaxis, and opsonization.

▶ Regulatory proteins may be cell bound or in the plasma, and may act on all three pathways or be limited in action to only one pathway.

▶ Complement receptors react with fragments of complement molecules, and include CR1, CR2, CR3, and CR4.

▶ Microbial organisms may use complement receptors as a means of entering cells or to evade complement mediated lysis.

▶ Diseases linked to complement deficiencies are usually the result of an autosomal recessive inheritance pattern. A deficiency in MAC leads to recurrent *Neisseria* sp. infections while a deficiency in C1, C2, or C4 leads to immune complex diseases. Deficiencies in C3 may result in recurrent infections.

▶ Hereditary angioedema (HAE) results from continual activation of the complement pathway due to lack of C1INH.

▶ Paroxysmal nocturnal hemoglobinuria (PNH) is the result of increased sensitivity to complement lysis.

▶ Hemolytic uremic syndrome (HUS) is due to mutation of Factor H or to a MCP defect.

▶ Immune deficiencies due to complement disorders may be assessed by a quantitative immunoglobulin test, a total hemolytic assay (CH_{50}), or by quantitation of individual complement proteins.

▶ The complement fixation test is used in a variety of applications and is based on lysis of antibody coated cells.

▶ Treatment of complement deficiencies is in the early stages of development, and may involve monoclonal antibody or recombinant forms of complement regulator proteins.

LEARNING ASSESSMENT QUESTIONS

1. The primary function of C1INH is to
   a. dissociate C1 r and s from C1q.
   b. prevent binding of Ca++ to C1qrs.
   c. dissociate the individual molecules of C1q.
   d. irreversibly bind factor H to C1qrs.

2. The reaction that signifies a *positive* reaction in a complement fixation test is
   a. agglutination.
   b. no agglutination.
   c. lysis.
   d. no lysis.

3. Hereditary angioedema is associated with a deficiency of which factor?
   a. Cr1
   b. Factor I
   c. S protein
   d. C1INH

4. The major function of CR1 is to:
   a. serve as a receptor for C1qrs.
   b. help transport C3b coated immune complexes to the liver.
   c. increase the "tickover" mechanism of C3 in the alternate pathway.
   d. serve as a cofactor for C3b inactivation.

5. The protein responsible for stabilizing the complement cascade is
   a. Factor I.
   b. properdin.
   c. MASP1.
   d. C4 binding protein.

6. Which of the following is a membrane bound regulator protein?
   a. C4BP
   b. S protein
   c. DAF
   d. Factor H

7. Activities of C5a include all of the following except:
   a. chemotaxis.
   b. degranulation of basophils.
   c. opsonization.
   d. increased expression of CR1.

8. Which of the following factors is not involved in the activation of the alternate pathway?
   a. C2
   b. C3
   c. Factor B
   d. Factor D

9. The regulatory protein that acts on the MAC is:
   a. Factor I.
   b. S protein.
   c. DAF.
   d. Factor H.

10. When complement proteins such as C4 or C3 are cleaved, what is the term applied to the fragment deposited on the cell membrane?
    a. anaphylotoxin
    b. chemotaxin
    c. convertase
    d. opsonin

11. Where on the immunoglobulin molecule does C1q bind?
    a. Fab fragment domain
    b. hypervariable region
    c. heavy chain domain
    d. light chain disulfide bond

12. Which of the following activated molecules is known as C3 convertase?
    a. C4b2a
    b. C3bP
    c. C14a
    d. C4d2b

REFERENCES

Atkinson J. P. 2003. Complement system on the attack in autoimmunity. *J Clin Invest* 112:1639–41.

Barilla-LaBarca, M. L. and J. P. Atkinson 2003. Rheumatic syndromes associated with complement deficiency. *Current Opinion in Rheumatology* 15:55–60.

Barrington, R., M. Zhang, M. Fischer, and M. C. Carroll. 2001. The role of complement in inflammation and adaptive immunity. *Immunological Reviews* 180:5–15.

Bhole, D. and G. Stahl. 2003. Therapeutic potential of targeting the complement cascade in critical care medicine. *Critical Care Medicine* 31:S97–104.

Boackle, S. A. 2003. Complement and autoimmunity. *Biomedicine & Pharmacotherapy* 57:269–73.

Carroll, M. A. and M. B. Fischer. 1997. Complement and the immune response. *Current Opinion in Immunology* 9:64–69.

Davis, A. E. 2003. The pathogenesis of hereditary angioedema. *Transfusion and Apheresis Science* 29:195–203.

Dempsey, P. W., S. A. Vaidya, and G. Cheng 2003. The art of war: Innate and adaptive immune responses. *Cell Mol Life Sci* 60:2604–21.

Ember, J. A. and T. E. Hugli. 1997. Complement factors and their receptors. *Immunopharmacology* 38:3–15.

Epstein, J., Q. Eichbaum, S. Sheriff, and R. A. B. Ezekowitz. 1996. The collectins in innate immunity. *Current Opinion in Immunology* 8:29–35.

Fleer, A. 2000. Cellular and humoral defence mechanisms against bacteria. *Paediatric Respiratory Reviews* 1:235–40.

Fleisher, T. A. and R. H. Tomar. 1997. Introduction to diagnostic laboratory immunology. *JAMA* 278:1823–34.

Garred, P., F. Larsen, Madsen, and C. Koch. 2003. Mannose-binding lectin deficiency—revisited. *Molecular Immunology* 40:73–84.

Hart, S. P., J. R. Smith, and I. Dransfield. 2004. Phagocytosis of opsonized apoptotic cells: Roles for "old-fashioned" receptors for antibody and complement. *Clin Exp Immunol* 135:181–85.

Holers, V. M. 2003. The complement system as a therapeutic target in autoimmunity. *Clinical Immunology* 107:140–51.

Krauss, J. S. 2003. Laboratory diagnosis of paroxysmal nocturnal hemoglobinuria. *Annals of Clinical & Laboratory Science* 33:401–6.

Landau, D., H. Shalev, G. Levy-Finer, et al. 2001. Familial hemolytic uremic syndrome associated with complement factor H deficiency. *Journal of Pediatrics* 138:412–17.

Leendert, A. T., A. Roos, and M. R. Daha. 2001. Autoantibodies to complement components. *Molecular Immunology* 38:199–206.

Lin, F., H. J. Kaminski, B. M. Conti-Fine, et al. 2002. Markedly enhanced susceptibility to experimental autoimmune myasthenias gravis in the absence of decay-accelerating factor protection. *J Clin Investigation* 110:1269–74.

Manuelian, T., J. Hellwage, S. Meri, et al. 2003. Mutations in factor H reduce binding to C3b and heparin and surface attachment to endothelial cells in hemolytic uremic syndrome. *Journal of Clinical Investigation* 111:1181–90.

Meri, S. and H. Jarva. 1998. Complement regulation. *Vox Sang* 74S2:291–302.

Morgan, B. P. and C. L. Harris. 2003. Complement therapeutics: History and current progress. *Molecular Immunology* 40:159–70.

Nauta, A. J., L. A. Trouw, M. R. Daha, et al. 2002. Direct binding of C1q to apoptotic cells and cell blebs induces complement activation. *Eur J Immunolo* 32:1726–36.

Noris, M., S. Brioschi, J. Caprioli, et al. 2003. Familial haemolytic uraemic syndrome and an MCP mutation. *Lancet* 362:1542–47.

Parker, C. J. 2002. Historical aspects of paroxysmal nocturnal haemoglobinuria: "Defining the disease." *British J of Haematology* 117:3–22.

Perdriger, A., S. Werner-Leyval, and K. Rollot-Elamrani. 2003. The genetic basis for systemic lupus erythematosus. *Joint Bone Spine* 70:103–8.

Peterson S. V., S. Thiel, L. Jensen, et al. 2000. Control of the classical and the MBL pathway of complement activation. *Molecular Immunology* 37:803–11.

Pickering, M. C., M. Botto, Taylor P.R., et al. 2001. Systemic lupus erythematosus, complement deficiency, and apoptosis. *Adv Immunol* 76:227–332.

Richards, A., J. A. Goodship, and T. H. Goodship. 2002. The genetics and pathogenesis of haemolytic uraemic syndrome and thrombotic thrombocytopenic purpura. *Current Opinion in Nephrology & Hypertension* 11:431–35.

Richards, A., E. J. Kemp, M. K. Liszewski, et al. 2003. Mutation in human complement regulator, membrane cofactor protein (CD46), predispose to development of familial hemolytic uremic syndrome. *Proceedings of the National Academy of Sciences of the United States of America* 100:12966–71.

Sahu, A. and J. D. Lambris. 2001. Structure and biology of complement protein C3, a connecting link between innate and acquired immunity. *Immunological Reviews* 180:35–48.

Sanchez-Corral, P., D. Perez-Caballero, O. Huarte, et al. 2002. Structural and functional characterization of factor H mutations associated with atypical hemolytic uremic syndrome. *American Journal of Human Genetics,* 71:1285–95.

Sheerin, N. S. and S. H. Sacks. 1998. Complement and complement inhibitors: Their role in autoimmune and inflammatory diseases. *Curr Opin Nephrol Hypertens,* 7:305–10.

Sturfelt, G. 2002. The complement system in systemic lupus erythematosus. *Scand J Rheumatol,* 31:129–32.

Tangsinmankong, N., S. L. Bahna, and R. A. Good. 2001. The immunologic workup of the child suspected of immunodeficiency. *Ann Allergy Asthma Immunol;* 87:362–70.

Turner, M. W. 2003. The role of mannose-binding lectin in health and disease. *Molecular Immunology,* 40:423–29.

Walport, M. 2001. Advances in immunology: Complement (first of two parts). *NEJM* 344:1058–66.

Walport, M. 2001. Advances in immunology: Complement (second of two parts). *NEJM* 344:1140–44.

Wen, L., J. P. Atkinson, and P. C. Giclas. 2004. Clinical and laboratory evaluation of complement deficiency. *J Allergy Clin Immunol,* 113:585–93.

Yazdanbakhsh, K., S. Kang, D. Tamasauskas, et al. 2003. Complement receptor 1 inhibitors for prevention of immune-mediated red cell destruction: Potential use in transfusion therapy. *Blood* 101:5046–52.

Zhang Y, Suankratay C, Zhang X, and others. Lysis via the lectin pathway of complement activation: Mini-review and lectin pathway enhancement of endotoxin-initiated hemolysis. *Immunopharmacology.* 1999;42:81-90.

PART II • CLINICAL AND LABORATORY DIAGNOSIS

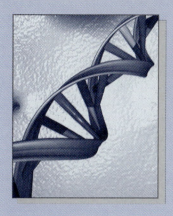

6

Hypersensitivity

■ CHAPTER CHECKLIST

After reading and studying this chapter, the reader will be able to:

1. Define hypersensitivity.

2. Differentiate the types of hypersensitivity reactions.

3. Differentiate between immediate and delayed-type hypersensitivity reactions.

4. Describe the basic mechanisms underlying hypersensitivity, and identify the positive and negative effects of hypersensitivity reactions to an individual.

5. Discuss the immunologic mechanisms underlying each type of hypersensitivity reaction, indicating the involvement of various cell types, antibody (specifying the classes involved), and complement, where applicable.

6. Given a clinical manifestation, associate the clinical condition with the type of hypersensitivity reaction.

7. Differentiate between the hypersensitivity reactions in terms of their onset, immunologic mechanism, and the role of antibody, complement, or T cells.

8. Describe the RIST and RAST procedures and indicate what each test is designed to measure.

9. Explain how laboratory methods are used to detect and evaluate disorders involving Type II or Type III hypersensitivity.

10. Discuss the purpose of skin testing for Type IV hypersensitivity.

@ CASE IN POINT

A clinical laboratory science student developed a rash on her hands one day while performing a procedure in the student laboratory. The rash consisted of small, slightly red papules and itched intensely. The student noticed that the rash appeared about fifteen minutes after she had put on her gloves. She suspected that she might be allergic to the gloves since she had a history of hayfever and food allergies.

CASE IN POINT *(continued)*

ISSUES TO CONSIDER

After reading this patient's case history, consider

- The material(s) in the gloves that likely cause this reaction

- The type of hypersensitivity reaction responsible for the student's rash

- The immunological mechanism responsible for this reaction

- The types of testing that can be done to verify the student's suspicion of allergy

- Treatments to be recommended for this student

IMPORTANT TERMS

Allergen
Allergic rhinitis
Anaphylaxis
Arthus reaction
Atopy
Cell-mediated
Contact dermatitis
Delayed hypersensitivity
Granulomas
Hemolytic disease of the newborn (HDN)
Humoral

Hyperacute graft rejection
Hypersensitivity
Immediate hypersensitivity
Intravascular hemolysis
Radioallergosorbent test (RAST)
Radioimmunosorbent test (RIST)
Serum sickness
Type I hypersensitivity (anaphylactic hypersensitivity)

Type II hypersensitivity (antibody-dependent cytotoxic hypersensitivity)
Type III hypersensitivity (immune complex–mediated hypersensitivity)
Type IV hypersensitivity (cell-mediated or delayed hypersensitivity)

▶ INTRODUCTION

Hypersensitivity reactions are exaggerated immune responses. These reactions involve immune responses that would normally protect the host, but instead cause inflammation and tissue damage because they are prolonged or directed against an antigen that would otherwise cause no harm.

Hypersensitivity reactions involve either humoral or cell-mediated responses, depending on their type. The British immunologists, Gell and Coombs, classified the hypersensitivity reactions into four major groups on the basis of their specific immunological mechanisms. They are as follows:

Type I hypersensitivity (anaphylactic hypersensitivity)

Type II hypersensitivity (antibody-dependent cytotoxic) hypersensitivity

Type III hypersensitivity (immune complex–mediated hypersensitivity)

Type IV hypersensitivity (cell-mediated or delayed hypersensitivity)

A fifth type of hypersensitivity, called stimulatory hypersensitivity, was added later but is most commonly classified under the Type II responses. Even though the hypersensitivities are conveniently classified into separate groups to facilitate their understanding, two or more types of hypersensitivity may occur simultaneously in some conditions.

Types I, II, and III are caused by **humoral** immune mechanisms. Because they occur within a few minutes to several hours after contact with the inducing antigen, they can also be classified as **immediate hypersensitivity** reactions. Type IV hypersensitivity reactions are the result of **T cell-mediated responses,** and occur 24–72 hours after antigen contact; thus, they are also known as **delayed type hypersensitivity.** The major features of the hypersensitivity reactions are summarized in Table 6-1✪. This chapter discusses the different types of hypersensitivity and the clinical manifestations in the affected individual. In addition, this chapter discusses how various cell types, antibody, and comple-

✪ TABLE 6-1

Major Features of the Hypersensitivity Reactions

	Type I	Type II	Type III	Type IV
Synonym	Anaphylactic hypersensitivity	Antibody—dependent cytotoxic hypersensitivity	Complex-mediated hypersensitivity	Cell-mediated, or delayed type hypersensitivity
Antibody involvement	IgE	IgG, IgM	IgG, IgM	None
Complement involvement	No	Yes	Yes	No
Timing	Immediate	Immediate	Immediate	Delayed
Immunologic mechanism	Allergen-specific IgE antibodies sensitize mast cells and basophils; cross-linking of surface IgE's by allergen causes release of histamine and other chemical mediators, causing increased vaso-permeability smooth muscle contractions, and mucous secretion	IgG or IgM antibodies directed against a cell surface antigen promote opsonization and ADCC, or activate complement, resulting in cell lysis; in some cases, the antibodies stimulate cell function rather than destroy the cell	Antigen-antibody complexes activate complement, resulting in anaphylatoxin activity, chemotaxis, and opsonization; neutrophils are attracted to the site of the immune response and release lysosomal enzymes, which cause tissue damage and inflammation	Antigen-specific T cells become activated and release cytokines which cause hematopoiesis and chemotaxis of monocytes and PMN and enhancement of macrophage activity; granulomas form and release lytic enzymes which cause damage to surrounding tissues
Clinical examples	Allergic rhinitis, allergic asthma, atopic dermatitis, urticaria, gastrointestinal reactions, systemic anaphylaxis	Transfusion reactions, hyperacute graft rejection, hemolytic disease of the newborn, drug reactions, autoimmune hemolytic anemia, autoimmune thrombocytopenic purpura, Hashimoto's disease, Goodpasture's syndrome, Grave's disease	Arthus reaction, serum sickness, systemic lupus erythematosus, rheumatoid arthritis, drug reactions, poststreptococcal glomerulonephritis, allergic bronchopulmonary aspergillosis	*Mycobacterium tuberculosis* infection, contact dermatitis, Hypersensitivity pneumonitis, Mantoux skin test

ment, where applicable, are involved in hypersensitivity reactions. Clinical diagnosis, laboratory methods, and treatment used to evaluate each type of hypersensitivity reaction are presented as appropriate.

► TYPES OF HYPERSENSITIVITY

TYPE I HYPERSENSITIVITY: ANAPHYLACTIC HYPERSENSITIVITY

Type I hypersensitivity reactions are commonly referred to as allergies. They are an immediate type of hypersensitivity that occurs very rapidly—usually within 2–30 minutes after exposure to the inducing antigen,

which is called an **allergen.** These reactions are also referred to as **atopy** (from the Greek word, *atopos,* which means "out of place," and individuals who experience these reactions are said to be "atopic.") Type I hypersensitivity has also been called anaphylactic hypersensitivity, to reflect one of its major clinical manifestations.

Immunologic Response Mechanisms

The key immunologic components of the Type I hypersensitivity mechanism are IgE antibodies, mast cells, and basophils. The response begins when the individual is first exposed to an allergen. Common allergens include certain foods (e.g., nuts, seafood, eggs), pollens from plants (e.g., timothy grass, ragweed), drugs (e.g., penicillin, sulfonamides), insect venoms (e.g., bee venom, wasp venom), dust mites, mold spores, and animal hair/dander (e.g., dog, cat). The allergen elicits the production of specific IgE antibodies. These antibodies bind to high-affinity receptors for the Fc portion of the ε heavy chain (FcεRI) on the surface of mast cells and basophils (Figure 6-1■). Mast cells and basophils with surface-bound IgE are said to be sensitized, and can persist in the body for several weeks.

A subsequent exposure of the sensitized individual to the same allergen results in the binding of that allergen to the surface-bound IgE molecules, with cross-linking of adjacent FcεRI receptors. This cross-linkage stimulates a series of biochemical events that results in mast cell activation and degranulation, with release of chemical mediators. Two types of chemical mediators are involved: primary mediators, such as histamine, which were made before the response occurred and stored in the granules, and secondary mediators, such as leukotrienes and prostaglandins, which are synthesized quickly after the mast cells are activated. Histamine binds to specific receptors on various target cells in the body and causes an increase in vascular permeability, smooth muscle contractions in the bronchial and intestinal tracts, and increased mucus secretion by goblet cells. Other primary mediators, Eosinophil Chemotactic Factor and Neutrophil Chemotactic Factor, attract eosinophils and neutrophils to the site of the immune response. The effects of histamine and other primary mediators are sustained following the release of leukotrienes and prostaglandins, which are more potent stimulators of

vascular permeability, smooth muscle contractions, and mucus secretion.

Finally a late phase response results from the release of various cytokines (e.g., Il-4, IL-5, IL-6, and TNF-α) from the mast cells and eosinophils. These cytokines induce leukocyte migration and activation and an inflammatory response that can persist for 1–2 days after allergen exposure.

Clinical Manifestations

The clinical consequences of Type I hypersensitivity range from mild allergic reactions to life-threatening anaphylaxis. Examples of clinical manifestations associated with Type I hypersensitivity include allergic rhinitis, allergic asthma, atopic dermatitis, gastrointestinal reactions, and systemic anaphylaxis.

Allergic Rhinitis.   The most common atopic disorder in the United States affecting 10–15% of individuals in this country is **allergic rhinitis.** It is characterized by a runny nose, nasal itching and congestion, sneezing, and watery eyes, and is elicited by airborne allergens such as pollens, molds, dust mites, and animal dander. It may be seasonal or perennial in nature.

Allergic Asthma.   Allergic asthma is characterized by bronchial hyperresponsiveness, recurrent cough, wheezing, and shortness of breath due to partial airway obstruction. It is caused by many of the same antigens that induce allergic rhinitis, and the two conditions commonly occur together. The incidence of allergic asthma is on the rise, and appears to be associated with environmental factors such as viral infections, exposure to cigarette smoke, and air pollution.

Atopic Dermatitis.   Atopic dermatitis, an itchy red rash with tiny papules, is a skin reaction associated with Type I hypersensitivity. The papules in atopic dermatitis may lead to a thickening and hardening of the skin in chronic lesions. Acute lesions may become superinfected with staphylococci and develop weeping and crusting. Atopic dermatitis may be triggered by a variety of factors, including contact with irritating substances such as soaps and detergents, airborne allergens, microbial agents, or certain foods.

Urticaria.   Urticaria, also known as hives, is also associated with Type I hypersensitivity. This type of dermatitis is widespread, intensely itchy, with well-marked edematous plaques that are white with surrounding erythema, or red with blanching upon pressure. These eruptions have thus been called a "wheal and flare re-

Sensitization of mast cells and basophils
1st exposure to allergen production of allergen-specfic IgE

Y Y Y Y Y Y

IgE binds to mast cells and basophils

Mast cells or basophils
sensitized with IgE

Activation of mast cells and basophils
Subsequent exposure to allergen

Cross-linking of surface
IgEs by allergen

■ FIGURE 6-1 Immunologic mechanism of Type I hypersensitivity.

action." Urticaria may appear as a localized reaction or as one of the manifestations of systemic anaphylaxis. Urticaria are most commonly associated with allergies to foods, drugs, and latex.

Gastrointestinal Reactions.

Gastrointestinal reactions, such as nausea, vomiting, abdominal pain, and diarrhea, may be associated with food allergies or may appear as one of the manifestations of systemic anaphylaxis.

Systemic Anaphylaxis.

A potentially life-threatening allergic reaction, systemic **anaphylaxis** involves multiple organ systems, especially the skin, respiratory tract, gastrointestinal tract, and cardiovascular system. Common causes of anaphylaxis are sensitivities to food, drugs, insect venom, or latex. Observation of this reaction was first documented in the early 1900s by Portier and Richet, after testing their jellyfish toxin vaccine in dogs. A variety of symptoms are seen in anaphylaxis, including hypotension and shock, acute airway obstruction, laryngeal edema, pruritis, urticaria, and abdominal pain that may be accompanied by nausea and diarrhea. The reaction begins within seconds or minutes after exposure to the allergen and may be fatal if the patient is not treated promptly. Treatment involves intramuscular or subcutaneous injection with epinephrine, which rapidly reverses the action of histamine.

Multiple factors appear to be involved in the development of allergic diseases. Family studies have indicated that genetic factors play a role in predisposing individuals to atopy: the risk of a child developing an allergy has been noted to be 13% when neither parent is atopic, 29% when one parent is atopic, and 50% when both parents are atopic. Genetic studies have provided evidence for linkage of atopic genes to multiple chromosomes, and positional cloning studies suggest that there is linkage of asthma and atopy to chromosomes 2q, 5q, 6q, 12q, and 13q.

Analysis of the immune response involved in Type I hypersensitivity indicates that it is shifted so that a Th2 helper T cell response predominates, in which production of the cytokines IL-3, IL-4, IL-5, and IL-10 is favored. IL-4 plays a critical role in Type I hypersensitivity by inducing immunoglobulin class switching to IgE, while IL-3, IL-4, and IL-10 stimulate mast cell production, and IL-3 and IL-5 enhance eosinophil maturation and activation. Knowledge of this immunologic mechanism has stimulated research on the development of therapies to better regulate this response.

Clinical Diagnosis

Diagnosis of Type I hypersensitivity begins with a physical examination and clinical history of the patient. This is followed by allergy testing to confirm reactivity to clinically suspected allergens. The most widely used allergy tests are skin tests, whose basic underlying principle is to determine the degree of sensitization by detection of mast cell-bound allergen-specific IgE following the introduction of specific allergens into the skin. These tests are performed by experienced medical personnel and are most helpful in the identification of allergies associated with rhinitis, asthma, stinging-insect reactions, drug sensitivities, and food reactions.

Three routes of allergen administration have been developed for skin testing: epicutaneous or patch testing (on the skin surface), percutaneous (through the top layers of the skin), and intradermal (into the dermis layer of the skin). The epicutaneous and intradermal routes are not used routinely, since the former is ineffective in promoting allergen access to the mast cells and the latter poses a higher risk of inducing systemic allergic reactions. Percutaneous injection is therefore the method of choice, and can be performed by scratching, or pricking/puncturing the skin with special devices.

Prick testing is the main diagnostic procedure used in the initial screening for allergies. Prick tests are routinely performed by applying a drop of allergen to the skin surface of the inner forearm or the upper back. A device such as a hypodermic needle, plastic pricking device, metal lancet, or bifurcated scarifier is then used to deliver the antigen into the topmost layers of the skin. A panel of allergens is usually used, each applied to separate sites 2–2.5 cm apart. Also included are a negative control site to which the diluent used in the allergen extract is applied, and a positive control site, to which a histamine base is applied. The patient's response at each site is measured and recorded 15–30 minutes after application of the allergen. A positive result at a test site is indicated by the development of a wheal and flare reaction equal to or larger than the response seen with the histamine control; specific recommendations for interpretation of results have been published by professional American and European allergy organizations. The reliability of the test results depends on a number of factors, including the stability of the allergen extract, the type of device used to deliver the allergen, and the depth, force, duration, and angle of allergen administration. Intradermal tests are more sensitive than prick tests because they involve injection of a larger amount of allergen with a syringe and needle, and may be performed when prick testing is not sensitive enough to detect a reaction.

Skin tests are usually the method of choice for initial testing for allergies because they are relatively inexpensive, convenient to perform, provide immediate results, and have a higher sensitivity than in vitro tests. However, they have some limitations. First, they cannot be performed on sites in which there is active dermatitis. Second, because antihistamines and other allergy medications can inhibit skin test responses, they should be discontinued prior to testing; however, some patients may be unable to do so. A third disadvantage of skin tests is their potential to induce large local reactions or, rarely, severe systemic allergic reactions (more commonly seen with intradermal tests).

Laboratory Diagnosis

For those allergic patients who cannot discontinue medications prior to testing, who have severe eczema, or nearly fatal reactions to an allergen, in vitro IgE tests may be performed. There are two major types of IgE tests: those that quantitate total serum IgE and those that measure allergen-specific IgE levels. The first test developed to measure total serum IgE was the **radioimmunosorbent test (RIST)** (Figure 6-2a■). This is a radioimmunoassay capable of detecting nanogram (ng) levels of total IgE. In this method, patient serum is incubated with a solid phase (agarose beads or paper disks) coated with rabbit-anti-IgE antibodies. Excess serum is removed in a washing step, and ^{125}I-labeled anti-IgE conjugate is added. Excess conjugate is removed by washing, and the amount of radioactivity bound to the solid phase is measured by a gamma counter. The total level of IgE is proportional to the amount of radioactivity. IgE values are reported in international units per milliliter of serum (IU/mL), where one IU is equal to 2.4 ng/mL. Although total IgE levels may indicate atopy, they do not always correlate with allergic disease and cannot aid in the identification of the responsible allergens.

Tests for allergen-specific IgE have more clinical value. The immunoassay for specific IgE antibodies is called the **radioallergosorbent test (RAST).** The first RAST test developed used a radioactive label. The basic principle of this test involves incubating patient serum with a solid phase precoated with a specific allergen (Figure 6-2b). After a washing step, ^{125}I-labeled anti-IgE conjugate is added. Following a second incubation period and wash, the amount of bound radioactivity is measured. The level of radioactivity is proportional to the concentration of allergen-specific IgE in the patient sample. Patient serum can be tested for reactivity to a variety of allergens with this method.

The RAST assays are useful in situations in which skin testing cannot be performed (as discussed), in detecting food allergies in infants, and in monitoring IgE levels after therapy or antigen avoidance. In general, however, they have been found to be more expensive and less sensitive than skin tests. In recent years, many improvements to the IgE immunoassays have been made, including the use of enzyme-labeled conjugates instead of radio-labeled reagents, the use of monoclonal antibody reagents, and the development of solid phases which are better able to bind allergens. With these improvements, RAST tests are showing comparable sensitivity to skin tests for some allergens.

The case of the clinical laboratory science/medical technology student presented earlier in this chapter is a likely manifestation of Type I hypersensitivity to latex in the gloves she was wearing. This type of hypersensitivity is indicated by the rapid nature of the response (15 minutes after donning the gloves) and the

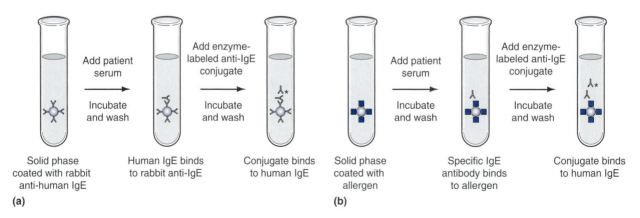

■ FIGURE 6-2 (a) Principle of radioimmunosorbent assay (RIST). (b) Principle of radioallergosorbent assay (RAST).

nature of the rash (urticaria, or intensely itchy, small red papules). Allergy to latex, a natural material derived from the *Hevea brasiliensis* rubber tree, has become an important problem among health care professionals, as the use of gloves increased to provide necessary barrier protection against bloodborne pathogens such as HIV and hepatitis B. Health care professionals with latex allergy are now being provided with gloves made of nonlatex materials in order to prevent the development of more serious consequences of Type I hypersensitivity (e.g., asthma, systemic anaphylaxis) upon repeated exposures. Latex allergies are commonly diagnosed by obtaining a detailed medical history of the individual. These allergies can be confirmed by a variety of diagnostic tests, including skin tests (patch, prick, or intradermal), latex-specific RAST, or a latex challenge test involving inhalation of airborne latex particles.

Treatment

Treatment for allergies involves avoidance of the allergen whenever possible, administration of drugs that block various steps in the biochemical mechanism of Type I hypersensitivity, and immunotherapy to redirect the immune response away from allergy. Avoiding or reducing contact with the offending allergens may be accomplished in certain situations by removing responsible foods from the diet, giving away household pets, and implementing dust-control procedures, for example. When it is not possible to avoid contact with the allergen, drug therapy is usually initiated. One group of drugs that have been useful, especially in the treatment of allergic rhinitis, are the antihistamines, which block the binding of histamine to receptors on target cells. Several other drugs interfere with biochemical steps in mast cell activation and degranulation. Cromolyn sodium, for example, prevents calcium influx into mast cells. Theophylline, which may be given to asthma patients to prevent wheezing, blocks degranulation by inhibiting the breakdown of cAMP (cyclic adenosine monophosphate). Epinephrine injections, as mentioned earlier, are administered to persons experiencing systemic anaphylaxis, and act by rapidly increasing cAMP levels, which block mast cell degranulation and relax bronchial smooth muscles. Corticosteroid drugs reduce inflammation by blocking the synthesis of histamine and other chemical mediators and can be administered orally or topically, in the case of skin reactions.

When drug therapies do not sufficiently control symptoms, allergen immunotherapy may be indicated. Allergen immunotherapy, or desensitization, involves administering gradually increasing doses of allergens to the allergic patient with the goal of alleviating symptoms by naturally altering the course of disease. Although the mechanisms by which allergen immunotherapy works are not completely understood, it is believed to induce tolerance by a number of ways, most notably, by shifting the immune response from a predominantly Th2 response to a Th1 response, with a concomitant decrease in IL-4 and IgE production. This form of therapy has been effective in treating allergic rhinitis, allergic asthma, and allergic reactions to insect venoms. While immunotherapy is typically administered by parenteral injection, other forms of administration are being investigated, such as oral, sublingual swallow, and nasal administration.

TYPE II HYPERSENSITIVITY: ANTIBODY-DEPENDENT CYTOTOXIC HYPERSENSITIVITY

Immunologic Response Mechanisms

Type II hypersensitivity, also known as antibody-dependent cytotoxic hypersensitivity, is an immediate form of hypersensitivity which is caused by IgG and IgM antibodies directed against cell surface or tissue antigens. These antibodies can promote damage to the target cells containing these antigens by a variety of mechanisms in the absence or presence of complement (Figure 6-3■):

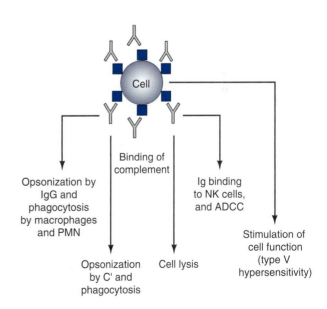

■ FIGURE 6-3 Immunologic mechanism of Type II hypersensitivity.

- Activation and completion of the classical pathway of complement, resulting in lysis of the target cells

- Opsonization of the target cells, either through the binding of antibody to Fc receptors, or the binding of complement fragments to C3b receptors on the surface of phagocytic cells, with subsequent phagocytosis of the target cells

- Induction of antibody-dependent cell-mediated cytotoxicity (ADCC), a mechanism in which NK (natural killer) cells bind to the Fc portion of the antibody coating the target cells, and release enzymes that destroy the cells

In some cases, binding of the antibody to the target cells results in stimulation of the cells' function instead of destruction of the cells. Some sources classify these situations under a separate category, called type V hypersensitivity or stimulatory hypersensitivity.

Clinical Manifestations

The clinical manifestations, treatment, and laboratory detection of Type II hypersensitivity vary tremendously, and depend on the specific antigen/target cell toward which the antibody is directed. The following section describes the clinical manifestations of Type II hypersensitivity reactions.

Transfusion Reactions.   Transfusion with donor blood that is incompatible for ABO or other blood group antigens leads to destruction of red blood cells. Antibodies against red blood cell antigens may be present naturally in the recipient (such as antibodies to the A or B antigens of the ABO system), depending on his/her blood type, or may be induced by prior exposure to foreign erythrocytes. These antibodies can produce massive **intravascular hemolysis** of the transfused erythrocytes or destruction of the erythrocytes at extravascular sites through opsonization and phagocytosis by macrophages. Treatment of patients involves prompt termination of the transfusion. Transfusion reactions can be prevented by performing compatibility (cross-match) tests to ensure that the recipient does not contain antibodies to the donor's major blood group antigens prior to performing the transfusion.

Hyperacute Graft Rejection.   Another form of type II hypersensitivity reaction is **hyperacute graft rejection.** In this reaction rapid destruction of a graft (e.g., a kidney transplant) occurs if the recipient has preformed antibodies against major histocompatibility (MHC) antigens on the graft tissue due to prior exposure to those antigens. These reactions can be prevented by performing cross-match tests to detect the antibodies in the recipient prior to selection of the organ donor.

Hemolytic Disease of the Newborn (HDN). **Hemolytic disease of the newborn (HDN)** is a disease that develops in infants whose mothers have produced antibodies to a fetal blood group antigen. The antigen most commonly implicated in HDN is the Rhesus D (RhD) antigen. An Rh-negative mother can become sensitized when she delivers her first Rh-positive child, as large numbers of fetal red blood cells enter her circulation at that time. In response to the exposure, the mother produces IgG antibodies to the D antigen and memory B cells specific for that antigen. The risk of HDN arises during a subsequent pregnancy of the mother with an Rh-positive infant, when her antibodies can cross the placenta and cause damage to the fetus's red blood cells. A mild to severe, potentially fatal anemia can develop in the fetus. In addition, hemoglobin released from the red blood cells is converted to bilirubin which can accumulate in the brain and cause brain damage. Sensitization of the mother can be detected by testing her serum for antibodies to the Rh antigen during her pregnancy. Sensitization can be prevented by administering RhoGAM, a solution of preformed anti-Rh antibodies, to the mother within 48 hours after her first delivery. These antibodies are thought to bind to the fetal red blood cells, clear them from the maternal circulation, and thus inhibit production of the antibody by the mother.

Drug-Induced Hypersensitivity.   Certain drugs can induce Type II hypersensitivity reactions through their ability to nonspecifically bind to proteins on red blood cells or platelets. Destruction of these red blood cells or platelets can occur if the patient produces antibodies to the drug, which subsequently bind to the drug molecules attached to the cell surface. Hemolytic anemia or thrombocytopenic purpura result. Drugs that can induce these reactions include certain antibiotics (e.g., penicillin, cephalosporin, and streptomycin), quinidine (a drug used to treat cardiac arrhythmia, and methyldopa (a drug used to lower blood pressure). Clinical symptoms improve shortly after treatment with the drug is stopped.

Autoimmune Diseases.   Type II hypersensitivity is a major pathologic mechanism in a variety of autoimmune diseases including autoimmune hemolytic anemia, autoimmune thrombocytopenic purpura, Hashimoto's disease, Goodpasture's syndrome, and Graves' disease. Patients with autoimmune hemolytic anemia spontaneously produce antibodies to their own erythrocytes. These "auto" antibodies may be either warm-reacting (IgG) or cold-reacting (IgM), and can be identified by performing an indirect antiglobulin test. In autoimmune thrombocytopenic pupura, patients spontaneously produce antibodies to their own platelets. The antibody-coated platelets are destroyed primarily by phagocytic cells in the spleen; treatment thus involves surgical removal of the spleen.

Hashimoto's disease is an autoimmune disease of the thyroid gland, a gland in the neck that plays a central role in regulating metabolism. In this disease, damage to the thyroid gland is caused by cell-mediated immune mechanisms and by autoantibodies produced against thyroid proteins, most notably thyroglobulin (a glycoprotein involved in the synthesis and storage of thyroid hormones) and thyroid peroxidase (an enzyme that mediates oxidation of iodine and its incorporation into thyroglobulin). These antibodies are thought to participate in the type II hypersensitivity reaction, and can be detected in the sera of patients with the disease. Damage to the thyroid results in symptoms of hypothyroidism, such as dry skin, intolerance to cold temperatures, fatigue, and weight gain. Patients are treated with thyroid hormones.

Patients with Goodpasture's syndrome produce antibodies against specific basement membrane antigens. These antibodies bind to basement membranes in the kidneys and lungs. Damage to these organs results in progressive renal damage and pulmonary hemorrhage. Early diagnosis is essential in preventing permanent kidney damage and death. Immunologic tests key to the diagnosis are detection of circulating antiglomerular basement membrane (anti-GBM) antibody and detection of IgG and C3b in the basement membranes of renal biopsies from patients with the syndrome. Treatment involves administration of corticosteroids and other drugs to suppress the immune response, plasmapheresis to remove the anti-GBM antibodies from the blood, and kidney dialysis as needed.

Graves' disease is an autoimmune disease in which the thyroid gland is stimulated to increase its function. Patients with this disease produce antibodies against the thyroid receptor for the pituitary hormone, thyroid stimulating hormone (TSH, or thyrotropin), which are thought to participate in a mechanism of stimulatory hypersensitivity. Binding of these antibodies to the TSH receptor mimics the action of TSH, resulting in overstimulation of the thyroid gland and production of a condition known as hyperthyroidism. Symptoms of increased metabolism result, such as sweating, nervousness, weight loss, intolerance to

heat, and heart palpitations. Other clinical manifestations include an enlarged thyroid gland, or goiter, and exophthalmos, or a bulging of the eyes to give a staring expression. Laboratory detection involves measurement of TSH and T4 serum hormone levels.

TYPE III HYPERSENSITIVITY: IMMUNE COMPLEX-MEDIATED HYPERSENSITIVITY

Type III hypersensitivity is another form of immediate hypersensitivity which occurs a few hours after antigen exposure. It is also known as immune complex-mediated hypersensitivity because the underlying pathology involves immune complexes containing IgG or IgM antibodies and complement. Normally, immune complexes are effectively cleared by the mononuclear phagocyte system. However, in chronic conditions such as certain autoimmune diseases and persistent infections, the complexes can persist, deposit in the tissues, and cause damage.

Immune Response Mechanism

Type III hypersensitivity begins with the formation of antibodies to the inducing antigen, such as a foreign protein, agent of infectious disease, or self-antigen (Figure 6-4■). Large numbers of antigen-antibody complexes form; under conditions of antigen excess, these complexes are small and cannot be effectively cleared from the body. The complexes may remain at a localized site in the body, or may circulate in the blood, then deposit in blood vessel walls and various tissues, particularly the skin, joints, kidneys, and brain. These

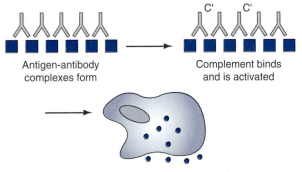

Antigen-antibody complexes form

Complement binds and is activated

Complement proteins attract macrophages and PMN, which degranulate, releasing proteolytic enzymes that destroy surrounding tissues and cause inflammation

■ FIGURE 6-4 Immunologic mechanism of Type III hypersensitivity.

immune complexes bind complement and activate the complement cascade, resulting in the production of various complement proteins with important biologic activities. C3a and C5a are anaphylatoxins that stimulate the release of histamine from mast cells, resulting in increased vascular permeability. Vascular permeability is also increased through the action of vasoactive amines released from platelets, following their interaction with the immune complexes. The complement fragments C3a, C5a, and C5b67 are chemotaxins that attract large numbers of neutrophils to the sites of immune complex deposition, and C3b is an opsonin that promotes phagocytosis. As the neutrophils attempt to ingest the immune complexes, they release their lysosomal enzymes, which damage the surrounding tissues and cause inflammation. The resulting inflammatory response can either be localized or generalized, depending on the sites of immune complex deposition.

Clinical Manifestations

Arthus Reaction.   The classic example of a localized Type III hypersensitivity response is the **Arthus reaction.** The Arthus reaction is a localized skin reaction that was discovered by Nicholas Maurice Arthus in the early 1900s. Arthus demonstrated this reaction by performing intradermal or subcutaneous injections of antigen into rabbits that had been previously immunized with the antigen and produced high levels of specific circulating antibody. Three to eight hours after the skin injection, an area of redness and edema developed, which later progressed to a necrotic, hemorrhagic lesion. These reactions are rare in humans, but may develop after an insect bite or sting or after injection with certain drugs or vaccines.

Serum Sickness.   **Serum sickness,** the classic example of generalized Type III hypersensitivity, is caused by exposure of a host to proteins from animal serum. The reaction was first recognized before the discovery of antibiotics, when horse antitoxins were used in passive immunization to treat various infections such as diphtheria and tetanus. In modern times, these antisera have been used less often. Serum sickness reactions also develop in response to antilymphocyte or antithymocyte serum used in immunosuppressive therapy and to mouse monoclonal antibodies used in cancer immunotherapy. In serum sickness, immune complexes are formed between the foreign serum proteins and antibodies produced to them, and deposit in the blood vessel walls and tissues. An inflammatory response develops days to weeks after antigen exposure, and produces a number of symptoms, including fever,

lymphadenopathy, skin rashes, painful joints, nausea/vomiting, and, possibly, glomerulonephritis. Serum sickness is usually a self-limiting condition, with recovery occurring in 7–30 days.

Other Manifestations.   Other diseases that are characterized by the formation of immune complexes and generalized Type III hypersensitivity reactions include certain autoimmune diseases (e.g., systemic lupus erythematosus, rheumatoid arthritis), drug reactions (e.g., allergies to penicillin and sulfonamides), infectious diseases (e.g., poststreptococcal glomerulonephritis, viral hepatitis, mononucleosis, malaria), and allergic bronchopulmonary aspergillosis. Since these conditions are diverse in nature, methods of laboratory diagnosis and treatment vary widely.

TYPE IV HYPERSENSITIVITY: CELL-MEDIATED OR DELAYED HYPERSENSITIVITY

Type IV hypersensitivity is also known as cell-mediated hypersensitivity or delayed-type hypersensitivity. This type of hypersensitivity, in contrast to the others, involves a cell-mediated immune response. This reaction typically takes 24 hours to appear after contact of sensitized T lymphocytes with antigen, and peaks at 48–72 hours.

Immune Response Mechanism

The immunologic mechanism of Type IV hypersensitivity consists of two phases: a sensitization phase, and an effector phase (Figure 6-5■). The sensitization phase occurs within 1–2 weeks after initial contact with the antigen. During this phase, the antigen is processed by antigen presenting cells (APCs), most notably, macrophages and Langerhan's cells, and presented to antigen-specific T helper cells (T_H) in the context of an MHC Class II molecule. These antigen-sensitized T_H become activated and proliferate to form a clone of identical T_H, some of which become memory cells. The activated T_H are thought to be mainly of the T_H1 subset of T helper cells and are often referred to as delayed-type hypersensitivity T cells (T_{DTH}) to reflect their function in Type IV hypersensitivity.

The effector phase of the response begins after a second or subsequent exposure to the antigen, which stimulates the memory T_{DTH} to produce a variety of cytokines and chemokines. These include interleukin 3 (IL-3) and granulocyte-monocyte colony stimulating factor (GM-CSF), which induce hematopoiesis of

Sensitization Phase

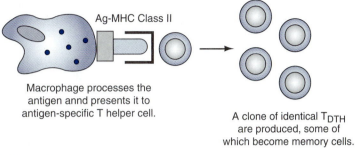

Macrophage processes the antigen annd presents it to antigen-specific T helper cell.

A clone of identical T_{DTH} are produced, some of which become memory cells.

Effector Phase

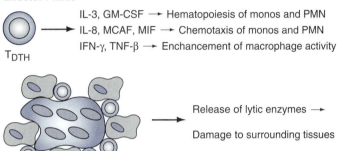

T_{DTH}

IL-3, GM-CSF ⟶ Hematopoiesis of monos and PMN
IL-8, MCAF, MIF ⟶ Chemotaxis of monos and PMN
IFN-γ, TNF-β ⟶ Enchancement of macrophage activity

Release of lytic enzymes ⟶

Damage to surrounding tissues

Granuloma formation

■ **FIGURE 6-5** Immunologic mechanism of Type IV hypersensitivity.

monocytes and neutrophils; interleukin 8 (IL-8), monocyte chemotactic and activating factor (MCAF), and migration inhibition factor (MIF), which attract monocytes and polymorphonuclear neutrophil cells (PMNs) to the site of the immune response; and interferon gamma (IFN-γ) and tumor necrosis factor beta (TNF-β), which enhance macrophage activity. While both monocytes and PMNs are attracted to the site of the immune response, the PMNs migrate out of the area quickly. Meanwhile, monocytes develop into activated tissue macrophages to serve as the primary effector cells of the inflammatory response that follows. These macrophages have an increased ability to phagocytize and kill microorganisms and are therefore an important defense against intracellular pathogens. However, in situations where the antigen is not easily cleared, the prolonged delayed type hypersensitivity response can lead to intense inflammation and tissue damage. The activated macrophages adhere closely to each other and may fuse to form multinucleated giant cells, which associate with T_{DTH} and modified macrophages to form large clusters of cells called **granulomas.** Granulomas form in an attempt to wall off sites of persistent infection from the rest of the body,

but they can displace normal tissue, and they can release high concentrations of lytic enzymes, which damage surrounding tissues and lead to extensive tissue necrosis.

Clinical Manifestations
Clinical conditions of Type IV hypersensitivity include chronic infections with intracellular pathogens, contact dermatitis, and hypersensitivity pneumonitis.

Chronic Infections Caused by Intracellular Pathogens. Type IV hypersensitivity reactions can be induced by a variety of intracellular pathogens. *Mycobacterium tuberculosis, Mycobacterium leprae, Pneumocystis jeroveci, Candida albicans, Leishmania* species, herpes simplex virus and measles virus are typical examples. Immune reactions develop as a defensive response to the pathogen, but often culminate in tissue damage due to persistence of the response. In tuberculosis, for example, granulomatous lesions called tubercles form around the pathogenic mycobacteria in the lungs in attempt to prevent spread of the organism throughout the body. Lytic enzymes released from macrophages in the tubercles, however, can damage the surrounding lung tissue and lead to the formation of pulmonary cavities.

Contact Dermatitis. **Contact dermatitis** is an eczematous skin reaction caused by delayed type hypersensitivity which has been provoked by contact with a variety of environmental chemicals or metals, including detergents and soaps, hair dyes, cosmetics, certain plants such as poison ivy and poison oak, and nickel salts in jewelry. These materials contain allergens that are thought to act as haptens by binding to carrier proteins in the skin and activating specific memory T cells to mediate a delayed type response. The resulting skin reaction appears from six hours to several days after contact with the allergen and is characterized by redness, swelling, and blistering. The lesions may be itchy or painful, depending on their severity. Contact dermatitis can be treated with systemic or topical corticosteroids, and antibiotics may be given if the lesions contain secondary bacterial infections.

Hypersensitivity Pneumonitis. Hypersensitivity or extrinsic allergic alveolitis is an allergic disease of the lungs caused by inhalation of allergens that sensitize T cells and provoke a delayed type hypersensitivity reaction. Inflammation of the lung alveoli and interstitial spaces result, producing shortness of breath, cough, malaise, fever, and chest pain. The onset of these symptoms may be abrupt or gradual. A number of antigens have been found to induce hypersensitivity pneumonitis, including bacterial and fungal spores, animal and plant proteins, and industrial chemicals. Most cases of hypersensitivity pneumonitis have been occupational in nature, and have been given specific names, such as farmer's lung, which is associated with exposure to contaminated hay or grains, and pigeon fancier's disease, which is associated with exposure to proteins in bird droppings. Early diagnosis of hypersensitivity pneumonitis is important if the prognosis is to be favorable. Treatment involves avoidance of fur-ther exposure to the responsible allergen and administration of corticosteroid drugs.

Clinical Diagnosis

Delayed type hypersensitivity reactions can be detected by performing skin tests that measure the memory response of T_{DTH} previously sensitized with specific antigen. In these tests, antigen can be applied to the skin either by intradermal injection or by patch testing, where suspected allergens are applied to separate sites on the skin surface. Patch testing has been used mainly in the detection of allergic contact dermatitis. Intradermal injections are used to detect exposure to intracellular pathogens such as *Mycobacterium tuberculosis,* or to detect immunodeficiency by checking for the ability to mount cell-mediated immune responses to commonly encountered antigens such as *Candida albicans* extracts and streptococcal enzymes. The skin is examined for the development of redness and a firm, hard swelling called induration 48–72 hours after antigen application.

A commonly performed skin test is the Mantoux test which detects exposure to *Mycobacterium tuberculosis.* It is commonly used to screen health care workers and other high-risk individuals. In this test, 0.1 ml of PPD, a purified protein derivative from cultures of the bacterium, is injected intradermally into the inner surface of the forearm with a disposable tuberculin syringe. A positive skin test is indicated by the presence of erythema and induration at the injection site 48–72 hours later. The diameter of induration is measured and compared with cut-offs established for the appropriate category of individuals, depending on age, HIV status, and other factors. A positive test result indicates exposure to *Mycobacterium tuberculosis,* but cannot differentiate between exposure and active tuberculosis.

Laboratory isolation and identification of *M. tuberculosis* from clinical samples confirm the presence of active disease. Similarly, in cases where a microbial etiology is suspected (i.e, *P. jeroveci, C. albicans*), laboratory diagnosis may include recovery of the agent in culture or microscopy.

SUMMARY

Hypersensitivity reactions are enhanced immune responses triggered by an antigen. Depending on the type of reaction, the immune response may involve either humoral or cell-mediated responses. The four major types of hypersensitivity, based on their immunological mechanisms, include Type I or anaphylactic, Type II or antibody-dependent cytotoxic, Type III or immune-complex mediated, and Type IV, cell mediated or delayed hypersensitivity.

Humoral immune mechanisms are involved in Types I, II, and III, whereas cell-mediated response is associated with Type IV hypersensitivity reactions. Although there are certain laboratory tests available to detect and evaluate these reactions, most are diagnosed clinically. Treatment modalities vary depending on the clinical manifestations presented by the patient.

POINTS TO REMEMBER

▶ Immunologic mechanisms underlying each type of hypersensitivity reaction

▶ Clinical manifestations and symptoms associated with each type of reaction

▶ The role of antibody, complement, and T cells

▶ The laboratory tests and other measures used to detect and evaluate hypersensitivity reactions

LEARNING ASSESSMENT QUESTIONS

1. A young boy experiences a runny nose and itchy eyes within 15 minutes of playing with his neighbor's cat. His case would be an example of what type of hypersensitivity reaction?
   a. Type I
   b. Type II
   c. Type III
   d. Type IV

2. The Arthus reaction is an example of what type of hypersensitivity?
   a. Type I
   b. Type II
   c. Type III
   d. Type IV

3. Suppose a health care worker who underwent the Mantoux skin test two days earlier developed redness and swelling at the PPD injection site. This reaction indicates that the health care worker:
   a. has active tuberculosis.
   b. has been exposed to *Mycobacterium tuberculosis* and has developed antibodies against the organism.
   c. has been exposed to *Mycobacterium tuberculosis* and has developed a cell-mediated immune response against the organism.
   d. is HIV-positive.

4. Suppose a woman develops hives a few minutes after eating a cookie, which, unknown to her, contains trace amounts of peanuts. Her reaction is mediated by:
   a. antigen-specific T cells and cytokines.
   b. mast cells and basophils sensitized with IgE antibodies.
   c. complexes of IgG antibodies and peanut proteins.
   d. lysis of antigen-sensitized skin cells by antibodies and complement.

5. Complement activation plays a key role in the pathology of which type(s) of hypersensitivity?
   a. Type I only
   b. Type III only
   c. Types II and III
   d. Types I, II, III, and IV

6. The RAST test measures:
   a. skin reactions to allergens.
   b. total serum concentration of IgE.
   c. levels of antigen-specific IgG.
   d. levels of allergen-specific IgE.

7. An infant born to an Rh-negative mother develops hemolytic disease of the newborn. This condition is due to which type of hypersensitivity?
   a. Type I
   b. Type II
   c. Type III
   d. Type IV

8. T cell–mediated hypersensitivity responses typically take how long after exposure to the inducing antigen to develop?
   a. 10–15 minutes
   b. 30–60 minutes
   c. 8–10 hours
   d. 1–3 days

9. The preferred method of screening for allergies mediated by Type I hypersensitivity is:
   a. prick skin testing.
   b. skin testing by intradermal injection.
   c. the RIST test.
   d. the RAST test.

10. In serum sickness, exposure to foreign proteins in animal serum produces inflammation by:
    a. inducing the production of IgE antibodies.
    b. stimulating the production of granulomas.
    c. phagocytosis of cells in the body that bind the proteins.
    d. inducing the production of immune complexes that activate complement.

REFERENCES

Centers for Disease Control and Prevention. Core Curriculum on Tuberculosis. Chapter 4- Testing for TB disease and infection. http://www.cdc.gov/nchstp/tb/pubs/corecurr/Chapter_4_Skin _Testing.htm. Accessed February 15, 2002.

Feijen, M., J. Gerritsen, and D. S. Postma. 2000. Genetics of allergic disease. *Br Med Bull* 56:894–907.

Goldsby, R. A., T. S. Kindt, and B. A. Osborne, J. Kuby. 2003. *Kuby Immunology,* 5th ed. New York, NY: W. H. Freeman and Co., pp. 361–388, 460–466.

Hamilton, R. G. and A. Kagey-Sobotka. 2000. In vitro diagnostic tests of IgE-mediated diseases. *Clin Allergy and Immunol* 15:89–110.

Hammett-Stabler, C. 1998. Update on thyroid testing. *ADVANCE for Medical Laboratory Professionals* 11–16.

Huss, K. and R. W. Huss. 2000. Genetics of asthma and allergies. *Nursing Clinics of North America* 35:695–705.

Kay, A. B. 2001. Allergy and allergic diseases: First of two parts. *N Eng J Med* 344:30–37.

Kay, A. B. 2001. Allergy and allergic diseases: Second of two parts. *N Eng J Med* 344:109–13.

Kay, A. B. 2000. Overview of "Allergy and Allergic Diseases: With a View to the Future." *Br Med Bull* 56:843–64.

Larson, L. E. 1998. Latex allergy: How a protective material threatens some of its users. *Lab Medicine* 29:278–85.

Leicht, S. and M. Hanggi. 2001. Atopic dermatitis. *Postgraduate Medicine* 109:119–27.

Nimmagadda, S. R. and R. Evans. 1999. Allergy: Etiology and epidemiology. *Pediatrics in Review* 20:111–15.

Patel, A. M., J. H. Ryu, and C. E. Reed. 2001. Hypersensitivity pneumonitis: Current concepts and future questions. *J Allergy Clin Immunol,* 108:661–70.

Roitt, I. 1997. *Roitt's Essential Immunology,* 9th ed. London, England: Blackwell Science Ltd., pp. 328–52.

Skoner, D. P. 2001. Allergic rhinitis: Definition, epidemiology, pathophysiology, detection, and diagnosis. *J Allergy Clin Immunol* 108:S2–8.

Terr, A. I. 2001. Anaphylaxis and urticaria. In T. G. Parslow, D. P. Stites, A. I. Terr, and J. B. Imboden, eds. *Medical Immunology.* 10th ed. New York, NY: Lange Medical Books/McGraw-Hill, 370–379.

Terr, A. I. 2001. The atopic diseases. In T. G. Parslow, D. P. Stites, A. I. Terr, and J. B. Imboden, eds. *Medical Immunology,* 10th ed. New York, NY: Lange Medical Books/McGraw-Hill, 349–369.

Terr, A. I. 2001. Cell-mediated hypersensitivity diseases. In T.G. Parslow, D.P. Stites, A.I. Terr, J.B. Imboden, eds. *Medical Immunology.* 10th ed. New York, NY: Lange Medical Books/McGraw-Hill, 386–393.

Terr, A. I. 2001. Immune complex allergic diseases. In T. G. Parslow, D. P. Stites, A. I. Terr, J. B. Imboden, eds. *Medical Immunology.* 10th ed. New York, NY: Lange Medical Books/McGraw-Hill, 380–385.

Theodoropoulos, D. S. and R. F. Lockey. 2000. Allergen immunotherapy: Guidelines, update, and recommendations of the World Health Organization. *Allergy and Asthma Proc* 21:159–66.

Turkeltaub, P. C. 2000. Percutaneous and intracutaneous diagnostic tests of IgE-mediated diseases (immediate hypersensitivity). *Clin Allergy and Immunol* 15:53–87.

Volcheck, G. W. 2001. Which diagnostic tests for common allergies? *Postgrad Med* 109:71–85.

Watts, P. H. and A. D. Cornetto. 1999. Latex sensitivity: Could it affect you? *Advance/Laboratory* 63–66.

Yunginger, J. W., S. Ahlstedt, P. A. Peyton, et al. 2000. Quantitative IgE antibody assays in allergic diseases. *J Allergy Clin Immunol* 105:1077–84.

7

Immunologic Detection of Infectious Diseases

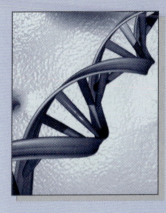

■ CHAPTER CHECKLIST

After reading and studying this chapter, the reader should be able to:

1. Describe the principles of the following antigen detection methods:
   • precipitin tests
   • particle agglutination
   • immunofluorescent assays
   • enzyme immunoassays
2. Differentiate each of the following immunoassay methods:
   • direct and indirect EIA
   • direct and indirect FA
   • optical immunoassay
3. Describe the current clinical applications of direct antigen detection methods in each of the following infectious diseases:
   • respiratory tract infections
   • meningitis and sepsis
   • gastrointestinal tract infections
   • sexually transmitted diseases
   • blood-borne and body fluid-borne diseases

℮ CASE IN POINT

Sandy, an incoming freshman at a local college, did not understand why her classes were on a "medical hold." Her immunizations were up to date, and she had been to her physician and laboratory for all of the necessary tests. She was told that she didn't have an adequate rubella titer. Sandy was still confused—she knew that she had never had the disease, but her immunization records showed that she had been immunized against rubella.

⊚ CASE IN POINT *(continued)*

ISSUES TO CONSIDER

After reading this patient's case history, consider

⊚ Reasons that might account for Sandy's low rubella titer

⊚ Reasons why it is considered important for young adults to have been adequately immunized against rubella

⊚ Tests that might have been used to determine the titer to rubella

⊚ The expected results if Sandy had actually had the disease rather than being vaccinated

IMPORTANT TERMS

Accuracy
Agglutination reaction
Analyte
Analytic sensitivity
Analytic specificity
Antigen-antibody complex
Antigen binding site
Antigenic determinant
Clinical accuracy
Clinical sensitivity
Clinical specificity
Coagglutination
Cross-reacting antigens

Electrochemiluminescence
Epitope
False-negative reaction
False-positive reaction
Gold standard
Home-brew test
Immunodiffusion
Immunofluorescence (IFA)
Liposomes
Microbial antigen
Monoclonal antibody
Negative predictive value
Polyclonal antibody

Positive predictive value
Precipitin reaction
Precision
Predictive value
Prevalence
Sensitivity
Specificity
Technical accuracy
Titer
Validation
Verification

▶ INTRODUCTION

In the early 1900s, investigators determined that body fluids such as blood, urine, and cerebrospinal fluid (CSF) of patients with typhoid fever, pneumococcal pneumonia, and meningococcal meningitis contained soluble substances (precipitins) that would precipitate when mixed with antiserum from animals inoculated with the microorganisms responsible for the disease. These events marked the beginnings of **microbial antigen** detection.

Around 1950, direct smear visualization of whole organisms in specimens became practical when fluorescent-labeled antibody tests were developed. By the mid 1970s, rapid diagnosis of infectious diseases by direct antigen detection had caught the interest of clinicians for a number of very practical reasons. First, access to testing dramatically increased with the commercial availability of highly specific diagnostic test kits approved by the Food and Drug Administration (FDA) for detection of disease. Concurrently, infectious disease therapies became increasingly available for therapeutic intervention of bacterial infections. By the 1990s, clinicians had the ability to detect, and, in some cases, treat viral respiratory infections.

The increase of commercially available diagnostic test kits was directly related to the ability to produce large quantities of highly specific antibodies, or **monoclonal antibodies**, to detect the etiological agent. The development of cell hybridoma technology led to monoclonal antibody production (Figure 7-1■). A hybridoma results from fusing a single plasma B cell that produces an antibody of interest with a mouse myeloma cell. The transformed myeloma cells are able to grow and divide in culture indefinitely. The progeny of these cells, if appropriately selected, can be grown in culture or in animals and can secrete large amounts of the target antibody. Because it originates from a single B cell or clone and is thus chemically homogeneous, the antibodies produced by these cells are referred to as monoclonal. Monoclonal antibodies are highly specific for a single antigenic determinant and less likely to cross-react with chemically related antigens than polyclonal antibodies. **Polyclonal antibodies** recognize multiple antigenic determinants because they are usually produced by immunizing animals with an antigen of interest and then isolating and purifying the antibody from the animal's serum. These antibodies are generally heterogeneous in nature because of the vari-

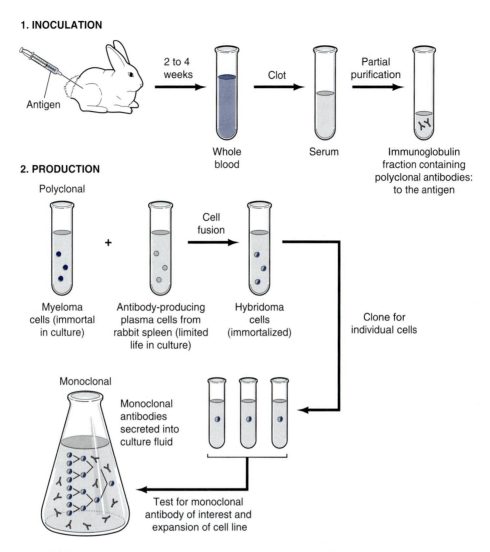

1. INOCULATION

Antigen

2 to 4 weeks

Whole blood

Clot

Serum

Partial purification

Immunoglobulin fraction containing polyclonal antibodies: to the antigen

2. PRODUCTION

Polyclonal

Myeloma cells (immortal in culture)

+

Antibody-producing plasma cells from rabbit spleen (limited life in culture)

Cell fusion

Hybridoma cells (immortalized)

Clone for individual cells

Monoclonal

Monoclonal antibodies secreted into culture fluid

Test for monoclonal antibody of interest and expansion of cell line

■ **FIGURE 7-1** Monoclonal and polyclonal antibody preparation.

ability associated with the immune response. Therefore, unlike monoclonal antibodies, polyclonal antibodies may lack avidity or specificity.

This chapter presents a variety of methods, clinical applications, and commercial products that utilize antibodies and antigens for the detection of clinically significant bacteria, fungi, parasites, and viruses in patient specimens.

► PRINCIPLES OF IMMUNOLOGICAL DETECTION METHODS

Antigen or antibody detection in a clinical sample offers the capability to detect and rapidly identify the infectious agent without culture. In the clinical labora-

tory, the basic process involves reacting a target antigen or antibody in the patient specimen with a specific antibody or antigen preparation of interest. The antibodies or antigens in the preparation recognize and combine specifically with the target antigen or antibody in the patient's specimen to form a stable product. This product, an **antigen-antibody complex,** is then detected utilizing detection methods such as antibody conjugated enzymatic cleavage of substrate, fluorochrome excitation, or chemiluminescence.

A microorganism contains many antigens, either on its surface (bacterial capsular polysaccharide or viral glycoprotein) or internally (bacterial enzymes or viral nucleocapsids). The diagnostic test interaction occurs between the antigenic determinant and the **antigen binding site** on the antibody. **Antigenic determinants** contain chemically unique areas known as

epitopes. There may be many epitopes, either identical or different in chemical composition, on a large antigen molecule. As a result, these tests often yield very specific (high **positive predictive value** or **specificity**) results, but generate varying levels of **sensitivity (negative predictive value)**, depending on the amount and type of specimen, collection, and transport conditions to the laboratory.

An advantage of antigen detection is that etiologic agents can be detected in specimens obtained from an infected host without the inherent delay of the immune response, one of the historical limitations of serological or antibody detection testing. These methods also allow for rapid reporting of test results to the clinician and may lead to more appropriate and less empirical therapeutic decisions. Diagnostic evaluation criteria should include **accuracy, precision,** sensitivity, specificity, and positive and negative predictive values. Clinical and diagnostic assessment criteria used to justify, verify, and validate new technology in the laboratory is discussed at the conclusion of this chapter.

Antigen detection has other important roles in the clinical laboratory. For previously cultured clinical specimens, these methods can be used to confirm the identity of an isolated colony on the primary culture plate. Examples include confirmation of *E. coli* 0157:H7 colony phenotypes on sorbitol MacConkey agar and serotyping of confirmed isolates of *Salmonella, Shigella,* and *Legionella* sp. Outside of the diagnostic microbiol-ogy or immunology laboratory, these techniques are also broadly applicable to a number of analytes, such as serum proteins, hormones, and drugs, as well as for the detection and quantitation of serum antibodies.

MANUAL METHODS OF DETECTION

Precipitin Tests

The basic type of antigen-antibody reaction is the **precipitin reaction.** Found in test systems, this reaction allows the free diffusion of soluble antigen and soluble antibody fronts toward one another; at a point of interface where the concentrations are optimal, a visible precipitate forms. These reactions are most stable when performed in an agarose gel (Figure 7-2■).

The double **immunodiffusion,** or Ouchterlony gel diffusion, is a classic example of antigen-antibody reaction in agarose gel. This technique is most often used to detect fungal exoantigens or serum antibodies. To perform this procedure, cylindrical holes or wells are cut out of an agarose gel in a small petri dish and spaced appropriately. The specimen containing the unknown soluble antigen is placed in one well, and a known antibody-containing solution is placed in an adjacent well. The antigen and antibody molecule in solution diffuse out of the wells and through the porous agarose. If antigen specific for the known antibody is present, the two components combine and produce a visible precip-

---

✳ Box 7-1   Evaluation of Rapid Diagnostic Tests

A word of caution should be considered before undertaking a rapid diagnostic test evaluation. First, each new test should be evaluated in the clinical environment in which the patient, provider, and laboratory will interact. Second, it's important to assess patient outcome of a newly proposed laboratory test algorithm with the clinicians who see that patient population and influence the therapeutic impact of the test result. For example, a rapid group A streptococcus (GAS) test may show high analytical sensitivity and specificity in your laboratory evaluation versus a gold standard technology such as culture. But if the majority of acute care providers in your institution will make a therapeutic decision and prescribe antibiotics for acute pharyngitis before the test results are known (strongly discouraged!), then offering the test will provide no additional benefit or "favorable outcome" to the patient or the clinician. Similarly, if the laboratory is not staffed 24 hours, seven days a week for a one-hour turnaround time, rapid test implementation will not lead to rapid test reporting and timely interpretation by the clinician. As a result, the patient may go home and wait for test results, potentially having to return to the facility for a prescription. Conversely, the facility stands to lose money by sending the patient home on empirically prescribed antibiotics if the GAS test results are not reported before the patient is sent home. Since the outcome of rapid testing ends up being the same as when utilizing traditional bacterial culture, there is no clinical reason to change to a rapid test. These types of evaluations for positive patient outcome are now a major criterion utilized by laboratory and residency program accreditation agencies and must be considered in each individual institution's plan for clinical support services.

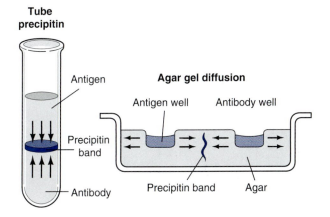

■ FIGURE 7-2 Tube and agar gel diffusion precipitin tests.

itin band, or line of precipitation, at a point of optimal concentration of each component.

Counterimmunoelectrophoresis

A modification of the immunodiffusion principle, counterimmunoelectrophoresis (CIE), greatly speeds up migration of soluble antigens and antibodies by applying an electric current. Antigen and antibody preparations are placed in adjacent wells cut out of an agarose gel. A glass or plastic surface supports the gel. The gel is placed in an alkaline buffer-containing electrophoresis chamber and the electric field is applied (Figure 7-3■). Under the buffer conditions chosen, most microbial antigens have a net negative charge (anions) and therefore migrate in the gel toward the positively charged electrode (anode). Antibody molecules, on the other hand, are very weakly negatively charged or neutral under alkaline buffer conditions. They do not migrate significantly in the charged field, but rather are carried toward the negatively charged electrode (cathode) by the effect of buffer ions. This phenomenon is known as electroendosmosis. If target antigen and antibody are present, at some point of optimum proportion or equilibrium, they will meet and form a visible precipitin band. The process may occur in one hour or less, compared with 24 hours required for precipitin bands to form in gels by passive diffusion.

Counterimmunoelectrophoretic plates are generally read immediately after electrophoresis, again after washing to remove nonspecific precipitins, and once again after overnight refrigeration to allow the specific bands to intensify.

Although very popular in the 1970s for a number of applications, CIE has been replaced by particle agglutination tests and immunoassays for rapid microbial antigen detection.

Complement Fixation (CF)

Similarly, complement fixation tests are performed mainly by public health laboratories for typing of viral isolates. Typically, the presence of antibody in a patient's serum is detected indirectly using carefully titered antigen, complement, and red blood cells (RBCs). If antibody is present, it will bind to the specific viral antigen. When complement is added, a complex forms. The formed complex allows RBCs to settle out of the serum as a pellet without being lysed by unbound complement. If the patient's serum does not have the antibodies specific for the antigen, a complexes will not form, and the complement will be free to lyse the RBCs when they are added (Figure 7-4■).

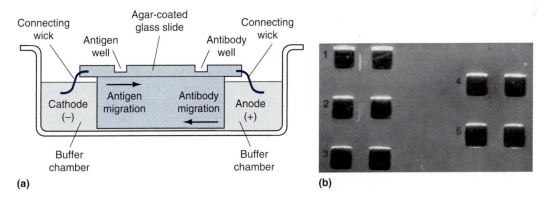

(a) **(b)**

■ FIGURE 7-3 (a) Illustration of counterimmunoelectrophoresis. (b) Precipitin band formed between antigen and antibody wells of CIE test: (1) Strong band (2) weak band, 3, 4, 5 no bands.

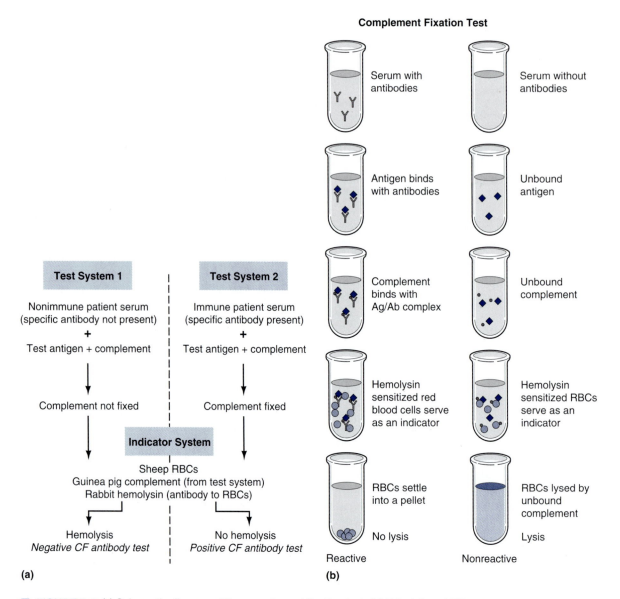

Complement Fixation Test

Test System 1

Nonimmune patient serum
(specific antibody not present)
+
Test antigen + complement

↓

Complement not fixed

↓

Test System 2

Immune patient serum
(specific antibody present)
+
Test antigen + complement

↓

Complement fixed

Indicator System

Sheep RBCs
Guinea pig complement (from test system)
Rabbit hemolysin (antibody to RBCs)

Hemolysis
Negative CF antibody test

No hemolysis
Positive CF antibody test

(a)

Serum with antibodies

Serum without antibodies

Antigen binds with antibodies

Unbound antigen

Complement binds with Ag/Ab complex

Unbound complement

Hemolysin sensitized red blood cells serve as an indicator

Hemolysin sensitized RBCs serve as an indicator

RBCs settle into a pellet

No lysis

RBCs lysed by unbound complement

Lysis

Reactive   Nonreactive

(b)

■ **FIGURE 7-4** (a) Schematic diagram of the complement fixation test. (b) Principles of CF test.

The difficulty of this test lies in the careful titration of reagents necessary for consistent results. Each component must be standardized before a test can be run, and it can take up to two days to complete just one test.

Hemagglutination

Hemagglutination inhibition (HI) assays are affected and interpreted by the same titration issues encountered in CF tests. Once the serum samples are serially diluted using a microtiter plate, the viral antigen is added at a very specific four hemagglutination units (HUs), incubated with RBCs and then interpreted. The last serial dilution that yields total inhibition of agglutination is the serum **titer** for the patient. Limitations of the procedure include (1) nonspecific inhibitors present in serum and the age of the erythrocytes used that may also present technical problems; (2) the antigen titrations must be done each time the test is performed and are only good for that day; and (3) the test requires some experience to interpret correctly.

Particle Agglutination

The basic chemical principle in **agglutination reaction** is similar with precipitin reactions with one exception. In agglutination reactions, the antigen or antibody is bound to a particulate carrier. Monoclonal or polyclonal antibody molecules can be bound to the surface of latex (polystyrene) beads. Beads measure about one micron in diameter (Figure 7-5■) and enhance the visible agglutination reaction. Each bead can be charged with thousands of antibody molecules. The antibody-charged latex beads form a homogeneous milky suspension that, when mixed with a specimen containing specific antigen, results in antigen-antibody binding. However this primary binding between antigen and antibody molecules does not produce a visible agglutination (clumping) reaction. Only if the antigen molecules contain multiple antigenic determinants, as is commonly the case for high molecular weight (HMW) polysaccharides, proteins, or microorganisms, will antigen molecules be cross-linked by the antibody coated latex beads. It is this secondary cross-linking of antigen and antibody, resulting in a macromolecular lattice, that precipitates out of solution and results in a visible agglutination reaction.

Latex Agglutination Latex agglutination is generally conducted on a treated cardboard or glass slide using liquid specimen and latex volumes of about 50 μl each. The reagents are mixed thoroughly, and then the slide is rocked or rotated by hand or with a mechanical device for two to three minutes before being read using appropriate lighting and the naked eye. The reaction depends on many variables and therefore must be carefully standardized. Variables include latex particle size, avidity of antibody, type of antibody (mono- or polyclonal), reaction temperature, pH, ionic strength, and concentration of antigen in the specimen. Levels of detection of microbial polysaccharide or protein can be as low as 0.1 ng/ml. The strength and rapidity of the reaction varies depending on all these test conditions and, most important, on the concentration of antigen in the specimen. With high antigen

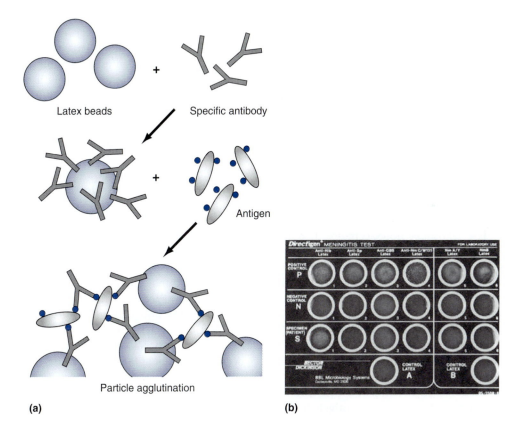

(a)

(b)

■ FIGURE 7-5 (a) Schematic diagram of agglutination reaction. (b) An example of latex agglutination slide test showing positive and negative reactions.

concentration, a maximum agglutination reaction (4+ on a 1+ to 4+ scale) may occur in only a few seconds. In the absence of specific antigen, the latex suspension remains homogeneous and milky, that is, no agglutination. Although most applications of latex agglutination use white latex beads, colored latexes are also available to enhance visual detection.

Because nonspecific agglutination reactions occur, it is important to incorporate the following controls when testing a patient specimen. These controls include (1) a positive antigen control (a solution containing the known antigen of interest), (2) a negative antigen control (a solution not containing the antigen), and (3) a control latex suspension to detect the presence of nonspecific agglutination reactions. The control latex involves testing the patient specimen with latex beads coated with an immunoglobulin whose specificity is not directed to the test antigen. This nonimmune serum is generally obtained from the same animal species in which the specific antibody was provided. A nonspecific agglutination reaction occurs when the patient's specimen reacts with both the test and the control latex. When such reactions occur, the test cannot be interpreted. A positive test result requires that the test latex, but not the control latex, agglutinate the patient specimen.

A number of specimen pretreatment procedures can be used to eliminate or minimize nonspecific agglutinations, presumably by removing or inactivating factors in the specimen responsible for these reactions. These procedures include specimen centrifugation to remove particulate material, boiling to inactivate protein constituents (acceptable when test antigen is a heat-stable polysaccharide), and passing the specimen through a membrane filter. Specimens such as serum contain very high protein concentrations. If the antigen of interest is a heat-stable polysaccharide, it is necessary to first treat the specimen with ethylenediamine tetraacetic acid (EDTA) or a proteolytic enzyme before heating. Otherwise the polysaccharide antigen may be trapped in the coagulated protein, leading to false negative test results. Furthermore, if the specimen is centrifuged, the polysaccharide may be completely removed from the test supernatant.

Latex agglutination tests for microbial antigens, like other laboratory tests, are subject to false-negative and false-positive reactions when compared with culture. **False-negative reactions** (negative antigen test result, positive culture) may be due to the presence of antigen in the specimen at concentrations below the test detection limit. **False-positive reactions** (positive antigen test result, negative culture) are more diffi-

cult to explain; they may be due to the presence of **cross-reacting antigens** or nonviability of organisms in the original specimen. It is important to remember that antigen detection tests do not require viable microbes. Antibody-coated latex suspensions can agglutinate viable or nonviable organisms, microbial components such as cell wall or membrane fragments, or soluble antigen such as bacterial capsular polysaccharide. Thus, an apparent false-positive latex test result may represent a true-positive result for disease in a patient with a negative culture.

Some specimens, such as urine, may be concentrated by centrifugation or membrane filtration before testing. Filters typically hold back or exclude HMW antigenic materials while allowing water and small compounds to pass through. These concentration methods increase the sensitivity of the test.

The advantages of commercially available latex agglutination tests are the availability of good quality reagents in complete kit form, good sensitivity, relative rapidity, and ease of performance. Disadvantages include subjectivity in reading endpoints, nonspecific reactions due to interfering substances in clinical samples, and the fact that some tests are not as "rapid" as an ordering physician might expect. In many clinical laboratories, culture confirmation and serotyping are routinely performed using latex agglutination test kits. Recently, detection of altered penicillin binding proteins that predict for bacterial resistance in gram positive cocci to beta lactam antibiotics (such as penicillin) have become commercially available.

Staphylococcal Coagglutination   Similar to latex agglutination, **coagglutination** utilizes particle-bound antibody to enhance the visibility of antigen-antibody reactions. Instead of a latex bead, intact formalin-killed *Staphylococcus aureus* cells (typically Cowan 1 strain) are utilized. The cell wall of this strain of *S. aureus* contains a large amount of protein A that has the capacity to bind antibody molecules in the Fc portion (base of the heavy immunoglobulin chain) of the IgG antibody. This leaves the antigen-binding sites of the molecule (Fab portion) available to react with specific antigens (Figure 7-6■). It has been estimated that each staphylococcal cell has about 80,000 antibody binding sites. The actual number of antibody molecules bound to the staphylococcal cell is limited by steric hindrance. Coating is sufficient, however, to render the product of clinical utility in direct antigen tests.

Most of the observations made regarding latex agglutination are also true for coagglutination. Reactions are prepared by mixing antibody-sensitized staphylo-

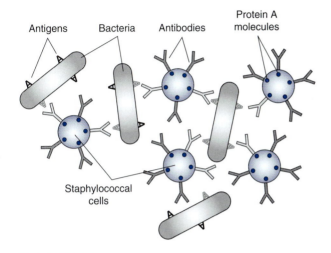

■ **FIGURE 7-6** Schematic diagram of coagglutination reaction.

coccal cells with a solution containing the antigen of interest on a slide or card. Coagglutination procedures appear more susceptible to nonspecific agglutination reactions, and thus specimen preparation is important. This is particularly true for testing serum specimens, because staphylococcal cells may bind human IgG in test serum specimens and subsequently be agglutinated by the presence of rheumatoid factor (IgM anti-IgG) in the serum. Coagglutination is highly specific but may be less sensitive in detecting small quantities of antigen than latex agglutination. Therefore, these reagents are often used to confirm the identification of bacterial colonies on culture plates, but not for rapid antigen detection from clinical specimens.

Liposome-Mediated Agglutination A recent development in agglutination technology involves the use of **liposomes,** single-lipid bilayer membranes that form closed vesicles under appropriate conditions. In their manufacture, antigen or antibody molecules may be incorporated into the surface of the membrane and thus be available for interaction with the corresponding molecule. In addition, the liposome vesicle may be constructed with a chemical dye or bioactive molecule trapped in the interior. The colored dye allows easy visual detection of lattice formation and agglutination between liposome-bound antibody and antigen. Alternatively, combining dye-containing liposomes and latex beads, both of which contain the reactive antibody on the surface, may increase the sensitivity of latex agglutination. Perhaps the greatest potential advantage of liposome technology is in its application to immunoassays other than particle agglutination that

make use of the ability of the liposome to carry reactive chemicals. Liposomes have yet to reach their full potential as diagnostic reagents in the clinical laboratory.

Immunofluorescent Assays

The principles of fluorescent antibody methods are also applied to other immunologic assays. In fluorescent antibody (FA) assay, or **immunofluorescence** (IFA), specific monoclonal or polyclonal antibodies are conjugated with fluorescent dyes (fluorochromes). They are then visualized with a fluorescent microscope. Detection techniques may be direct or indirect. For both techniques, a counterstain is often used as a last step to quench background nonspecific fluorescence.

In the *direct fluorescent antibody* (DFA) test, the antigen-specific labeled antibody is applied to the fixed specimen on a microscope slide, incubated, washed, and visualized using a fluorescent microscope. In the *indirect fluorescent antibody* (IFA) test, an unlabeled antigen-specific antibody is applied, incubated, and washed. A second fluorochrome labeled antibody specific for the first antibody is applied, washed, and read using a fluorescent microscope (Figure 7-7■). The microscopy utilizes an epi-illuminescent (incident) light system of vertical illumination, wavelength filters, and a dichroic mirror. The dichroic mirror allows passage of

FLUORESCENCE ANTIBODY TESTS

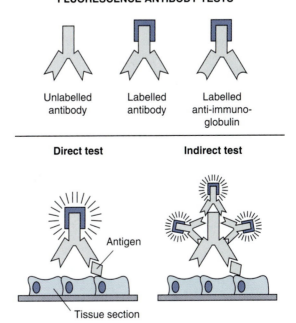

■ **FIGURE 7-7** A schematic representation of direct and indirect fluorescence antibody tests.

light at an excitation wavelength from the light source to the specimen. The mirror also allows passage of the emission (longer) wavelength light from the labeled source to the objective. This emitted, or excited, wavelength light appears as a bright color based on the dye used (Figure 7-8■). A very popular fluorochrome is fluorescein isothiocyanate (FITC) which upon excitation emits a bright apple green fluorescence.

There are advantages as well as limitations in using immunofluorescent methods. Immunofluorescent staining allows for rapid visualization of infected tissue, cell culture, body fluids, and swab specimens. This allows for an increased specificity since the desired morphology can be visualized through the microscope. However, the requirement for a fluorescent microscope and the significant subjective interpretation involved in reading the slides are limitations. In addition, the procedure may not be very rapid (1–4 hours) and is not easily automated. Last, fluorescence fades over time. Because of these, the newer colorimetric labels use conjugated enzymes instead of fluorochromes to detect the presence of antigen by converting a colorless substrate into a colored end product. Even with storage, these products do not fade and can be detected with the naked eye.

As will be described, fluorescent antibody tests are commonly used in the clinical laboratory to detect bacterial, viral, parasitological, and fungal infections.

Enzyme Immunoassays

Enzyme immunoassay (EIA) provides another option to FA for detecting antigens in clinical samples. EIA utilizes enzyme molecules conjugated to specific monoclonal or polyclonal antibodies in such a way that

both enzymatic and antigen-binding activities are preserved. The enzymes used are often alkaline phosphatase or horseradish peroxidase. When the appropriate substrate is added to the antigen-conjugated antibody complex, the enzyme catalyzes the production of a visible (colored) end product that can be visualized or quantitated spectrophotometrically. These procedures are adaptable to automated platforms and testing large volumes of samples (see the Automated Platforms Section).

Most commercially developed EIA systems for detection of infectious agents require physical separation of the specific antigens from nonspecific complexes found in clinical samples. Such systems are called solid-phase immunosorbent assays (SPIA); see Figure 7-9■. Separation is achieved through binding the antigen specific antibody to a solid phase or matrix. A variety of solid matrix platforms are commercially available to include individual wells of polystyrene microtiter trays, spherical plastic beads, or magnetic beads. This solid matrix allows for separation, or washing, of sample and reagent to decrease nonspecific binding or background activity.

When performing an EIA, a clinical sample is first added to the solid matrix. If the antigen of interest is present in sample, it will form a stable complex with the antibody bound to the matrix. Unbound sample is removed by washing, and a second antibody specific for the antigen is added. In the *direct method,* this second antibody is conjugated to an enzyme. In the *indirect method,* a second nonconjugated antibody is added and washed; a third antibody specific for the second is added. The third antibody is conjugated to the enzyme and is directed against the Fc portion of the unlabeled second antibody. In either method, once the conjugate is added and washed, then a specific substrate is added. The amount of colored end product measured is directly proportional to the amount of enzyme-bound conjugate, and, therefore, antigen is present in the original clinical sample. The methods just described are often called *direct sandwich* and *indirect sandwich* immunoassays (Figures 7-9a and b). The advantage of the indirect sandwich immunoassay is the need for only one enzyme conjugated anti-immunoglobulin antibody (3rd antibody) that can be used for the detection step for a variety of antigen detection kits.

Commercial companies have produced good quality EIA kits for detection of a variety of microbial antigens. Conjugates can be inexpensively prepared, are stable for up to six months, and have reasonably good sensitivity in most applications. The use of microtiter plates and

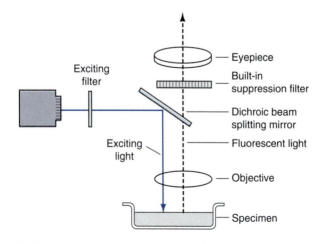

■ **FIGURE 7-8** A diagram of incident light microscope showing the light path.

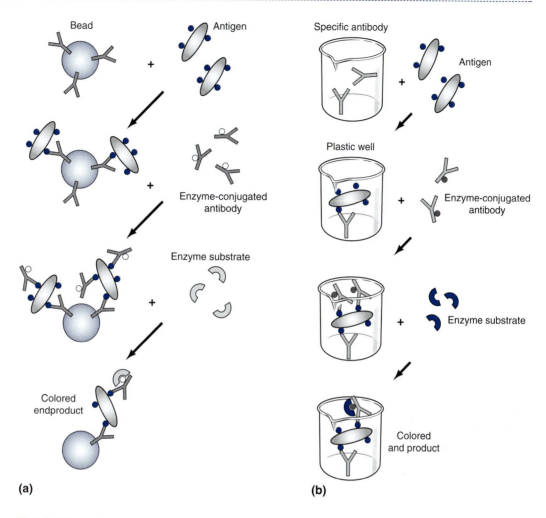

■ FIGURE 7-9 Schematic flow diagram of direct sandwich immunassay.

instrumentation for dispensing reagents, wash procedures, and automated optical reading of reactions have greatly facilitated EIA methods to allow large volumes to be batch tested. Some methods are time consuming, however, and may not be practical for low-volume labs or STAT runs. Thus, they cannot always be considered rapid tests when compared with other procedures such as latex agglutination. Enzyme immunoassay kits are commonly used for the detection of bacteria and their toxins, viruses, yeasts, and parasites.

A variation of enzyme labeling involves coupling a reactive molecule such as biotin to the primary antibody. Binding of antibody to specific antigen is then detected by reacting with enzyme-labeled streptavidin, which binds very tightly and specifically to biotin by one of four reactive sites on each streptavidin molecule. The avidin-biotin interaction takes the place of

primary antibody-secondary antibody interaction. This method tends to increase the amount of signal detected (increased sensitivity) for the following reasons: (1) multiple biotin molecules may be bound to the primary antibody, and (2) each avidin molecule has four reactive sites to biotin. In combination, avidin-biotin interactions allow for multiple complexes with enzyme to bind and cleave substrate.

Newer formats for rapid EIAs are constantly being developed, resulting in greater speed and simplicity of EIAs. The most popular methods are described as follows.

Membrane-Bound EIA The flow-through and large surface area characteristics of nitrocellulose, nylon, or other membranes have been demonstrated to enhance the speed and sensitivity of EIA reactions. The improvements associated with membrane bound

EIAs are largely the result of immobilizing antibody onto the surface of porous membranes. This modification of SPIA utilizes a disposable plastic cassette consisting of the antibody-bound membrane and a small chamber to which the clinical sample can be added. An absorbent material is placed below the membrane to pull, or wick, the liquid reactants through the membrane. This helps to separate nonreacted components from the antigen-antibody complexes of interest bound to the membrane and thus simplify washing steps. Incubation times are also decreased because the rate of antigen binding is proportional to its concentration in solution near the membrane surface; this action increases the rate and extent of binding. These "flow-through" EIAs have become popular because they can easily be performed as rapid single tests and because positive and negative controls can be incorporated at different sites on the same membrane used for clinical samples. These tests are easily incorporated into stand-alone kits and may be used in a laboratory environment. If cleared by the FDA as a "waived test," it may be performed in a physician's office or other non-laboratory setting. Membrane-bound EIA tests are commonly used for the rapid detection of viruses, bacteria and their toxins, and parasites.

Optical Immunoassay   Optical immunoassay (OIA) relies on the interaction of antigen-antibody complexes on inert surfaces. Specific antigen-antibody interaction alters the thickness of the reactants on the test surface. Light reflecting off the surface film containing antibody only is viewed as one color. However, when specific antigen is bound to antibody, it increases the thickness of the film. This causes the surface to appear a different color to the naked eye. An optical immunoassay is used in many laboratories to detect group A *Streptococcus* (GAS) in pediatric populations and respiratory viruses.

Electrochemiluminescence   **Electrochemiluminescence** is a process in which certain chemical compounds emit light when electrochemically stimulated. Such chemical compounds can be used for detection in the same way conjugates and fluorochromes are used in EIA and IFA. By applying an electrical potential, the excited chemicals serve as a detection signal for specific antigen-antibody reactions. These reactions are highly specific. In contrast to fluorescent methods, assay samples typically contribute little or no native background chemiluminescence (i.e., equivalence of autofluorescence).

Hybrid Capture   Hybrid capture is an interesting combination of antigen-antibody, nucleic acid, and chemiluminescent technologies. Very briefly, DNA:DNA or DNA:RNA hybrids can be captured by nucleic acid hybrid specific antibodies attached to a solid phase. These complexes may then be detected by chemiluminescence markers. Such a system is commercially available from DiGene (Gaithersburg, MD) and is now the standard of care for the detection of human papilloma virus in cervical specimens collected for pap smear.

▶ AUTOMATED PLATFORMS

Several commercial companies offer free-standing or bench-top models of automated testing platforms. Selection of platforms is often based on test volume, turnaround time requirements, therapeutic impact of test results, and staffing of the laboratory. While large volume reference laboratories often utilize free-standing analyzers to batch test for a specific antibody or antigen, smaller bench-top analyzers are often selected for low-volume testing or dedication to a unique test method. The previously described methods, most frequently either EIA, IFA, or chemiluminescence, are supported by most testing platforms. Testing platforms will include hardware and software to support specimen processing, dilution, reagent delivery, incubation, washing, detection of signal, result analysis and reporting, and data management. The ability to interface large-volume testing platforms to the laboratory information system (LIS) is important to facilitate electronic transmission of results to clinicians without a manual intervention from the laboratory technologist. Platforms may support matrices such as microplates, carousels, or individual tubes and carriers for specimen testing.

Readers are referred to a very detailed tabular description of commercial test platforms that may be found in the *Manual of Commercial Methods in Clinical Microbiology,* 1st edition, ASM Press.

▶ IMMUNOLOGIC DETECTION OF BACTERIAL INFECTIONS

STREPTOCOCCAL PHARYNGITIS

First marketed in the 1980s, the rapid direct antigen testing for group A streptococci (GAS) in throat swab specimens provides an advantage over standard throat culture procedures; results are available while the patient waits in the clinician's office instead of waiting 24 to 48 hours for culture results. Antibiotic therapy is critical in preventing poststreptococcal pharyngitis syndromes such as rheumatic fever and glomerulonephritis. Therapy may also shorten the patient's illness, reduce secondary infections, or spread to close contacts.

There are several diagnostic test kits for direct GAS detection currently in the market. Most of these kits, either latex agglutination or some version of solid-phase immunoassay, require an initial extraction of the group A carbohydrate antigen from the cell wall of the organism. This is usually achieved by exposing the sample to nitrous acid or enzymatic digestion. Once the solubilized antigen preparation is completed, the specimen is tested following the directions provided by the manufacturer. A number of EIA tests have become popular, particularly those that use lateral flow membrane-bound antibody to speed up the reaction and facilitate the washing procedure. Because of the colored product, they are generally easier to read than latex agglutination tests.

The sensitivity and specificity of direct GAS tests, when compared with the gold standard–throat culture, vary by manufacturer, individual performing the test, and accuracy of the throat culture procedure used for comparison. A conservative estimate is in the range of 70% to 90% and 95% to 97%, respectively. Nevertheless, the sensitivities of the rapid GAS antigen tests are not high enough to permit their use in pediatric populations without an accompanying culture. The best overall approach for diagnosis of streptococcal pharyngitis would couple a rapid direct test with a throat culture performed when the direct test is negative. Positive direct test results would lead to immediate initiation of antibiotic therapy. It must be remembered that the most important reason for diagnosing and treating GAS pharyngitis is to prevent the nonsuppurative sequelae previously mentioned. Fortunately, a delay in initiation of therapy for 24–48 hours (while awaiting culture results) will not increase the patient's risk of developing such complications.

WHOOPING COUGH (PERTUSSIS)

The fluorescent antibody (FA) test to detect the presence of *Bordetella pertussis,* the agent of whooping cough, in nasopharyngeal swabs, or aspirates may result in early initiation of therapy and isolation of the patient to prevent secondary spread of this highly contagious organism. *Bordetella pertussis* are slow-growing, fastidious, gram-negative coccobacilli. It may take up to 10 days for organisms to appear in culture. Hence, a fluorescent test may be performed on smears prepared

from nasopharyngeal washings or swabs to facilitate diagnosis. Such smears are positive in up to 70% of culture-positive specimens. As in any FA performed on respiratory specimens, specificity is dependent on the expertise of a well-trained technologist. Thus, if using FA, a culture backup is recommended.

LEGIONNAIRES' DISEASE

Early diagnosis and therapy are important, particularly in immunosuppressed patients who acquire Legionnaire's disease. *Legionella pneumophila* and other *Legionella* sp. cause this acute lobar pneumonia with multisystem involvement. Disease may occur as community-acquired individual cases or outbreaks and as nosocomial infections. A variety of antigen detection methods have been evaluated and compared with culture isolation. A commonly performed test is the FA on respiratory specimens. A monoclonal antibody is usually directed against *L. pneumophila* serogroup 1 whereas polyclonal antibody may include other serogroups and, in some cases, other species of *Legionella.* Sensitivity of FA is approximately 70%. Specificity has been a problem with some reagents, owing to antigens shared with other gram negative rods. A number of immunoassays have been evaluated, including detection of soluble urinary antigen. These assays have sensitivities in the 85% to 95% range, with even higher specificity. Most recently an EIA for urinary antigen has become commercially available with published sensitivity of 80% and specificity of greater than 90%. The EIA test is limited to monoclonal antibody detection of *L. pneumophila* serogroup 1 only.

BACTERIAL MENINGITIS AND SEPSIS

Clinical laboratories have regularly used antigen detection testing of CSF and other body fluids to detect organisms causing bacterial meningitis for about 25 years. However, with the advent of *H. influenzae* type b vaccine, the incidence of *H. influenzae* meningitis of defined subtype and/or bacteremia has declined by 90%. For this and other reasons, the utilization of antigen tests for bacterial meningitis has declined sharply. Nevertheless, the clinical utility of antigen tests for diagnosing meningitis has not completely disappeared; rather it varies with a number of factors such as initiation of therapy, specimen type, etiologic agent, and the manufacturer of the kit. In many clinical laboratories, the use of these tests is reserved for very specific diagnostic testing requirements. Probably the greatest clinical significance of these antigen tests occurs when testing specimens from patients who have previously received antibiotic therapy before cultures were collected and in whom the gram stain was negative. In this situation the likelihood of recovering the organism in culture is dramatically decreased.

Latex agglutination tests are used when performing rapid antigen testing for bacterial meningitis. The bacterial agents detected in the commercially available kits include *Haemophilus influenzae* type b, *N. meningitidis, Streptococcus pneumoniae,* and *Streptococcus agalactiae* (group B streptococcus) and *E. coli.* Although antibodies in each kit vary, they are all designed to detect capsular polysaccharide antigens of the organisms.

These organisms often cause bacteremia before the organism invades the central nervous system. As these organisms multiply and cause infection, the antigens are shed into the body tissues and fluids. Thus, the organism and antigens may be detected in the serum before or at the same time they are found in the CSF in cases of meningitis. Furthermore, circulating organisms and soluble antigens are trapped, degraded, and released by phagocytic cells of the liver and spleen. These products are cleared from the body by filtration in the kidney and excreted in the urine; thus, urine can be examined for the presence of antigen in addition to CSF in suspected meningitis. Urine is also useful as a test specimen either alone or in addition to serum in cases of bacteremia and focal infections other than meningitis. Urine may be concentrated by ultrafiltration (removing water but not microbial antigens) to increase test sensitivity.

GASTROENTERITIS

Direct microbial detection methods have been applied to the diagnosis of bacterial, viral, and parasitic agents of gastrointestinal tract infections. Pseudomembranous colitis and antibiotic associated diarrhea caused by *Clostridium difficile* typically occur among hospitalized patients receiving antibiotics or other chemotherapeutic agents that alter bowel flora. The organism produces two exotoxins, toxin A and B. Toxin A functions as an enterotoxin that causes inflammation, increased vascular permeability, and fluid secretion. Toxin B is a cytotoxin that causes mucosal damage with 10-fold more potency than toxin A and causes hemorrhagic colitis and cytopathic effects.

Numerous EIA tests for toxin A have been evaluated with sensitivities that range from 75% to 95% or higher, and therefore negative predictive values may be close to 99%. Recent studies suggest the possible emergence of

toxin B producing and nontoxin A producing strains. There are now a number of commercially available products to detect the presence of both toxin A and toxin B.

Rapid EIA tests are also available for detection of shigalike producing and/or specific enterohemorrhagic strains of *E. coli* directly from stool samples. Enterohemorrhagic strains of *E. coli,* such as O157:H7 and others, secrete a verotoxin that causes endothelial injury that can result in the development of hemolytic-uremic syndrome (HUS). Rapid identification may prove useful in identifying exposed individuals in an outbreak situation. Those individuals can then be carefully watched for progression to systemic disease including HUS.

Another common cause of gastrointestinal infections is *Campylobacter* species. These organisms are capnophilic, gram-negative, curved rods that often take up to 72 hours to grow in culture on a selective agar medium in a microaerophilic environment. A two-hour EIA kit is commercially available to detect antigen directly from stool specimens.

NONTREPONEMAL TESTS FOR SYPHILIS

In 1906, Wasserman, Neisser, and Bruck were the first to develop the nontreponemal tests for the diagnosis of *T. pallidum* infection. In 1941 Pangborn further modified the antigen to increase its sensitivity and specificity. Today the flocculation test is used for the nontreponemal testing of syphilis. In this reaction, an infected patient's serum contains antibody to the cellular component of the inflammation associated with syphilis infection. That cellular component is the antigen used in the Venereal Disease Research Laboratory (VDRL) test and contains cardiolipin, cholesterol, and lecithin. The patient's serum is mixed with the test antigen, placed on a rotator for a specified time, then read microscopically for flocculation or granularity associated with specific antibody-antigen reaction.

The Rapid Plasma Reagin (RPR) 18 mm circle card test is a macroscopic flocculation test. It is performed on a disposable plastic-coated card, and uses charcoal size particles in the antigen. The RPR uses heated or unheated sera or unheated plasma specimens. Reagin screen test (RST) is another macroscopic card test. It uses a stabilized antigen stained with a lipid-soluble diazo dye, Sudan black B. Last, the toluidine red unheated serum test (TRUST) is another macroscopic flocculation test. Toluidine red is added to the TRUST antigen. The test is performed on a plastic-coated card.

The non-treponemal tests are most often used as a screening test for syphilis and are prone to false reactive

⁂ Box 7-2 Syphilis

Syphilis is a sexually transmitted disease caused by *Treponema pallidum,* a spiral shaped bacterium with 6 to 14 spirals and tapered ends which propels itself by spinning around its longitudinal axis. Nearly all cases of syphilis are acquired by sexual contact. The most common presentation is a skin lesion such as a chancre, mucous patch, or condyloma latum. The organism can also pass through broken skin on other parts of the body. In addition, a pregnant woman with syphilis can pass *T. pallidum* to her unborn child.

The initial infection causes the chancre at the primary infection site. The bacteria then move throughout the body and, if untreated, damage many organs over a period of time. The disease is divided into four stages: primary, secondary, latent, and tertiary (late). An untreated infected person can transmit the infection during the first two stages. These stages last approximately 1-2 years. Untreated syphilis in the later stages is not contagious, but can cause blindness, mental disorders, serious heart abnormalities, and even death in the host.

The first symptom of primary syphilis is a lesion called a chancre. It can appear within 10 days to 3 months after exposure, but generally will appear within 2 to 6 weeks. The chancre is usually painless and may be hidden inside the body. Approximately one-third of the people who are not treated during the primary stage will progress to the chronic stages.

In secondary syphilis, a skin rash with brown sores about the size of a penny will occur. This is attributed to systemic infection. The rash appears approximately 3 to 6 weeks after the chancre appears, and occurs primarily on the palms of the hands and the soles of the feet. This rash usually heals within several weeks or months. Fatigue, headache, mild fever, sore throat, patchy hair loss, and swollen lymph glands throughout the body are other symptoms during this stage. These symptoms may be very mild and will usually disappear without treatment. The signs of secondary syphilis may reoccur over the next 1 to 2 years.

To establish a diagnosis of latent syphilis, the following criteria must be met: (1) positive specific treponemal antibody test for syphilis, (2) a normal CSF examination, (3) no clinical manifestation of syphilis on a physical exam or chest x-ray, (4) a history of primary or secondary lesions, (5) history of exposure to syphilis, or (6) delivery of an infant with congenital syphilis. Left untreated, a person with syphilis may lapse into the latent stage. Latent syphilis is no longer contagious and is often asymptomatic.

In tertiary syphilis, lesions may be cardiovascular due to a hypersensitivity reaction. Treponemes are spread via the lymphatic system and lodge in the proximal aorta. The inflammatory response may continue for years. Neurosyphilis occurs when the spirochete crosses the blood-brain barrier, resulting in inflammation of the meninges. It may also cause lesions in the brain itself. Approximately one-third of people who have secondary syphilis go on to develop the complications of tertiary syphilis (i.e., damage to heart, brain, CNS).

The fourth month of gestation is when the fetus is at most risk to develop congenital syphilis because this is when the cell layers of the placenta are completed and the immune system begins to develop. Diagnosis of syphilis is conclusive in the neonate if demonstrated by direct examination of the umbilical cord, placenta, nasal discharge, or skin lesion material.

tests. Due to their lack of specificity, these tests are usually confirmed with a high-specificity treponemal test.

TREPONEMAL TESTS FOR SYPHILIS

In 1910, treponemes were first visualized in stained tissue sections by direct microscopy. As a result, darkfield microscopy was adapted to visualize motile spirochetes. If the patient had moist lesions and the specimen was immediately available for wet mount, this became the test of choice. Today, very few laboratories or clinicians perform darkfield microscopy due to the limited availability of darkfield microscopes and the expertise required for darkfield interpretation.

In 1949, the *T. pallidum* immobilization (TPI) test was first described. This test used the bacteria itself as the antigen, hence the "treponemal tests" for syphilis. Today there are three treponemal tests that are used as the standard: (1) the fluorescent treponemal antibody absorption (FTA-ABS), (2) the FTA-ABS double staining (DS), and (3) the microhemagglutination assay for antibodies to *T. pallidum* (MHA-TP). These tests use the antibodies directed against treponemal cellular components as their basis. Considered confirmatory tests due to increased sensitivity, specificity, and cost effectiveness, they have replaced the TPI as a routine clinical test.

The FTA-ABS test is an indirect immunofluorescent antibody test. The patient's serum is diluted in an adsorbent that binds potentially cross-reacting proteins and is placed on a microscope slide fixed with the antigen. The slide is then examined for fluorescent reactivity using a fluorescent microscope. The FTA-ABS DS simply adds a contrasting fluorochrome-labeled counterstain for *T. pallidum* as the final staining step. The MHA-TP is a qualitative hemagglutination test. It uses tanned formalinized sheep red blood cells (SRBCs) as the carrier for the *T. pallidum* antigen. Patient serum is serially diluted in the absorbing diluent and is added to SRBCs sensitized with *T. pallidum* and to unsensitized SRBCs. Results are reported as titers of the hemagglutination reaction. This test does not require the subjective expertise of a fluorescent microscopist or the microscope. It is however less sensitive than the FTA-ABS for lab diagnosis of primary syphilis. Last, a DFA for *T. pallidum* (DFA-TP) utilizes a fluorescent labeled anti-*T. pallidum* polyclonal or monoclonal immunoglobulin against lesion material fixed to a slide.

Of therapeutic importance, treponemal antibody persists for life and is a better indicator of previous infection than non-treponemal antibodies, which dissipate with time or therapy.

▶ IMMUNOLOGIC DETECTION OF VIRAL INFECTIONS

RESPIRATORY VIRUS INFECTIONS

Direct Antigen Detection

A number of respiratory viruses can be directly detected in both upper respiratory and lower respiratory specimens. Direct fluorescent antibody (DFA) is a common technique used for detecting respiratory syncytial virus (RSV), influenza A and B, parainfluenza 1, 2, and 3, and adenovirus in respiratory secretions. These reagents may be used for direct detection by FA or to confirm cytopathic effect in conventional tissue culture tubes or shell vials. When used for direct detection, these reagents are between 80% and 95% sensitive and 90% to 99% specific. Of particular importance, rapid detection of influenza and RSV by DFA or membrane-bound EIA in nasopharyngeal samples is common in the clinical laboratory. Rapid direct detection is important because RSV causes serious lower respiratory tract disease (bronchiolitis and pneumonia) in young children, often requiring hospitalization, and influenza may be now be treated if diagnosed within 48 hours of symptoms. Also, RSV is extremely labile, and it is difficult to maintain viral viability during transport, compromising recovery in cell culture.

Serodiagnosis of Respiratory Viral Infections

Serodiagnosis of respiratory viral infections is limited in clinical applications and usually provides retrospective evidence of infection without therapeutic impact.

There are methods for the serodiagnosis of adenoviruses, respiratory syncytial virus, parainfluenza viruses, and influenza viruses, but they are not commonly used due to the necessity of measuring acute and convalescent titers. The common methods of serological testing used are complement fixation (CF), EIA, serum neutralization (SN), and hemagglutination inhibition (HI). These tests all employ paired acute and convalescent sera to demonstrate the standard fourfold rise in antibody titer required to attribute illness to respiratory viruses. The acute phase serum should be taken as early in the course of the disease as possible and the convalescent serum between two and four weeks later. Usually IgG is the antibody of choice for this determination, however, IgM assays are also available but are less sensitive due to the more transient and often nonspecific nature of the IgM response.

EIA is an easy method for detection of respiratory viruses antibody in serum. As with many other tests for antiviral antibodies, results can be of limited use in the clinical treatment of the disease because by the time the paired sera are collected the patient has recovered. The information collected can be of use in epidemiologic studies and can monitor the spread of infection within a population. There are also numerous commercially marketed direct detection kits for respiratory viruses, with varying sensitivity and specificity depending on the collection site and quality of the sample.

Rhinoviruses (Picornaviridae) and Coronaviruses The rhinoviruses and coronaviruses are usually implicated in upper respiratory viral infections or the common cold. Coronaviruses are also causative agents of enteritis and more recently have been identified as the pathogen responsible for severe acute respiratory distress syndrome (SARS), referred to as the SARS-Covariant (CoV). Serological diagnosis of these two viruses is generally not available in clinical laboratories, and isolation by cell culture is usually not performed because other than SARS associated illnesses generally are nonlife threatening, self-limiting, and of relatively short duration. There are over 100 serotypes of rhinoviruses making isolation of a single source of infection both time consuming and costly. Additionally, it has been shown that by the age of two, up to 91% of children have rhinovirus-specific antibodies circulating, so unless a specific serotype is suspected there may be cross-reactivity issues in serological testing. Diagnosis may be made by methods such as cell culture, electron microscopy, or polymerase chain reaction (PCR). Cell culture is usually not practical from a clinical standpoint as the patient is usually recovered by the time results could be reported and both viruses are slow growing and difficult to isolate in this manner. Electron microscopy (EM) and nucleic acid amplification (NAA) are both definitive methods of identification but require expensive equipment and riprous validation studies. In the case of EM, a considerable amount of expertise and training is also needed, and NAA is rarely an FDA-approved testing method. Both of these methods are generally used more in the public health or research setting. Antigen suitable for serological detection can be isolated for use in complement fixation or EIA testing, but it is not widely available in a commercial form suitable for clinical use and is generally only applied in research settings.

The recent emergence of SARS-CoV as a human pathogen elicited a rapid response in the medical and epidemiology community. Testing methods were rapidly developed that could detect virus in culture, by NAA, and serologically. Serological diagnosis of the presence of anti-SARS IgG by IFA used infected cells from viral culture. EIA and Western blot assays were used to confirm diagnoses based on rises in both IgG and IgM titers. In SARS-CoV the major antigen expressed is the spike or S protein that stimulates neutralizing antibody. The N protein is also highly immunogenic. Interestingly one serological study showed that subclinical infection may be very rare with SARS-CoV. In health care workers from a SARS-affected facility, there was no evidence of antibody to the virus. Recombinant SARS-CoV antigens are now being produced and could be used in the production of standardized serological tests. Suspected diagnostic serology for SARS-CoV lies primarily in the realm of the public health laboratories, CDC, and research institutions.

GASTROENTERITIS

The most important identifiable agents of viral gastroenteritis are human rotaviruses, noroviruses, caliciviruses, and enteric adenoviruses. These agents are either very difficult or impossible to grow in cell culture and electron microscopy capabilities are rarely cost-efficient in a clinical microbiology laboratory. Therefore, antigen detection methods are very important for diagnosis. Rotaviruses are the most important agents in this group for a number of reasons. They commonly infect very young infants, often in day care settings, causing vomiting and diarrhea and resulting in dehydration. Rotavirus disease can also be severe and long lasting, while gastroenteritis due to these other viruses is usually much shorter in duration. Both EIA and Latex Latex agglutination (LA) tests are available for rotavirus detection in stool specimens,

EIA is generally more sensitive than LA. In either case, soluble antigen must be extracted from the particulate matter in stool before testing. This is generally accomplished by mixing the stool with extract buffer solution. At least one EIA is available for detection of enteric adenovirus types 40 and 41. There are no FDA approved rapid tests for the noroviruses or caliciviruses.

BLOOD-BORNE AND BODY FLUID-BORNE DISEASES

Viral Hepatitis
Hepatitis, an inflammation of the liver, may be the result of physical damage, exposure to toxins, or viral or bacterial infections. Infectious viral hepatitis is usually the result of infection with the hepatitis A virus (HAV), hepatitis B virus (HBV), hepatitis C virus (HCV), hepatitis D virus (HDV), hepatitis E virus (HEV), hepatitis G virus (HGV), or one of the other yet-to-be-classified hepatitis viruses. Nonculture methods are the mainstays for laboratory diagnosis of viral hepatitis.

Measurement of serologic response to viral antigens and direct viral antigen detection are important. For HBV, EIA methods have largely replaced RIA methods. Both hepatitis B surface antigen and hepatitis B e (capsid) antigen can generally be detected early in acute infection and may also be detected in patients who are chronically infected. These antigen tests, when performed concurrently with antibody detection tests, have important diagnostic and prognostic value in the workup of acute versus chronic disease.

Hepatitis A   HAV infection is most commonly associated with food-borne outbreaks of disease due to its fecal-oral route of transmission, and incidents are frequently traced to contaminated food or water. Large outbreaks due to contaminated water are usually not found in more developed countries with adequate water treatment facilities. Serological testing for anti-HAV antibodies are most often performed using an EIA method on an automated platform. Anti-HAV IgM begins to appear in the serum of infected persons five to 10 days before the onset of clinical symptoms, then decreases to undetectable levels after about six months. Anti-HAV IgG antibody is measured as part of the total serum anti-HAV antibody (both IgM and IgG) as an indication of lifelong immunity. Figure 7-10■ shows the antibody response during HAV infection.

Hepatitis B   HBV testing is one of the most common tests performed in a clinical immunology laboratory. Hepatitis B causes both acute and chronic conditions with approximately 10% of infected patients

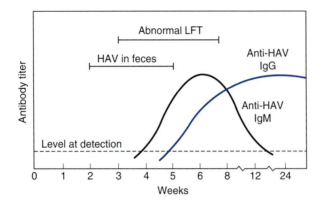

■ **FIGURE 7-10** Serologic response to HAV infection showing the rise and decline of detectable antibodies. LFT: liver function tests.

antigen (HBc) appears early, and indicates that the patient has an acute infection. Concentrations of anti-HBc IgG and IgM antibodies peak at approximately four months after clinical onset. Anti-HBc IgG reaches higher concentrations than IgM. The IgM begins to decrease thereafter, and generally decreases over the next four to six months and become undetectable. Anti-HBc IgG peaks and remains detectable at high concentration for life. The hepatitis B e-antigen indicates the potential for infection, and disappears with the production of anti-HBeAg. Levels of this antibody peak at fairly high concentration between five to six months postexposure and then slightly decline, but remain detectable for life. Figure 7-11■ shows the rise and fall of antibody levels in an HBV infection. Table 7-1✪ summarizes the hepatitis B serology profiles.

Unusual serological profiles can occur, including:

■ Chronic carrier—These patients are characterized serologically by persistently high titers of HBsAg and HBeAg, as the patients do not develop neutralizing antibodies to either of the viral antigens. Anti-HBc antibodies are also produced and patients in this category are chronic shedders of infectious virus.

■ Late seroconversion (also a chronic carrier)—Patients who are infected but fall into the category of late serconversion have a serological profile similar to the chronic carrier, in which levels of HBsAg increase and remain high throughout the chronic period. However, the levels of HBeAg in these patients will eventually decline as anti-HBe is produced.

becoming persistent carriers. Testing is usually performed by EIA designed to detect either antibody or antigen in the serum. Complete characterization of a patient's immune status with regard to exposure to HBV can provide a large amount of clinically relevant information to the physician. In the majority of patients, the first measurable serological marker is the hepatitis B surface antigen (HBsAg). The presence of HBsAg in the patient's serum indicates that the patient has either HBV infection, is an acute carrier, or is in an incubation period. The antigen becomes detectable in the acute infectious stage, which appears about two weeks after symptoms develop. Antigenemia peaks and then falls to undetectable levels generally within three months, with the appearance of anti-HBsAg antibody, usually six to seven months postexposure. Hepatitis B e-antigen (HBeAg) follows a similar rise to a peak beginning later than HBsAg and then falling to undetectable levels sooner. IgM antibody to the HB core

Hepatitis D HDV coinfection or superinfection (sometimes referred to as the delta agent) is a defective RNA virus that appears to infect only those already infected with HBV. There is well-characterized serological testing for diagnosis, disease management, and moni-

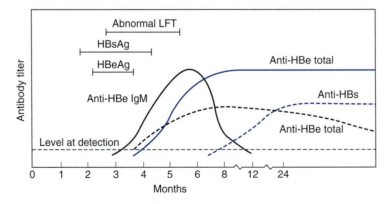

■ **FIGURE 7-11** Serologic response to HBV infection showing the rise and decline of detectable antibodies.

✪ TABLE 7-1

Summary of Hepatitis B Serology Profiles

Serologic Markers Present	Patient Status
None	Susceptible to infection
Anti-HBc total Anti-HBs	Immune—derived from past infection
Anti-HBs	Immune—derived from hepatitis B vaccine
HBe Ag (possibly) HBs Ag Anti-HBc Total Anti-HBc IgM	Acute infection
HBe Ag HBs Ag Anti-HBc total Anti-HBc IgM Anti-HBe Anti-HBs	Early to late recovery period. During early recovery immunity is not yet established.
HBe Ag HBs Ag Anti-HBc total	Chronic infection
Anti-HBc total	Several possibilities. Recovery from acute infection. Immune with anti-HBs levels too low to detect. Susceptible to infection with a false-positive anti-HBc total. Chronic carrier with HBs Ag levels too low to detect.

toring of vaccine status. HDV relies on HBV for maturation because the outer coat of the virus itself is made of HBsAg even though the HDV genome does not encode for it. Infections of HBV patients with HDV are categorized either as a superinfection or as a coinfection. Coinfection occurs when a patient is infected with both HBV and HDV at the same time. Superinfection occurs when an already infected HBV patient subsequently acquires HDV. The serological profiles can distinguish between the two types of infection. In coinfection, both the HBeAg and anti-HBe measurements are replaced by HDAg and anti-HD. HDAg is detectable in the patient serum for a short period at relatively low levels during the acute phase, and anti-HD begins to appear before the HDAg disappears. Anti-HD rises to fairly high levels then decreases slightly but remains detectable for years. In the case of superinfection of HDV, levels of HBsAg and anti-HBc total antibody are already elevated. When the HDAg levels rise to detectable levels early in the acute phase of HDV in-

fection, there is a corresponding dip in the level of HBsAg. This occurs as the HDV begins replicating and suppresses the replication of HBV. Antibody response to HDV infection is shown in Figures 7-12a■ and b.

Hepatitis C   In 1974, it became apparent that there was evidence of a non-A, non-B hepatitis (NANB) virus associated with transfusion-related hepatitis, which was predicted to be HCV. The genome of HCV was sequenced 15 years later, and shortly thereafter, the virus was seen on electron micrographs. This ss RNA virus accounted for approximately 90% of all previously detected NANB hepatitis cases. The virus is usually parenterally transmitted, although sexual and perinatal transmission may occur as well. Serological testing for the antibody to the hepatitis C virus (anti-HCV) began in the early 1990s. Since then screening has been done primarily using an anti-HCV ELISA. The profile for an HCV infected patient is relatively simple. Anti-HCV antibodies begin to appear in the serum sometime during the incubation period, which can last from two weeks to approximately six months. The titer rises fairly rapidly and, in the majority of patients, is present for life. In some cases, the titer may drop to undetectable levels years after infection. Figure 7-13■ shows the antibody response to HCV infection.

A positive EIA screening test for anti-HCV is confirmed by alternate tests. The confirmatory testing methods approved for are the recombinant immunoblot assay (RIBA) and NAA. The RIBA detects the presence of human antibody to four specific recombinant viral antigens on a solid phase strip. The NAA test detects the presence of HCV nucleic acid in the patient's serum. Recently the Centers for Disease Control (CDC) modified guidelines for confirming positive HCV EIAs test results by establishing a signal to cut-off ratio above which confirmatory testing is not required. In essence, establishing that if the signal is strong enough, RIBA confirmation is not necessary and the correlation should be ≥95% predictive for HCV exposure, regardless of the population being tested. This guideline, however, can result in incorrect reporting if the population being tested is low risk, since confirmation rates can vary from as low as 67% up to 97%.

Human Immunodeficiency Virus

HIV-1 the most prevalent serotype in the US, causes acquired immune deficiency syndrome (AIDS). For serodiagnosis, the important antigens of the virus are p24, gp41, gp120, and gp160. Immunologic markers of AIDS include decline in numbers of CD4+ T-cells, depression of the CD4+/CD8+ ratio, impairment of monocytes and macrophages, decrease in NK cell activity, and anergy.

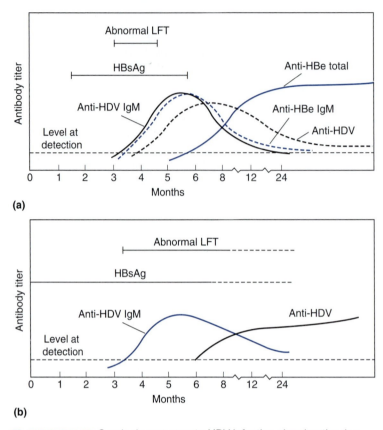

(a)

(b)

■ FIGURE 7-12 Serologic response to HDV infection showing the rise and decline of detectable antibodies. (a) Serologic profile in HDV coinfection. (b) Serologic profile in HDV superinfection.

Antigenic markers include detection of p24 antigen and HIV specific nucleic acid in blood.

The method for screening for HIV-1 is EIA using patient serum. Using the current third-generation EIA tests, antibody for HIV-1 is generally detectable within three weeks. By two months, almost all infected patients have detectable antibody. The high sensitivity of HIV EIAs results from very low positive/negative cutoff values and, by design, may yield falsely reactive results. This testing strategy requires that patient sera

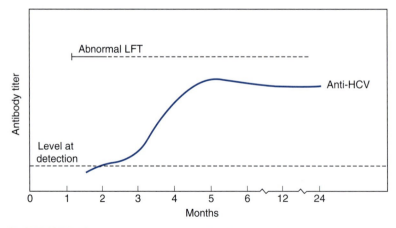

■ FIGURE 7-13 Serologic response to HCV infection showing persistence of detectable antibodies indicating continuous multiplication of HCV.

must be repeatedly reactive by EIA and then confirmed with another method of increased specificity, such as Western blot (WB). This immunoblot detects the viral envelope, core, and replication-associated antigens p17, p24, p31, gp41, p51, p55, p66, and gp120/gp160.

Commercially available HIV EIAs utilize indirect antibody capture and sandwich methodologies. The first generation indirect binding assays were nonspecific. These tests used antigen derived from cellular lysates containing impure mixtures of viral and cellular antigens. Improvements came in the second-generation assays by eliminating cellular lysates and using selected viral antigens made by recombinant technology, thereby improving specificity. This advance allowed the concentration of a few specific viral antigens, limiting interference of nonspecific antibody. Yet biological false-positives still resulted from the bacteria or yeast used in the recombinant technology and a decreased sensitivity to HIV-2 and some of the more divergent subtypes of HIV-1.

In the antibody capture method, anti-human IgG specific for the Fc region of anti-HIV antibody captures HIV specific IgG present in the patient serum. The secondary labeled antigen is derived from either HIV viral lysate or produced by recombinant methods as in the indirect binding assay. If human IgG is bound by the capture IgG, the Fab regions will be available to bind the labeled viral antigen. Essentially this assay is the indirect binding assay described earlier, but performed in reverse.

The third generation of serological testing for HIV-1 is the sandwich assay and is the most sensitive of those described here. This assay is able to detect all classes of antibody produced against HIV-1. There can be limitations in detection of some subtypes if the antigen (recombinant or infected cell lysate) is too specific. This problem can be remedied by using a wider variety of antigens for binding but may then compromise sensitivity.

Fourth-generation HIV tests were developed to address the problem of the window period after infection, that is, the time after exposure but before a detectable immune response in the patient. During this period there is active viral replication and thus the patient is highly infectious, but even the most sensitive antibody detection assays will not be reactive. The fourth-generation assays detect HIV-1 and HIV-2 viral antigen and antibody in various combinations and arrangements simultaneously in an EIA format. There are several different formats available that are being used for blood screening in Europe, but not yet FDA approved for use in the United States.

The standard confirmatory test for an anti-HIV reactive screening test result is the WB. Separation of viral proteins by molecular weight is done by electrophoresis. The resultant gel is then blotted onto a membrane such as nitrocellulose paper, allowing the transfer of viral proteins to the membrane. The membrane is then incubated with patient serum. HIV specific antibody binds to viral proteins on the membrane and may be detected using EIA or biotin-avidin detection systems. Although the test has gone through some advanced development, it still remains essentially a first-generation test with some well-described drawbacks. The use of recombinant antigens has improved the positive predictive value of the test. Interpretation of results is a source of variation due to visual subjectivity and an inability to standardize one interpretive criterion among recommending agencies such as the CDC, World Health Organization (WHO), and the American Red Cross.

Flow through or dot blot membrane HIV EIAs are now commercially available and are used by many laboratories that heretofore did have large volume platform-mediated HIV test capability. These tests have been justified in many laboratories when a rapid turnaround time is of utmost importance, such as in occupational exposure through a needle stick accident. These tests do not require complex laboratory equipment to perform and are suited for screening in remote areas that might not otherwise have access to modern lab services. Additionally, the tests come in multiple, easy-to-use formats with few steps and reagents and can give results in less than 10 minutes.

HIV-2 prevalence in the United States is low, but all blood and blood products must be screened for both HIV-1 and HIV-2. The third generation combined HIV-1/HIV-2 sandwich EIA test is used for screening. This test was modified from the HIV-1 assay by adding HIV-2 specific antigen to the solid phase of the assay. HIV-2 specific labeled antigen is also added to the final detection step so that sensitivity of detection using this combination assay has been shown to approach 99.5%. Confirmation of HIV-2 exposure may be performed using recombinant immunoblot strips similar to the HIV-1 WB.

Although diagnosis of HIV infection is generally accomplished by the detection of HIV specific antibody, an EIA for the viral p24 antigen has been used to detect active viral replication in blood. Its greatest value is in early detection for neonates where serologic diagnosis is of little value due to maternal anti-HIV IgG from a seropositive mother. It is also used in screening blood in transfusion medicine or blood bank laboratories.

Infections Caused by the Family of Herpesviruses

The viruses described here are those taxonomically designated as herpes viruses, and some are described in more detail elsewhere in this chapter. These viruses cause illness ranging from asymptomatic infection to rashes and cutaneous lesions and include serious neurological involvement such as meningitis. Human herpes viruses (HHV) are numbered from one to eight. HHV-1 and HHV-2 are sometimes more commonly referred to as the herpes simplex viruses (HSV). HHV-3 is otherwise known as varicella zoster virus (VZV) and is the causative agent of chicken pox in children and herpes zoster (shingles) in older adults. HHV-4 is the Epstein-Barr virus (EBV) and HHV-5 is cytomegalovirus (CMV). HHV-6, 7, and 8 are associated with childhood exanthem (rashes), Kaposi's sarcoma in AIDS patients, or reactivation in immunocompromised patients. Serological methods are often used to identify exposure to all of the members of the herpes viruses.

Herpes Simplex Viruses

HSVs are, for the most part, ubiquitous. Infections can be caused by either HSV-1 or HSV-2. HSV-1 is most commonly associated with oral lesions and HSV-2 with those found in the genital region; however, this is by no means a certainty. As many as a third of genital herpes isolates are HSV-1. Conversely HSV-2 can infect the oropharyngeal region, but the prevalence of such infections is much lower. As with the other herpes viruses primary infection is followed by latency in the sensory neurons, which may or may not result in periodic reactivation. Clinically, reactivation presents as mucocutaneous lesions (blisters) that rupture and then heal. Other manifestations can include ocular lesions and skin lesions, but the most serious complication is central nervous system involvement, either encephalitis due to HSV-1 or aseptic meningitis due to HSV-2. As with the other members of this family of viruses, reactivation can be much more serious in immunocompromised patients.

Direct culture of the virus from an active lesion is the primary method of diagnosis, but DFA is a rapid detection method for specimens obtained directly from lesions. There are HSV-specific EIA test kits available that are used for serological confirmation of exposure to the viruses. The testing of paired sera for a fourfold titer increase is not always reliable since a primary infection may not be discernible from an episode of reactivation. Because there is significant serological cross-reactivity with HSV, the most specific tests to distinguish HSV-1 from HSV-2 detect antibody to either glycoprotein G1 or glycoprotein G2. The immune response is differential for the two antigens, and can be used to diagnose an infection during the latent period.

Varicella Zoster Virus

A member of the herpesvirus group VZV is the cause of chicken pox in children and shingles in adults. Normally varicella is diagnosed clinically by its characteristic presentation of fever and vesicular rash in pediatric patients. Herpes zoster usually presents itself in older patients as rash spreading along the involved sensory ganglia and is the result of a reactivation of latent virus.

Serological diagnosis of VZV infection is not common. The disease is normally very recognizable by clinical symptoms and quickly confirmed by either viral culture or DFA of vesicular scrapings. HSV infection can complicate a diagnosis of VZV based on serology since the lesions can appear very similar and rises in the titer of antibodies to both viruses occur with coinfections. Current serological methods are very sensitive to the immune response following natural exposure resulting in chicken pox. However, only a glycoprotein specific method for the live viral vaccine strain is highly sensitive for detection of immune response to vaccine. Unfortunately, glycoprotein specific EIAs are not yet commercially available. Latex agglutination is the least sensitive method, while the fluorescent antibody membrane antigen (FAMA) test has been shown to be the most sensitive assay, but it is time consuming as it requires viral replication in cell culture to perform.

Epstein-Barr Virus

EBV is a member of the herpes viridae family, and anti-EBV antibody is associated with several clinical disease diagnoses. Infectious mononucleosis (IM) and Burkitt's lymphoma are two of the more familiar manifestations of infection. Characteristic of the herpes viruses, EBV can appear as both an acute and latent infection and may cause recurring infections in immunocompromised individuals. Serological diagnosis is most often utilized in detection, and there are several methods commercially available in standardized kits. The choice of which test to use depends on the information desired regarding the patient condition. Detection can be as simple as presence or absence of early antibody production to diagnose an acute case. Conversely an entire antibody panel may be needed to judge if a latent infection is involved in a chronic presentation, such as in chronic fatigue syndromes, or involved in malignant conditions such as Burkitt's lymphoma or nasopharyngeal carcinoma.

The earliest and strongest antibody response to EBV-caused infectious mononucleosis is the production of heterophile antibodies. These antibodies agglutinate sheep and horse erythrocytes (SRBC and HRBC) and are adsorbed by beef red blood cells (BRBC) but not guinea pig kidney cells (GPKC). The rapid spot test for IM is performed by mixing the patient serum with aliquots of GPKCs and BRBCs. Horse RBCs are then mixed with each spot. Agglutination present in the BRBC spot only indicates a positive test for heterophile antibodies. The antibodies are detectable in 80% to 90% of IM cases. The heterophile test is less predictive in young children, who often have EBV asymptomatically, as they are not as likely to produce a strong heterophile response. Assays such as the spot test that use animal cells are being replaced by tests with decreased biological cross-reactivity. The next generation of agglutination assays for detection of heterophile antibody is in the form of sensitized latex particle tests. Latex beads (usually colored) are coated with the IM antigen from bovine RBCs and used to test for agglutination in serum.

Antibody panels of patient serum are usually tested by IFA or EIA for the presence of various EBV-specific viral proteins, providing diagnostic information concerning acute or chronic disease. Individually these tests are used for the diagnosis of the approximately 10% of cases where the IM heterophile antibody is not detected. As a complete panel they may be used for epidemiological studies or for determining susceptibility to the infection. Viral capsid antigen (VCA), early antigen (EA) types D (diffuse) and R (restricted), as well as Epstein-Barr nuclear antigen (EBNA), all induce immunoglobulin production. After the appearance of heterophile antibody, there are sharp increases in both viral capsid antigen (VCA) IgM and IgG. The IgM begins to decrease soon after the onset of clinical symptoms and is detectable by approximately eight months after exposure. VCA IgG also begins to decrease after the acute phase but remains at detectable levels for life. EA begins to rise slowly at onset but does not peak until two to four months later when it begins a slow decline to low levels by one year; low titers of EA-R are indicative of a resolved past infection. An increase in the EA-R component can be a signal of either Burkitt's lymphoma or the reactivation of EBV in an immunocompromised patient. Elevation in the levels of VCA and EA IgA antibody in a patient suggests the early stages of nasopharyngeal carcinoma. Epstein-Barr nuclear antigen (EBNA) IgG antibodies typically develop gradually after the resolution of clinical symptoms and are sustained at low levels for life. Figure 7-14■ shows the antibody response to EBV infection.

Serological detection of the EBV-associated antibodies is often accomplished using IFA and reporting antiviral marker titers. These titers may help clinicians determine clinically significant immune reaction versus previous exposure. However IFA has been replaced in some laboratories by EIA utilizing automated platforms. There are numerous commercial manufacturers of both EIA and IFA kits. Sensitivity and specificity can vary considerably, requiring verification studies. Table 7-2✿ shows a summary of EBV serology profiles.

Cytomegalovirus For immunocompromised patients, reactivation of latent CMV associated with organ transplant immunosuppression can signal early progression to end organ disease. However, early CMV structural proteins can be monitored by the CMV antigenemia assay much quicker than by classical viral culture and recognition of cytopathic effect. In this procedure, buffy coats from whole blood specimens are stained by a fluorescent conjugated nonretonal antibody to early viral structural proteins. The number of

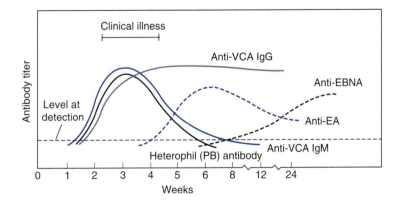

■ FIGURE 7-14 Serologic response to EBV infection showing the rise and decline of detectable antibodies.

⊗ TABLE 7-2

Summary of EBV Serology Profiles

Serologic Markers Present	Patient Status
None	Susceptible to infection
Heterophil antibody (80–90%)	Early primary infection
Anti-VCA IgM and IgG Anti-EA (usually)	Suffering from primary infection
EA-R (low titers) Anti-VCA IgG Anti-EBNA IgG	Past infection
Rise in EA-R	Burkitt's lymphoma or reactivation of EBV
VCA Anti-EA IgA	Possible indication of nasopharyngeal carcinoma

positive PMNs per 100,000 cells is counted. Increased numbers of fluorescently stained PMN nuclei are indicative of increased risk of developing CMV pneumonia or other end organ disease.

Serological testing for CMV is performed to detect IgM or IgG in patient serum but is not FDA approved for screening of blood donors. As with other members of the *Herpesviridae,* diagnosis based on serology alone can be problematic. Disease can be the result of reactivation of a latent infection in which case a rise in antibody titer may not be judged to be a seroconversion. Seropositivity could also be caused by a cross-reaction due to autoimmune disease or infection with another virus such as EBV. The serological profile of an otherwise healthy individual infected with CMV will show a rise in levels of IgM early in infection. Anti-CMV IgM will then decrease and disappear a few months later. CMV specific IgG becomes detectable soon after infection as well, rising, then declining but remaining detectable for life. There are also FDA-approved nucleic acid amplification and hybrid capture assays that can be used to rapidly detect CMV viremia in certain groups of immunocompromised patients. These tests detect viral nucleic acids found in leukocytes, whole blood or plasma and are detected by EIA or chemiluminescence.

Human Herpesviruses 6–8   HHVs 6–8 are the cause, like the other members of the herpesvirus family, of infections that have a primary stage followed by latency that can be reactivated particularly if the patient becomes immunocompromised. The three known HHVs that are not otherwise named are HHV-6, HHV-7,

and HHV-8. The viruses are morphologically similar to the other members of the herpes viruses but are genetically distinct and result in differential immune responses. HHV-6 is implicated in roseola (*exanthem subitum*) in young children. HHV-7 infects children at a slightly later age than HHV-6 and also manifests as exanthem subitum, but can cause disease similar to infection with EBV. HHV-8 is associated with Kaposi's sarcoma in AIDS patients and multicentric Castlemans disease. Infection with HHV-6 and 7 has been shown to cause seroconversion in young children. Detection of serum antibodies is by IFA or EIA, but test kits are not widely commercially available. The same methods have been used to demonstrate seropositivity in most adults, many of whom show no sign of disease. HHV-8 is less common but has been shown to have a higher prevalence in the male population living around the Mediterranean Sea or immunosuppressed populations. Detection is by EIA or IFA for antibodies to both the lytic and latency-associated nuclear antigen (LANA) of HHV-8.

Measles

Measles (rubeola) is a member of the paramyxovirus family along with mumps and shares the droplet route of transmission. It has become difficult to distinguish early measles infection from other contagious droplet spread viruses due to the success of immunization efforts. While prevalence of the disease has decreased, acute infections in poorly vaccinated populations may cause epidemic spread. Adults may also contract the disease later in life when immunity wanes and the infection can be more serious. This same characteristic trend is seen for all three agents covered by the live MMR vaccine, measles, mumps, and rubella. The most devastating manifestation of measles virus infection is the geriatric disease, subacute spongiform pan-encephalitis (SSPE), a brain dementia in which measles viral RNA has been associated. Methods used to measure titers of IgG are CF, HI, or plaque reduction neutralization assays (PRNA). IgM EIA is the serological test used to diagnose recent acute infections. As with most viral infections, a recent infection can also be detected by detecting a fourfold increase in IgG in paired acute and convalescent sera. IgG EIA is used to assess a patient for immune status. Status can be important when it comes to large populations of young adults such as in college or military environments where an underimmunized community could be at risk. Pregnant women also should be evaluated if at increased risk for exposure.

Mumps

Another member of the paramyxovirus family, mumps usually causes generalized, mild disease. The characteristic symptom of swelling of the salivary glands (parotitis) is present in two-thirds of cases, but infections can be subclinical and result in aseptic meningitis or inflammation of other organs. Methods of serological testing for exposure to the mumps virus include CF, HI, SN, IF, and EIA. As with many of the serological assays mentioned previously, the most commonly used method is EIA. As for measles and rubella, the availability of reliable and simple commercial assays has made this the method of choice. EIA procedures for mumps can measure both IgG and IgM antibodies. Mumps-specific IgM suggests recent exposure.

Rubella

Rubella, or German measles, presents clinically as a mild fever and transient rash usually in children. Concern for infection of young adult populations comes from the tendency of the virus to cause congenital defects in fetuses when the nonimmune mother is exposed during pregnancy. Anti-rubella IgG is a good indicator of the immune status of a patient and diagnosis of acute disease can be made by detection of IgM antibody. In postnatal rubella, IgM may be present during the period 1–20 days post-onset, and IgG may be detectable starting approximately eight days following the appearance of the rash. In congenital-related syndrome, IgM can often be detected at birth, with titers declining at approximately 6–12 months. These patients often have consistently high IgG levels, with the maternal IgG being replaced by the infant's. Historically, immunity was detected using sensitive assays, such as passive hemagglutination (PHA) or HA. Detection of antibody can also be rapid and simple, using antigen-coated latex beads, although this is not quite as sensitive. Solid phase capture EIA for IgG and IgM are efficient tests to detect immunity and to aid in serodiagnosis of acute infection.

Parvovirus B19

Parvovirus B19 can cause asymptomatic to potentially fatal infections. The most common manifestation of this virus is the so-called fifth (infectious rash) disease of childhood, named because it was discovered after measles, rubella, varicella, and roseola (HHV-6). This infection is also called erythema infectiosum (EI). Parvovirus B19 can also cause fetal hydrops, sometimes resulting in abortion and fetal death, as well as transient aplastic crisis. The structural VP1 and VP2 antigens are used in most serological assays for the detection of parvovirus B19 antibodies. Nucleic acid testing for viremia and dot-blot immunoassays can be used for research purposes, but neither are FDA-approved diagnostic tests. Detection of IgM using capture assays is the most common method for diagnosing infections. IgM antibody appears within 12 days of infection and may remain detectable for more than six months. IgG, on the other hand, can routinely be detected long-term using an indirect ELISA.

Viral Encephalitis (Arboviruses)

Arboviruses encompass a wide range of morphologically and taxonomically different viruses. The name arbovirus is a shortened version of the common feature of these viruses, their route of transmission. They are commonly spread by arthropod vectors, hence the name *arthropod-borne viruses*. The illnesses resulting from arboviral infection include nondescript fevers, fevers with rashes, arthritis, respiratory distress, pneumonia, hepatitis, encephalitis, and hemorrhagic fevers. Etiological agents represent many viral families, with specific viruses to include West Nile (WNV), rabies, yellow fever, Dengue, St. Louis encephalitis (SLE), Eastern and Western equine encephalitis (EEE, WEE), LaCrosse virus, and the hantaviruses. WNV, hantavirus, and rabies are briefly discussed here.

Most common serological methods (HI, HA, CF, IFA, and EIA) can be used for evaluation of patients suspected of suffering from arboviral infections but with differing degrees of success. IgM and IgG responses in patients follow the typical fourfold increase in titer seen for most viruses. For simple detection, there are FDA-approved testing kits that provide slides fixed with cells infected with several of the more common arboviruses for use with IFA. Unfortunately, with most of these methods there is considerable cross-reactivity between some of the viruses and the possibility of interference from autoimmune conditions. Virus neutralization testing is less prone to cross-reactivity but the availability of suitable test virus can be a problem with the more obscure agents. This capability may be limited to state public health or reference labs.

West Nile Virus   WNV is an arbovirus recently introduced to the United States. The *Culex* mosquito is the vector, and birds are the natural reservoir for the virus. Although most cases are subclinical in presentation with seroprevalence in certain endemic areas near 40%, serious disease can result from infection. The most sensitive detection assay for symptomatic patients is the detection of anti-WNV IgM antibody. It has been shown, however, that IgM antibody may persist and potentially confound acute diagnosis. There are two commercially available FDA-approved IgM capture antibody detection kits.

Hantavirus   Although hantaviruses belong to the family *Bunyaviridae* whose members are frequently arthropod borne, the New World pulmonary hantavirus is spread to humans through the inhalation of viral particles from infected rodent excreta. New World hantavirus or Sin Nombre virus infection became known in the four corners area of the desert southwest in the 1990s after an El Nino year. The abundant rainfall caused an explosion in the rodent population such that humans came into much closer contact than normal with the deer mice harboring the virus. Diagnosis by serology has been performed using EIA for IgM and IgG antibodies specific for Sin Nombre virus, as well as HI, SN, and WB. Commercial serologic assays for Sin Nombre virus antibodies have yet to be marketed, but reagents for testing can be obtained from the CDC. N and G1 viral proteins are the antigen basis for EIA and immunoblot testing. The N protein is highly antigenic and can give cross-reactive results with other hantaviruses while the G1 protein is more specific.

Rabies   Testing for an immune response to rabies is unusual since the disease is almost always fatal once symptoms appear and postexposure immune globulin therapy and vaccine are not always successful treatments. Rabies antibody may be found in serum but usually only after the onset of clinical symptoms and postvaccination. The rapid fluorescent-focus inhibition test (RFFIT) or fluorescent antibody virus neutralization (FAVN) for rabies antibody can be performed on serum. RFFIT can be used on human serum; however, the more recently developed FAVN test is a modified version of the RFFIT used to test antibody titer in animals. In those workers vaccinated for rabies, an EIA is available and sensitive for immune status determination.

▶ IMMUNOLOGIC DETECTION OF FUNGAL AND PARASITIC INFECTION

PNEUMONIA IN IMMUNOCOMPROMISED PATIENTS

Cryptococcus neoformans, cytomegalovirus (CMV), and *Pneumocystis jiroveci* (previously *P. carinii*) are important pulmonary pathogens in transplant, cancer, or AIDS patients. Those with cryptococcal pneumonia or meningitis can be quantitatively monitored for pres-

ence of antigen in serum or CSF by latex agglutination or EIA. A DFA procedure for *P. jiroveci* is approved for use on induced sputum and bronchoscopy specimens. In patients with a high probability of pneumocystis pneumonia, a negative FA on induced sputum should be followed by FA on a bronchoscopically obtained specimen. *P. jiroveci* culture is not widely available, making FA the only reliable method available for its detection in the clinical microbiology laboratory.

CRYPTOCOCCAL MENINGITIS

Cryptococcus neoformans is an important fungal pathogen causing meningitis, pneumonia, and disseminated disease. Antigen testing of CSF, performed by EIA or LA, is considerably more sensitive than direct examination of CSF using India ink. In addition, semi-quantitative antigen detection by LA may be determined by serially diluting CSF or serum. Following the rise or fall of titers is an important prognostic indicator of clinical response to antifungal therapy. An EIA test is also available for detection of *C. neoformans* and can be mathematically equated to serial dilution titers historically performed using LA.

GIARDIASIS AND CRYPTOSPORIDIOSIS

The classical work up for ova and parasites (O&P) requires chemical extraction, concentration, and microscopy of stool specimens. These methods are technically demanding and time consuming. In settings not including areas endemic for certain parasites, a number of studies have been published suggesting that 95% of all clinically important parasites detected in the continental United States are either *Giardia lamblia* or *Cryptosporidium parvum*. Direct FA and EIA kits are available for detection of soluble antigen of these agents directly from stool. Some formats include one monoclonal antibody to detect one organism, while other formats include separate monoclonal antibodies for both organisms. When DFA is utilized, the difference in size between these two parasites allows the technologist to visually distinguish the two organisms using one procedure. Many laboratories offer these tests to screen patients with apparent community acquired diarrhea who are otherwise healthy. Testing algorithms are designed so that only those patients with a history of travel or immunosuppression require a full O&P workup when the screen by EIA/FA is negative. A membrane EIA is FDA approved for the simultaneous detection of *G. lamblia, C. parvum,* and *Entamoeba histolytica* in stool samples.

▶ FUTURE TRENDS

One classical immunology technique that may soon find rapid antigen detection application in the clinical microbiology laboratory is flow cytometry. Recent developments in flow cytometry analysis are utilizing multiple monoclonal antibodies attached to different sized latex beads containing various amounts of different fluorochromes in a multiplex format. These multiplex assays provide the potential to detect up to 64 different antigens in a clinical sample. Currently a multiplex assay is commercially available for serological diagnosis of autoimmune disease.

▶ VERIFICATION AND VALIDATION OF TESTING METHODS

REGULATORY REQUIREMENTS

Clinical laboratories constantly face the challenge of introducing new technology or improving upon existing technology. In the diagnostic immunology or serology laboratory, this may include incorporating (1) a new test using the same diagnostic technology but from a different manufacturer, (2) a new test with the same diagnostic or clinical criteria but with a different methodology, or (3) a new method or technology that exceeds the diagnostic or clinical performance of the currently used test.

Historically, the introduction of new technology into the clinical laboratory was not regulated. Since the 1940s, federal regulations designed to oversee consumer safety have placed increasingly more burden on commercial vendors and diagnostic laboratories to validate the manufacture and use of clinical laboratory tests for patient care. Oversight of manufacturing processes and marketing of product has largely fallen

on the FDA. The use of diagnostic tests in the clinical laboratory involves both federal oversight of good laboratory practice (HHS, FDA, OSHA, CMMS), standardized criteria by which new test introduction must be evaluated (CMMS, NCCLS), and criteria for evaluation of continued performance or proficiency testing (CAP, COLA, CLIA). A list of agencies of legislation with regulatory roles in clinical laboratory medicine is located in Box 7-4✳.

Among the many regulatory recommendations and guidelines, a most practical resource for test method selection and evaluation is Cumitech #31, Verification and Validation of Procedures in the Clinical Microbiology Laboratory. According to Cumitech #31, clinical laboratories are required to establish policies and procedures to maintain or improve the reliability, efficiency, and clinical utility of laboratory tests. This document offers information concerning analytical definitions, federal regulations, test method (selection, verification, and validation), training, and competency.

STATISTICAL ANALYSIS

Definition of the most commonly used terms used in statistical analysis and quality control also describes well how tests may be verified and validated:

Verification. The claims stipulated by the manufacturer in the package insert can be met. Includes performance characteristics such as sensitivity, specificity, positive and negative predictive values, precision, and accuracy. A one-time only process that is achieved before the test is implemented for patient care.

Validation. Once a test is verified, the test is repeatedly giving the expected results over a period of time. This is an ongoing process that generates data to substantiate test algorithms or suggest modifications based on patient population or unique in vitro findings.

Technical Accuracy. The nearness of an individual measurement to the true value, as determined

✳ Box 7-3 Evaluation of Test Methodology	
Current	**Proposed**
Rubella IgG (EIA—Manufacturer A)	Rubella IgG (EIA—Manufacturer B)
Syphilis Ab, nontreponemal (RPR)	Syphilis Ab, nontreponemal (VDRL)
HIV antibody detection (EIA, WB)	HIV antigen detection (Viral load)

✳ Box 7-4   Agencies of Legislation with Regulatory Roles in Clinical Laboratory Medicine

	Agency/Legislation		Agency/Legislation
Oversight	Department of Health and Human Services (HHS)	Evaluation, accreditation, and proficiency	College of American Pathologists (CAP)
	Food and Drug Adminstration (FDA)		Joint Commission on Accreditation of Health Organizations (JCAHO)
	Occupational Safety and Health Association (OSHA)		Commission on Laboratory Accreditation (COLA)
	Centers for Medicare and Medicaid Services (CMS), formerly known as the Health Care Financing Agency (HCFA)		Clinical Laboratory Improvement Acts of 1967 and 1988 (CLIA)
Standardization	National Committee for Clinical Laboratory Standards (NCCLS)		
	Centers for Disease Control and Prevention (CDC)		

by a reference method. Sometimes referred to as test efficiency.

$$\frac{\text{Number of correct results}}{\text{Total number of results}} \times 100$$

Clinical Accuracy. The overall ability of a test to both rule in and rule out an analyte or specific disease.

Analyte. The component of a specimen or organism that is to be measured or demonstrated. In the diagnostic immunology or serology laboratory, the analyte is usually an antibody specific to an antigen of interest.

Precision. Quantitative agreement between replicate analysis using identical procedures. Precision in qualitative analysis is often referred to as reproducibility. Both terms imply freedom from inconsistency and random error but do not guarantee accuracy.

$$\frac{\text{Number of repeated results in agreement}}{\text{Total number of results}} \times 100$$

Analytic Sensitivity. The measurement of the smallest amount of an analyte or a specific disease.

Clinical Sensitivity. The percent test positivity in a population of affected patients.

$$\frac{\text{Number of true positive results}}{\text{Number of true positive plus false negative results}} \times 100$$

Analytic Specificity. The ability to detect only the analyte for which the test is designed.

Clinical Specificity. The percent of negative test results in a population without the specified disease.

$$\frac{\text{Number of true negative results}}{\text{Number of true negative plus false positive results}} \times 100$$

Predictive Value. The Probability that a positive result (positive predictive value, or PPV) accurately indicates the presence of an analyte or specific disease or that a negative result (negative predictive value, or NPV) accurately indicates the absence of an analyte or specific disease.

Prevalence. The pretest probability of a particular clinical state in a specified population; the frequency of a disease in the population of interest at a given point in time.

Gold Standard. The best available approximation of the truth, either a clinical diagnosis or a reference test method.

Home-Brew Test. A procedure developed in-house that uses commercially available or in-house prepared reagents, or any procedure that incorporates modifications of the manufacturer's package insert instructions.

On February 28, 1992, HHS published the final regulation implementing CLIA 88. This legislation extended the federal regulatory mandates of CLIA 67 to cover all laboratories that examine human specimens for the diagnosis, prevention, or treatment of any disease or impairment or for the assessment of the health of human beings. For commercially produced, FDA-approved, nonwaived tests of moderate or high complexity, quality control requirements were established. (Waived tests were exempt from quality control guidelines.) These requirements are addressed in the manufacturer's package insert and must be verified before use in patient testing. For non-FDA approved tests, documented quality control requirements were established to verify and validate performance specifications prior to reporting patient results. Quality control performance characteristics include accuracy, precision, analytical sensitivity and specificity, reportable ranges of patient test results, and reference ranges. The College of American Pathologists (CAP) has recently adopted a molecular checklist that may be used in preparation for accreditation of their molecular laboratories utilizing home-brew, or non-FDA approved, test methods. These test results must be reported with a disclaimer such as "this test was developed and its performance characteristics determined by (laboratory name); it has not been cleared or approved by the U.S. Food and Drug Administration."

ADOPTING A SEROLOGICAL TEST FOR USE IN THE CLINICAL LABORATORY

Once a decision is made to offer a new test capability, the laboratory must select the method by which the test will be performed. The following questions and suggestions are designed to serve as a guide for the initial selection of a laboratory method.

1. For what purpose will the lab test be used—screening, confirmation, or diagnosis?

2. What analyte will be detected, for example, detection of antigen specific antibody?

3. What is the reference method or gold standard?

4. Request input from the health care providers to determine medical usefulness and impact on patient outcomes.

5. Review the medical literature concerning the use of related laboratory test methods and impact on the related diagnosis.

6. Analyze laboratory management associated parameters such as cost effectiveness, practical performance, impact on work flow, shifting and staffing, turnaround time, batching, quality control, avail-

ability of proficiency test materials, special equipment, and adequate space.

7. Analyze technical requirements such as type of specimen, collection and transport, reagent availability and shelf-life, technical support, safety, and published reference ranges in patient populations.

Verification of an FDA Approved, Commercially Available Moderate or High-Complexity Test

Verification of a nonwaived, FDA-approved test is accomplished by performing the new method with known samples according to the manufacturer's package insert. The parallel study may be performed with existing validated technology or a known reference method. The evaluation should consist of at least 20 specimens containing the target analyte and at least 50 specimens that do not contain the target analyte.

Verification of a Non-FDA Approved, Commercially Available Test or In-House Home-Brew Test

Verification of a non-FDA approved test starts with performing the new method with known samples against an established reference method. The evaluation should consist of at least 50 specimens containing the target analyte and at least 100 specimens that do not contain the target analyte. Additionally, a non-FDA approved test, or home-brew test, must undergo continual validation and quality control assessment in the patient population. The parameters of such a validation have been discussed in this section.

Reporting of results for non-FDA approved tests can be confusing. In laboratories with a CLIA certificate or accredited by deemed organizations such as the CAP, results may be recorded in the laboratory information system (LIS) and posted to the patient record with a disclaimer of FDA approval. Non-FDA approved tests may be reported as investigational use only (IUO) under informed consent. If the test utilizes a research use only (RUO) technology, the results should not be recorded in the LIS nor posted to the patient's record, and should be used only in accordance with other clinical factors in making a diagnosis or therapeutic decisions. There are some exceptions to reporting RUO results, in which the commercial manufacturer and the FDA negotiate a specific test reagent and performance criteria. This situation occurs most frequently in viral load testing which is described in the chapter on molecular detection methodology.

SUMMARY

Significant progress has been made in the development and improvement of immunoassay testing. Direct detection of antigen, commercially available automated test platforms, and new test methodologies highlight the advances made in the infectious disease serological laboratory. Yet these advancements have not necessarily replaced older conventional technology, but are often used to supplement, efficiently increase test volumes, or detect newly described infectious agents of clinical significance. Of particular significance are the rapid detection immunoassays that immediately influence patient care management and therapeutic decisions. This capability is particularly important for those microorganisms that are difficult to culture by conventional methods. Such clinical impact ensures continued research and development of rapid diagnostic testing technologies. Other technologies that have been recently developed for similar reasons, such as nucleic acid amplification and detection, are discussed at length in a later chapter. There is little doubt that the variety and quality of immunoassay reagents and test platforms will increase in the future. Again, laboratory scientists will have to make wise choices regarding the most cost-effective and clinically relevant use of these reagents.

POINTS TO REMEMBER

▶ Antigen detection methods are based on precipitation, particle agglutination, complement fixation, immunofluorescence, or enzyme immunoassay.

▶ The increased number of diagnostic test kits commercially available is directly related to the ability to produce large quantities of monoclonal antibodies to many different organisms.

▶ Quality control requirements for commercially produced, FDA-approved, nonwaived tests of moderate or high complexity have been established and must be verified before use in patient testing.

▶ For non-FDA approved tests, documented quality control requirements must be established to verify and validate performance specifications prior to reporting patient results.

▶ Quality control performance characteristics include accuracy, precision, analytical sensitivity and specificity, reportable ranges of patient test results, and reference ranges.

LEARNING ASSESSMENT QUESTIONS

1. Bacterial capsular polysaccharide would be considered a(n)
   a. antibody.
   b. antigenic determinant.
   c. epitope.
   d. antigen binding site.

2. A latex bead test would be considered what type of assay?
   a. precipitation
   b. complement fixation
   c. coagulation
   d. agglutination

3. All of the following are disadvantages of immunofluorescent staining *except:*
   a. decreased specificity.
   b. subjective interpretation.
   c. lack of automation.
   d. fading of fluorescence over time.

4. The "gold standard" test for streptococcal pharyngitis is the
   a. membrane-bound EIA.
   b. latex agglutination test.
   c. optical immunoassay.
   d. throat culture.

5. Serological diagnosis of rhinovirus infections has proven to be difficult because
   a. rhinoviruses are only weakly antigenic.
   b. antibodies against rhinoviruses cross-react with adenoviruses.
   c. there are so many serotypes of rhinovirus.
   d. rhinoviruses induce production of noncomplement fixing antibodies.

REFERENCES

Aldeen, W. E., K. Carroll, et al. 1998. Comparison of nine commercially available enzyme-linked immunosorbent assays for detection of *Giardia lamblia* in fecal specimens. *J Clin Microbiol* 36:1338–40.

Ammons, B. S., D. L. Smalley, and B. M. Madison. 1994, Evaluation of a new, rapid latex test for the detection of heterophil antibody. *Clin Lab Sci.* 7:243–44.

Ashley, R. L., A. Wald, and M. Eagleton. 2000. Premarket evaluation of the POCkit HSV-2 type-specific serological test in culture-documented cases of genital herpes simplex virus type 2. *Sex Transm Dis.* 27:270–71.

Blomqvist, S., M. Roivainen, T. Puhakka, M. Kleemola, and T. Hovi. 2000. Virological and serological analysis of rhinovirus infections during the first two years of life in a cohort of children. *J Med Virol* 66:263–68.

Buck, G. E. 1989. Noncultural methods of detection and identification of microorganisms in clinical specimens. *Pediatr Clin North Am* 36:95.

Chan, P. K., M. Ip, K. C. Ng, et al. 2003. Severe acute respiratory syndrome-associated coronavirus infection. *Emerg Infect Dis* 9:1453–54.

Chan, P. K. S., W-K To, K-C Ng, et al. 2004. Laboratory diagnosis of SARS. *Emerg Infect Dis* 10:825–31.

Cliquet, F., M. Aubert, and L. Sagne. 1998. Development of a fluorescent antibody virus neutralisation test (FAVN test) for the quantitation of rabies-neutralising antibody. *J Immunol Methods* 212:79–87.

Constantine, N. T., and D. P. Lana. 2003. Immunoassays for the diagnosis of infectious diseases. In: *Manual of Clinical Microbiology*, 8th ed., ed. P. R. Murray, E. J. Baron, et al. American Society for Microbiology, Washington, DC, pp. 218–33.

Cook, L. 1998. New assays for infectious agents replacing traditional serologic methods. *Advance for Medical Laboratory Professionals* 12–15.

Corbett, J. V. 2000. *Laboratory Tests and Diagnostic Procedures with Nursing Diagnoses*, 5th ed. Prentice Hall Health, Upper Saddle River.

Craft, D. W. 2000. Emergent technologies. In: *Textbook of Diagnostic Microbiology*, 2nd ed., ed. C. Mahon and G. W. Manuselis. W. B. Saunders, Philadelphia, PA, pp. 130–90.

Craft, D. W., L. E. Williams et al. 1995. Rapid diagnostic testing for antibody to human immunodeficiency virus (HIV) in a deployed laboratory. *Mili Med Lab Sci* 24:16–21.

Dean, D., D. Ferrero, et al. 1998. Comparison of performance and cost-effectiveness of direct fluorescent-antibody, ligase chain reaction, and PCR assays for verification of chlamydial enzyme immunoassay results for populations with a low to moderate prevalence of *Chlamydia trachomatis* infection. *J Clin Microbiol* 36:94–99.

Elder, B. L., S. A. Hansen, J. A. Kellogg, et al. 1997. *Cumitech 31: Verification and Validation of Procedures in the Clinical Microbiology Laboratory*. American Society for Microbiology, Washington, DC.

Facklam, R. R. 1997. Screening for streptococcal pharyngitis: Current technology. *Infect Med* 14:891–98.

Forbes, B. A., D. F. Sahm, and A. S. Weissfeld, eds. 2002. Imunochemical methods used for organism detection. In: *Bailey and Scott's Diagnostic Microbiology*, 11th ed. C. V. Mosby, St. Louis, MO, pp. 189–201.

Forbes, B. A., D. F. Sahm, and A. S. Weissfeld, eds. 2002. Imunochemical methods used for organism detection. In: *Bailey and Scott's Diagnostic Microbiology*, 11th ed. C. V. Mosby, St. Louis, MO, pp. 324–55.

Gentilomi, G., M. Musiani, M. Zerbini, et al. 1997. Dot immunoperoxidase assay for detection of Parvovirus B19 antigens in serum samples. *J Clin Micro* 35: 1575–78.

Gerna, G. E., Percivalle, et al. 1998. Standardization of the human cytomegalovirus antigenemia assay by means of in vitro-generated pp65-positive peripheral blood polymorphonuclear leukocytes. *J Clin Microbiol* 36:3585–89.

Gray, L. D., and D. P. Fedorko. 1992. Laboratory diagnosis of bacterial meningitis. *Clin Microbiol Rev* 5:130–45.

Gupta, A. K., and G. S. Sarin. 1983. Serum and tear immunoglobulin levels in acute adenovirus conjunctivitis. *Br J Opthalmol* 67: 195–98.

Halsted, D. C. 1987. Noncultural methods for diagnosing respiratory syncytial virus infections. *Clin Microbiol Newsletter* 9:181–85.

Health Matters. 2002, November *Syphilis*. National Institute of Allergy and Infectious Disease, National Institute of Health.

Henrard, D. R., S. Wu, et al. 1995. Detection of p24 antigen with and without immune complex dissociation for longitudinal monitoring of human immunodeficiency virus type 1 infection. *J Clin Microbiol* 33:72–75.

Henry, J. B., 2001. *Clinical Diagnosis and Management by Laboratory Methods*, 20th ed. W. B. Saunders Company, Philadelphia, PA.

Ho, T. Y., S. L. Wu, S. E. Cheng, et al. 2004. Antigenicity and receptor-binding ability of recombinant SARS coronavirus spike protein. *Biochem Biophys Res Commun* 313: 938–47.

Hodinka, R. L. 2002. Automated immunoassay analyzers. In: *Manual of Commercial Methods in Clinical Microbiology*, ed. A. Truant. American Society for Microbiology, Washington, DC, pp. 324–55.

Julkunen, I., K. Lehtomaki, and T. Hovi. 1986. Immunoglobulin class-specific serological responses to adenovirus in respiratory infections of young adult men. *J Clin Micro.* 24: 112–15.

Kaier, B., and R. Wigand. 1986. Antigenic homogeneity of adenovirus types 1, 2, 5, and 6. *J Med Virol* 18: 283–87.

Kehl, K. S. C., H. Cicirello et al. 1995. Comparison of four different methods for detection of *Cryptosporidium* species. *J Clin Microbiol* 33:416–18.

Kim, M., and M. Wadke. 1990. Comparative evaluation of two test methods (enzyme immunoassay and latex fixation) for the detection of heterophil antibodies in infectious mononucleosis. *J Clin Micro* 28: 2511–13.

Kohler, R. B., ed. 1986. *Antigen Detection to Diagnose Bacterial Infections*. CRC Press, Boca Raton, FL.

Koneman, E. W., S. D. Allen, et al., eds. 1997. *Color Atlas and Textbook of Diagnostic Microbiology*, 5th ed. Lippincott-Raven, Philadelphia.

Larsen, S., E. Hunter, and S. Kraus. 1990. *A Manual of Tests for Syphilis*. American Public Health Association.

Limaye, A. P., D. K. Turgeon, et al. 2000. Pseudomembranous colitis caused by a toxin A-B+ strain of *C. difficile*. *J Clin Microbiol* 38:1696–97.

Mackenzie, A. M. R., P. Lebel, et al. 1998. Sensitivities and specificities of Premier E. coli O157 and Premier EHEC enzyme immunoassays for diagnosis of infection with verotoxin (shiga-like toxin)-producing *Escherichia coli*. *J Clin Microbiol* 36:1608–11.

Malan, A. K., T. B. Matins, H. R. Hill, and C. M. Litwin. 2004. Evaluations of commercial West Nile virus immunoglobulin G (IgG) and IgM enzyme immunoassays show the value of continuous validation. *J Clin Micro* 42:727–33.

Margalith, M., L. G. Chatlynne, E. Fuchs et al. 2003. Human herpesvirus 8 infection among various population groups in southern Israel. *J Acquir Immune Defic Syndr* 34:500–505.

Meurman, O., O. Ruuskanen, and H. Sarkkinen. 1983. Immunoassay diagnosis of adenovirus infections in children. *J Clin Micro* 18:1190–95.

Nasci, R. S. and C. Moore. 1998. Vector-borne disease surveillance and natural disasters. *Emerg Inf Dis* 4(2).

Needham, C. A., K. A. McPherson et al. 1998. Steptococcal pharyngitis: Impact of a high-sensitivity antigen test on physician outcome. *J Clin Microbiol* 36:3468–73.

Ni, A. P., Z. Wang, Y. Liu et al. 2003. [Isolation and Identification of SARS-coronavirus in nasal and throat swabs collected from clinically diagnosed SARS patients.] *Zhongguo Yi Xue Ke Xue Yuan Xue Bao* 25:520–24.

O'Connor, D., P. Hynes et al. 2001. Evaluation of methods for detection of toxins in specimens of feces submitted for diagnosis of *C. difficile*–associated diarrhea. *J Clin Microbiol* 39:2846–49.

Okano, M., G. M. Thiele, and D. T. Purtilo. 1990. Severe chronic active Epstein-Barr virus infection syndrome and adenovirus type-2 infection. *Am J Pediatr Hematol Oncol* 12:168–73.

Parslow, T. G., D. P. Stites, A. I. Terr, and J. B. Imboden. 2001. *Medical Immunology,* 10th ed. McGraw-Hill (Lange Medical Books), New York.

Payne, W. J., D. L. Marshall et al. 1988. Clinical laboratory applications of monoclonal antibodies. *Clin Microbiol Rev* 1:313–29.

Peace-Brewer, A., D. W. Craft, and J. L. Schmitz. 2000. Immunological techniques in the clinical microbiology laboratory. *Lab Medicine* 31:24–29.

Rose, N. R., R. G. Hamilton, B. Detrick et al., eds. 2002. *Manual of Clinical Laboratory Immunology,* 6th ed. American Society for Microbiology, Washington, DC.

Schwartz, E. J., R. F. Dorfman, and S. Kohler. 2003. Human herpesvirus-8 latent nuclear antigen-1 expression in endemic Kaposi sarcoma: An immunohistochemical study of 16 cases. *Am J Surg Pathol* 27:1546–50.

Sewell, D. L., and J. D. MacLowry. 2003. Laboratory management. In: *Manual of Clinical Microbiology,* 8th ed., ed. P. R. Murray, E. J. Baron et al. American Society for Microbiology, Washington, DC, pp. 4–21.

Sokhandan, M., E. R. McFadden, Y. Huang, and M. Mazanec. 1995. The contribution of respiratory viruses to severe exacerbations of asthma in adults. *Chest* 107:1570–75.

Svahn, A., M. Magnusson, L. Jagdahl et al. 1997. Evaluation of three commercial enzyme-linked immunosorbent assays and two latex agglutination assays for diagnosis of primary Epstein-Barr virus infection. *J Clin Micro* 35:2728–32.

Tilton, R. C., F. Dias, R. W. Ryan. 1988. Comparative evaluation of three commercial tests for detection of heterophile antibody in patients with infectious mononucleosis. *J Clin Micro* 26:275–78.

Uzieblo, A., G. Storch, and A. M. Gronowski. 2002. Diagnosis of cytomegalovirus infection. *Laboratory Medicine Newsletter–*Washington University School of Medicine 8(11).

Wang, J., J. Wen, J. Li et al. 2003. Assessment of immunoreactive synthetis peptides from the structural proteins of severe acute respiratory syndrome coronavirus. *Clin Chem* 49:1989–96.

Weber, B., E. L. M. Fall, A. Berger, and H. W. Doerr. 1998. Reduction of diagnostic window by new fourth-generation human immunodeficiency virus screening assays. *J Clin Micro* 36:2235–39.

Whittier, S., D. S. Shapiro et al. 1994. Evaluation of four commercially available enzyme immunoassays for laboratory diagnosis of *Clostridium difficile*–associated disease. *J Clin Microbiol* 31:2861–65.

Wolfson, J. S., M. A. Waldron et al. 1989. Blinded comparison of a direct immunofluorescent monoclonal antibody staining method for identification of *Pneumocystis carinii* in induced sputum and bronchoalveolar lavage specimens of patients infected with human immunodeficiency virus. *J Clin Microbiol* 28:2136–38.

Woods, G. L. and J. A. Washington. 2004. The clinician and the microbiology laboratory. In: *Principles and Practice of Infectious Disease,* 6th ed., ed. G. L. Mandell, J. E. Bennett et al. Churchill Livingstone, New York.

Zimmerman, S. K. and C. A. Needham. 1995. Comparison of conventional stool concentration and preserved-smear methods with Merifluor *Cryptosporidium/Giardia* direct immunofluorescence assay and ProSpectT *Giardia* ED microplate assay for detection of *Giardia lamblia. J Clin Microbiol* 33:1942–43.

8

Autoimmune Diseases and Immunodeficiency Disorders

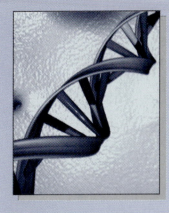

CHAPTER CHECKLIST

After reading and studying this chapter, the reader should be able to:

1. List and explain the major factors that may stimulate production of autoantibodies.

2. Differentiate between organ-specific and systemic autoimmune diseases.

3. For each disease in the chapter explain:
   - clinical manifestations.
   - mechanism of destruction.
   - self-antigens involved.
   - diagnostic testing.
   - treatment.

4. Differentiate between primary and secondary immunodeficiencies.

5. Discuss the utility of research on immunodeficiency disorders as it relates to an overall understanding of immune function.

6. For each immunodeficiency disorder in the chapter explain the:
   - clinical presentation and manifestations of the disorder.
   - defect in the immune system responsible for the disorder.
   - diagnostic testing.
   - treatment.

CHAPTER OUTLINE

CASE IN POINT #1

A 35-year-old female visited her physician complaining of fatigue, myalgia, and joint pain. Her history was unremarkable, and she had had no transfusions or surgeries. She had delivered a healthy male infant after her last pregnancy five years ago. Her CBC showed a hemoglobin of 10.9 g/L and a slightly decreased platelet count. All other values were within normal range.

ISSUES TO CONSIDER

After reading the patient's case, consider

- The diagnostic tests that should be performed

- The possible diagnoses and why should these diagnoses be considered

- Treatment of the disease

CASE IN POINT #2

An 18-month-old girl was taken to her pediatrician complaining of fever, chills, myalgia, nausea, and vomiting. Because she had a history since birth of multiple viral, bacterial, and fungal infections, many of them requiring hospitalization combined with intensive antibiotic therapy, she was hospitalized and referred to a pediatric hematologist. A differential count showed profound lymphopenia, with fewer than 500 lymphocytes/ml. Further analysis showed that she lacked B lymphocytes, T lymphocytes, and natural killer cells. Her parents were extremely disturbed because an older sister had died at the age of three after a similar clinical course. An older sister and brother have had no evidence of serious illness.

ISSUES TO CONSIDER
After reading the patient's case history, consider

- Whether this is a primary or secondary immunodeficiency
- The branch of the immune system that is affected
- The most probable type of immunodeficiency
- If this disorder is most likely to arise from a spontaneous mutation or as an inherited disease; if inherited, the mode of inheritance
- How this disorder might be treated

IMPORTANT TERMS

Acquired immunodeficiency syndrome (AIDS)
Adenosine deaminase
Anergy
Anti-idiotypic antibody
Antinuclear antibody
Antinuclear Antibody (ANA) Test
Ataxia telangiectasia
Autoantibody
Autoimmune disease
Autoimmune hepatitis
Bare lymphocyte syndrome
Bruton's agammaglobulinemia
CD3 complex deficiency
CD5+ cells
Central tolerance
Chediak-Higashi syndrome
Chronic granulomatous disease (CGD)
Common variable immunodeficiency (CVID)
Co-stimulatory signal
C-reactive protein (CRP)
CREST syndrome
Cross-reactive antibodies
Cyclic neutropenia

Cytokines
DiGeorge syndrome
Discoid lupus
Epitope spreading
Forbidden clone theory
Goodpasture's syndrome
Graves' disease
Hashimoto's thyroiditis
Heat shock proteins (HSP)
Highly active retroviral therapy (HART)
Horror autotoxicus
Immune complex
Immunologic deficiency theory
Immunologic ignorance
Job's syndrome
Leukocyte adhesion deficiency (LAD)
Molecular mimicry
Multiple sclerosis
Myasthenia gravis
Negative selection
Neoantigens
Omenn's syndrome
Paroxysmal nocturnal hemaglobinuria (PNH)

Peripheral tolerance
Pernicious anemia
Positive selection
Primary biliary cirrhosis
Primary immunodeficiency
Reticular dysgenesis
Reverse transcriptase
Rheumatoid arthritis
Rheumatoid factor
Scleroderma
Secondary immunodeficiency
Self-antigen
Sequestered antigen theory
Severe combined immunodeficiency (SCID)
Signal transduction
Sjorgen's syndrome
Superantigens
Systemic lupus erythematosus
Tolerance
Type I diabetes mellitus
Wiskott-Aldrich syndrome
X-inactivation
X-linked
X-linked hyper-IgM
ZAP-70

► INTRODUCTION

The body is uniquely programmed to recognize and respond through the immune system to foreign or non-self antigens. It routinely ignores or does not respond to those antigens that are self-antigens. In previous chapters, the role of the major histocompatibility complex (MHC) in recognition and processing of foreign antigens, the maturation and role of lymphocytes, the formation and characteristics of immunoglobulins, and the basic interaction between antigen and antibody were discussed.

The first sections of this chapter focus on what happens when the immune system responds, not to a foreign antigen, but to a self-antigen. This inappropriate response then leads to the development of autoimmunity. The major autoimmune diseases, including the humoral and/or cellular immune response underlying the disease, the clinical presentation, and the laboratory tests used for diagnosis are considered.

In the second portion of the chapter, failure of the immune system will be explored. Immunodeficiency disorders, whether primary or secondary, present with clinical symptoms reflective of the portion of the immune response affected. Defects may occur in lymphocytes, the MHC, the complement pathway, phagocytes, or a combination. Recurrent viral, fungal, and/or bacterial infections, depending on where the defect lies, are the hallmark of an immunodeficiency. Investigation of these disorders has led not only to some successful treatments, but also to a greater understanding of the immune system as a whole.

► AUTOIMMUNE DISEASES

DEFINITION OF AUTOIMMUNITY

The origins of the concept of autoimmunity go back to the early 1900s when Paul Ehrlich proposed **horror autotoxicus**—the idea that the body does not normally respond to its own antigens, but, if it does, the individual is harmed. Autoimmunity can, therefore, be broadly defined as the immune system's failure to recognize **self-antigens** followed by an immune response against those antigens. There may be activation of, and invasion by, T cells or increased production of **autoantibodies** by B cells with no identifiable underlying cause. During the early study of immunology, there were several theories that attempted to explain the mechanisms behind the development of autoimmunity. These included the

forbidden clone theory, the sequestered antigen theory, and the immunologic deficiency theory. Very simplistically, the forbidden clone theory proposed that if a clone of lymphocytes reactive with self-antigen was not destroyed, the immune system could react with self-antigen and cause disease. The sequestered antigen theory stated that some antigens were hidden from the immune system recognition. If, by accident, an antigen was to be released to interact with lymphocytes, the antigen would not be recognized as "self," and an immune response would be initiated. The immunologic deficiency theory addressed the balance between T suppressor lymphocytes, T helper lymphocytes, and B lymphocytes. It suggested that, as an individual ages, suppressor T lymphocytes decline in number and can no longer control the interaction between T helper and B lymphocytes. One consequence is the increased production of autoantibodies. As knowledge of the immune system has increased, each of these ideas has been refined and now explains a small part of the complex immunological response. These concepts will be alluded to in later parts of the chapter to show how the underlying premise has developed.

More than 40 diseases, affecting 5% to 7% of the U.S. population, have been identified as having an underlying autoimmune etiology. Some diseases such as **systemic lupus erythematosus** (SLE) show strong evidence of an autoimmune response, but for others the evidence is less convincing. **Autoimmune diseases** cause significant morbidity and mortality due to their chronic nature. The overall rate at which women are affected is higher than men (i.e., average of 2.7 females to 1 male). Although for some diseases such as SLE, it is even higher. Most autoimmune diseases occur in adults, but **Type 1 diabetes mellitus** is common in children. Onset of autoimmune diseases typically occurs between the ages of 20–40 years (as suggested in Case Study #1), although a few such as rheumatoid arthritis may occur later in life with onset up to age 60.

In the initial stage of some diseases, infiltration by T lymphocytes may induce inflammation and tissue damage, leading to alterations in self-antigens and subsequent production of autoantibodies. In others, there does not appear to be initial tissue damage, only production of autoantibody. These autoantibodies have a wide range of immune activities that cause damage to tissue. They attack cell surface antigens or membrane receptors or combine with antigen to form immune complexes that are deposited in tissue, subsequently causing complement activation and inflammation.

NORMAL ROLE OF AUTOANTIBODIES

The presence of autoantibodies in an individual does not mean that the person has an autoimmune disease. For autoimmune disease to occur, there must not only be the presence of autoantibodies, but there must also be damage to specific organs or organ systems. Knowledge about, and recognition of, the normal role of autoantibodies in the functioning of the immune system has evolved over a number of years. Some autoantibodies that are present in low titers function in clearing dead cells and defective self-antigens or in removing injured cellular components by binding to these molecules. It is now known that there is a subpopulation of **CD5+ cells** that normally produce autoantibodies responsible for the "cleanup" mechanisms in the body. Autoantibodies can also regulate the immune response by forming immune complexes. When a new epitope forms on an immunoglobulin (Ig) molecule, it can act as a stimulus to production of antibodies directed against it (anti-idiotype). Once the **anti-idiotypic antibody** binds to its corresponding Ig molecule, an **immune complex** is formed. This complex is cleared by phagocytosis in the reticuloendothelial system, thus eliminating excess antibody. These beneficial activities of autoantibodies serve in some measure to regulate immune response to self-antigens.

DEVELOPMENT OF CENTRAL AND PERIPHERAL TOLERANCE

The discussion of the normal immune response in previous chapters indicated that there are two signals required for the immune response—one from the presentation of the foreign antigen by an antigen-presenting cell (APC) and another from the appropriate MHC molecule on the host's cells. Without both signals, there is no immune response. To understand autoimmunity, knowledge of how the body develops nonresponsiveness (tolerance) to self-antigens is necessary.

Tolerance is the lack of immune response to self-antigens and is initiated during fetal development (**central tolerance**) by elimination of those cells with the potential to react strongly with self-antigens. **Peripheral tolerance,** which is a process involving mature lymphocytes, occurs in the circulation. The following section provides a brief review of the relationship between tolerance and autoimmunity.

Central Tolerance

As you learned in a previous chapter, central tolerance develops in the thymus during fetal life. This process, in which self-antigens are presented by dendritic cells to self-reactive T cells, is responsible for both positive selection and **negative selection** of specific lymphocytes. Its ultimate purpose is to remove those T cells that respond strongly to self-antigens. As genes rearrange and code for antigen receptors, the T cell receptors (TCRs) that are produced may or may not be specific for the MHC expressed on that individual's cells. In **positive selection,** those cells that have T cell receptors capable of responding with self-antigens MHC low level affinity are selected for continued growth.

The immature T cells (thymocytes) first encounter Class I and II self-MHC molecules when they are presented by thymic epithelial cells. Those thymocytes that are not MHC-restricted (able to react with that individual's self-MHC) cannot bind and die by apoptosis. This ensures that cells can respond when antigens are presented by these particular self-MHCs.

Cells that survive positive selection but express high-affinity receptors for self-MHC molecules undergo negative selection. In this process, the T lymphocytes interact with dendritic cells and macrophages that possess class I and II MHC. If the cells react with self-MHC molecules or with a combination of self-antigen and self-MHC, they are eliminated because they show potential for autoreactivity and could, in turn, initiate autoimmunity. Therefore, self-tolerance is initiated. The process of negative selection, however, does not eliminate those T cells that have receptors for self-peptides that are present specifically on tissue other than those present in the thymus.

B cells may also receive either stimulation or deletion signals in the bone marrow, but the process is less well understood. As discussed in Chapter 3, it appears that nonhematologic cells (dendritic cells) present the self-antigen to immature B cells. Without T cell costimulation, the clone is eliminated.

Peripheral Tolerance

Some potentially self-reactive lymphocytes are not eliminated in the thymus and enter the peripheral circulation. For these cells to be activated, self-antigen must be presented by cells with a high density of MHC complexes to cross-link with TCR, or the T cell must receive costimulatory signals from an APC with HLA-B7. Despite the potential exposure to self-antigens in the peripheral circulation, several processes may intervene to prevent this interaction. These include sequestration of self-antigen (**immunologic ignorance**), anergy, or active termination by immune regulation. In sequestration, self-reactive lymphocytes do not respond because the self-antigen is normally anatomically sequestered, preventing interaction with the lymphocyte. Cells do not encounter the antigen and therefore remain "ignorant" of it. In addition, MHC expression may be too low to activate the cells. Examples of this type of self-antigen include the lens protein of the eye, antigens on spermatozoa, and the myelin basic protein of the central nervous system. If the antigen is released as a result of injury, cells respond as if it is a foreign antigen. In the cases of spermatozoa and lens protein, the immune response is relatively short-lived, but in the case of myelin basic protein, the development of multiple sclerosis may occur.

In T cell anergy one or the other of the **co-stimulatory signals** (HLA-B7 on the APC or Class II MHC on a CD 38+ T cell) is absent. Without these, the T lymphocyte becomes functionally inactive and dies by apoptosis. B cell anergy in the peripheral circulation is due to increased immunoglobulin expression on the cell surface and cell signaling inhibition. Other active termination processes include apoptosis of self-reactive T cells or B cells by *Fas*-mediated activation, negative signaling, anti-idiotypic antibodies, and IL-2 mediated feedback.

Predisposing Factors

Why does the immune system lose tolerance to self-antigen? It is now believed to be not only a combination of genetic, hormonal, and environmental factors, but also failure of some regulatory sequence in the immune response.

Genetic Individuals may inherit genes that predispose them to autoimmune disease or may lack genes that confer protection against autoimmune diseases. Genes of the MHC complex are linked to susceptibility to autoimmune diseases. A number of HLA class I molecules as well as class II molecules are associated with specific autoimmune diseases. These HLA antigens are not directly responsible for autoimmune disease but may alter the host response to environmental factors or predispose the host to an immune system imbalance. The correlation between the presence of HLA B-27 and ankylosing spondylitis has been the most frequently cited example of this relationship. More than 90% of the patients with ankylosing spondylitis have the HLA B-27 gene. However, this HLA phenotype is not the direct cause of the disease because only 2% of people with HLA B-27 have ankylosing spondylitis. The association between some common autoimmune diseases and HLA antigens is shown in

Table 9-6 (Chapter 9). Alterations in the CD4+25+ regulatory cells may also predispose an individual to autoimmune diseases. Individuals with first generation relatives with an autoimmune disease are also more likely to develop either that disease or another autoimmune disease.

Hormonal Autoimmune diseases occur more frequently in women than in men. Although the exact role of sex hormones is not known, most autoimmune diseases have an onset in women during childbearing years when estrogen production is at its peak. This was evident in Case in Point 1. Studies on the animal model (NZB/NZW mouse) of systemic lupus erythematosus show that the severity of the disease was decreased when female mice were treated with androgens, which are known to enhance CD8+ cell function. In contrast, male mice treated with estrogens, which can suppress CD8+ cell function, had a more severe form of the disease.

Environmental Infectious agents including bacteria and viruses have long been proposed as a possible stimulus for developing autoimmune diseases. These organisms cause inflammatory conditions that can lead to changes in self-antigens. These changes may in turn provoke an autoimmune response. Some of the mechanisms involved include **molecular mimicry,** alteration of self-antigens, physical trauma leading to release or exposure of sequestered antigens, polyclonal activation of self-reactive lymphocytes, and altered expression of the MHC receptors. In addition, drugs such as penicillin can elicit production of autoantibodies. These drugs bind to the erythrocyte membrane to create **neoantigens.** In some cases, the antibodies produced are capable of reacting not only with the drug-coated cells, but also with normal erythrocyte membrane antigens.

Exposure of Sequestered Antigens As mentioned previously, tissues such as sperm-forming tissue in the testes, proteins of the anterior chamber of the eye, or the myelin basic protein of the central nervous system are not exposed to immune cells for recognition during the crucial periods of fetal development. They are not recognized as "self". In infections or as a result of trauma, injured or damaged cells die by the process of necrosis and release self-antigens that had not been previously presented to self-reactive T cells. These antigens are recognized as foreign and initiate an immune response leading to production of autoantibodies.

Molecular Mimicry and Cross-Reactive Antibodies   Viral or bacterial organisms may stimulate formation of autoantibodies by a number of related mechanisms including molecular mimicry, formation of superantigens, or epitope spreading. When an organism infects the host, the host's T lymphocytes are activated by antigenic determinants on the infectious agent. Alteration of self-antigens can also occur during the inflammation, resulting in the creation of neopeptides. During the immune response, antibodies are produced that are capable of reacting not only with the organism's antigenic determinants, but also cross-reacting with host antigenic determinants that closely resemble the organism's antigens. The development of these cross-reacting antibodies is the most likely mechanism involved in poststreptococcal rheumatic fever in which antibodies to Group A *Streptococcus* react with antigens on cardiac muscle. Studies have shown that T cell antigenic receptors may also recognize single shared peptides or structurally related peptides.

Evidence has linked bacterial **heat shock proteins (HSP)** to a role in autoimmunity. These antigens, which are known to be homologous with a number of tissue proteins are, however, foreign enough to stimulate an immune response. The resultant antibodies react not only with the HSP but also with host antigens that share the peptide sequences.

In **epitope spreading,** the reactions with self-antigens spread from the initial single antigen to many different ones. This type of reaction often occurs when self-antigen epitopes are exposed during inflammatory or infectious disease processes. A single auto-antigen initiates the process of autoantibody formation, but over time an increased number of previously nonreactive autoantigens interact with T cells which in turn help to stimulate formation of additional autoantibodies by B cells. The autoantibodies may react with different epitopes on the same protein that originally stimulated it or with epitopes on different proteins.

Another mechanism for development of **cross-reactive antibodies** is the expression of **superantigens** that are derived from bacterial proteins such as *Staphylococcus* enterotoxin or from proteins encoded by viruses. These proteins circumvent the specificity of the TCR and bind simultaneously to TCR and MHC Class II molecule without a specific peptide antigen present. The toxins bind to sites shared by many TCRs and are therefore capable of nonspecifically activating large numbers of T cells.

Polyclonal Activation   Normally only a single clone of B cells is stimulated to produce antibody following interaction with the T lymphocyte. In poly-clonal activation, viruses such as the Epstein-Barr virus may bypass the T cell interaction and directly stimulate the B cell resulting in stimulation of several clones.

Altered Expression of Class II MHC Molecules
A nonspecific mechanism by which organisms cause an autoimmune response occurs when the MHC molecules on APC are upregulated and therefore activated. The resulting inflammatory response produces increased levels of cytokines such as interferon-γ (IFN-γ) which induces expression of Class II MHC. The result is either increased numbers of MHC molecules on cells that already produce them or expression of molecules on cells that normally do not express them. This increases the number of peptides that can be presented by the APC and results in T-cell activation. The expression of Class II MHC molecules on cells which do not normally express them may initiate presentation of self-antigens for which no tolerance has been established.

Loss of Immune Regulation   Normally, if clones of B cells develop that cross-react with normal cells, the immune system responds by elimination or suppression of the clones. In some cases, the clone is not suppressed or eliminated, and autoantibody is produced unchecked. Therefore, in order for autoimmune disease to develop there must be interaction between T and B lymphocytes, MHC molecules able to present peptides from self-antigens, and environmental factors that disrupt normal immune tolerance mechanisms.

▶ CLASSIFICATION OF AUTOIMMUNE DISEASES

There are two ways to classify autoimmune diseases. One is by the effector mechanism or the underlying initiator. The other is by organ or organ-system. In autoimmune diseases classified by the effector mechanism, the initiation of damage is by either an antibody or a T cell mechanism. For example, in Type 1 diabetes mellitus or Hashimoto's thyroiditis, the initial tissue damage is due to invasion by T lymphocytes. In the antibody-mediated mechanism, the antibody may react with cellular components or form immune complexes that are deposited in tissue. In myasthenia gravis, the antibody reacts with receptors for acetylcholine whereas in (SLE) the immune complexes are deposited in various organs including the kidneys and skin. In many cases **cytokines** such as IFN-γ, tumor necrosis factor-α (TNF-α), and interleukin 2 (IL-2), which are produced during inflammation contribute to increased tissue damage.

In the second method of classification, by the organ or organ systems attacked, diseases are categorized as either organ-specific or systemic. The organ-specific diseases are characterized by damage to a single organ or organ system and by autoantibodies that react only with determinants on cells of that organ. A classic example of this is chronic lymphocytic thyroiditis (Hashimoto's thyroiditis) in which autoantibodies react with thyroglobulin. Systemic diseases, on the other hand, are characterized by the presence of autoantibodies to components shared by many cells that are capable of pathologic damage to multiple organ systems. An example is SLE in which the underlying autoantibodies react with nuclear components such as double-stranded DNA (dsDNA). There is another group of autoimmune diseases that exhibits characteristics of both organ-specific and systemic diseases. In this group the autoantibody has a specificity that is able to bind to epitopes found on many different organ system cells, but the damage is usually limited to a single organ/organ system. A classic example is primary biliary cirrhosis in which the autoantibody involved is directed against mitochondrial antigens, but organ damage is limited to the liver. Table 8-1✪ shows the classification of some of the more common organ specific and systemic autoimmune diseases. Table 8-2✪ identifies the underlying mechanism in several of the more common autoimmune diseases.

ORGAN-SPECIFIC AUTOIMMUNE DISEASES

As mentioned previously, there are many diseases that may have an underlying autoimmune etiology. The next section will highlight the more commonly encountered autoimmune diseases. For each there will be a brief description of the underlying etiology and clinical symptoms, as well as a discussion of the laboratory tests used for diagnosis.

Diseases of the Thyroid

The autoimmune conditions affecting the thyroid are typical of organ-specific diseases in which damage is confined to a single organ. There are two autoimmune conditions of the thyroid, each of which shows dramatically different clinical symptoms. One, **Hashimoto's thyroiditis,** also known as chronic lymphocytic thyroiditis, results in hypothyroidism; the other, **Graves' disease,** results in hyperthyroidism. A comparison of the clinical symptoms is given in Table 8-3✪. Keep in mind the basics of thyroid function as outlined as these two diseases are discussed.

✪ TABLE 8-1

Classification of Autoimmune Diseases

Target Organ/System	Disease
Endocrine glands	
Thyroid	Hashimoto's thyroiditis
	Graves' disease
Adrenals	Addison's disease
Pancreas	Type 1 diabetes mellitus
Nervous system	Multiple sclerosis
	Myasthenia gravis
Hematologic	Autoimmune hemolytic anemia
	Idiopathic thrombocytopenia
	Pernicious anemia
Blood vessels	Anti-phospholipid syndrome
	Wegener's granulomatosis
Hepatobiliary	Autoimmune chronic hepatitis
	Primary biliary cirrhosis
	Primary sclerosing cholangiitis
Gastrointestinal system	Ulcerative colitis
	Crohn's disease
Kidney and lung	Goodpasture's syndrome
Systemic	Rheumatoid arthritis
	Systemic lupus erythematosus
	Scleroderma
	Sjogren's syndrome
	Polymyositis /dermatomyositis

Hashimoto's Thyroiditis In Hashimoto's thyroiditis, the autoantibodies present are directed toward components of the thyroid, and tissue damage is confined to that organ. Destruction of the thyroid in Hashimoto's disease is characterized by both humoral and cellular responses. The first mechanism is a T cell response that targets thyroid antigens. This may occur due to a viral or bacterial infection in which a protein resembling thyroid protein activates these T cells. Presentation of cellular proteins to T cells and the resulting cytokine release causes an infiltration by CD4+ lymphocytes, macrophages, and plasma cells, resulting in direct cell damage and decreased production of thyroid hormones.

Microscopic examination of a biopsy specimen shows germinal centers of lymphocytes and the presence of plasma cells and few monocytes. The hypothyroidism is due primarily to direct killing of thyroid cells. Autoantibodies also contribute to the damage.

✪ TABLE 8-2

Underlying Effector Mechanisms for Autoimmune Diseases

Antibody to Receptors	
Disease	**Antibody Specificity**
Graves' disease	Acetylcholine receptor
Myasthenia gravis	Thyroid stimulating hormone receptor
Lymphocyte Infiltration Causing Initial Damage	
Type 1 diabetes mellitus	
Hashimoto's thyroiditis	
Rheumatoid arthritis	
Antibody to Cell Surface Antigens	
Autoimmune hemolytic anemia	RBC antigen
Idiopathic thrombocytopenia purpura	Platelet antigen
Hashimoto's thyroiditis	Thyroid peroxidase or thyroglobulin
Goodpasture's syndrome	Glomerular basement membrane
Type 1 diabetes mellitus	Native insulin
Immune Complex Deposition with Inflammation	
Rheumatoid arthritis	
Systemic lupus erythematosus	
Scleroderma	
Sjogren's syndrome	

✪ TABLE 8-3

Comparison of Graves' Disease and Hashimoto's Thyroiditis

Graves' Disease	Hashimoto's Thyroiditis
Clinical Symptoms	
Hyperactivity	Fatigue, lethargy
Weight loss/increased appetite	Weight gain
Heat intolerance	Cold intolerance
Thirst/polyuria	Dry, coarse skin
Diffuse goiter	Rubbery, nodular goiter
Ophthalmopathy	Facial edema
Eyelid retraction	
Exophthalmia	
Periorbital edema	
Treatment	
Antithyroid drugs	Thyroxine
Radioactive iodine	
Thyroidectomy	

Increased expression of HLA class I and class II antigens on follicular cells activates autoreactive T cells, which in turn stimulate B cells to produce antibodies.

The disease is characterized by anti-thyroglobulin antibodies and anti-thyroid peroxidase (anti-TPO) antibodies, formerly called antimicrosomal antibodies. The anti-thyroglobulin antibodies, which are found in over 90% of patients with Hashimoto's thyroiditis, are directed against the precursor of thyroglobulin in the thyroid follicles. Anti-TPO is directed against the thyroid peroxidase in the microsomal part of thyroid epithelial cells surrounding the follicle; increased levels of TPO generally correlate with active disease. Because TPO and thyroglobulin are involved in the uptake of iodine and subsequent production of thyroid hormone, these autoantibodies interfere with normal production of the hormone. When they bind to their respective antigens, iodine uptake is decreased. Hypothyroidism therefore results not only from outright destruction of hormone-producing cells but also from a decreased production of thyroid hormone by the remaining cells. Over 80% of patients with Hashimoto's thyroiditis have at least one of these antibodies present. A few patients may also have thyroid-stimulating hormone (TSH)-receptor blocking antibodies that bind to the TSH receptor sites and decrease stimulation to follicular cells or antibodies directed to thyrotropin receptor or second colloid antigen [CA-2].

Clinical Presentation Onset of the Hashimoto's thyroiditis is usually between 30–60 years of age; women are 5–7 times more likely to be affected than men. The onset in middle age may be linked to increased environmental insults and changes in immunoregulation. In the Caucasian population, HLA-DR3, -DR4, and -DR5 have been linked to a predisposition to develop the disease while the presence of HLA-DQB1 has been linked to protection from the condition. Patients with Hashimoto's thyroiditis have a rubbery and nodular goiter (enlargement of the thyroid) as a result of hyperactivity of the gland in order to compensate for decreased circulating levels of thyroid hormones. Onset of clinical symptoms is often insidious and may include alopecia; dry, coarse, cold skin; tiredness; intolerance to the cold; weight gain; mild depression; slow speech and movement; and facial puffiness (Table 8-3). In addition, some patients may develop elevated cholesterol or normocytic normochromic anemia. Myxedema, which is characterized by a pasty or doughy looking skin, puffy face, and a large tongue, is the result of prolonged hypothyroidism. Thyroid hormone replacement therapy is an effective treatment for Hashimoto's thyroiditis.

Laboratory Testing Patients have a low thyroxine (T4) level and an elevated TSH level (Table 8-4✪). Enzyme immunoassay, chemiluminescent assay, hemagglutination, or indirect immunofluorescence techniques can be used to detect either anti-thyroglobulin or anti-TPO autoantibodies. In the classic indirect immunofluorescence method primate thyroid cells are reacted with patient serum, then incubated with fluorescent labeled antihuman globulin. The resulting patterns of immunofluorescence correlate to the antibody present. Antithyroglobulin will demonstrate fluorescence on the interior of the follicular cell, while anti-TPO will cause granular fluorescence within the cytoplasm of the epithelial cells surrounding the follicle.

Graves' Disease **Graves' disease,** which results in hyperthyroidism, is due to antibodies that mimic TSH by binding to and activating receptors for TSH. This binding stimulates breakdown of thyroglobulin accompanied by production of T4 and triiodothyronine (T3). When the TSH receptor antibody occupies

✪ TABLE 8-4

Comparison of Laboratory Test Values in Graves' Disease and Hashimoto's Thyroiditis

Test	Graves' Disease	Hashimoto's Thyroiditis
TSH	D	I
Free T3	I	N to D
Free T4	I	D
Total T3	I	N to D
Total T4	I	D
Anti-thyroglobulin	N	I
Anti-TPO	N	I
Anti-TSHr	I	N

Key	
D	decreased
I	increased
N	normal
Anti-TPO	anti-thyroperoxidase antibody
Anti-TSHr	anti-thyroid stimulating hormone receptor antibody

TSH receptor sites, there is no negative feedback generated by increasing levels of T3 and T4. Therefore, the cells continue to produce thyroid hormones, resulting in hyperthyroidism. Figure 8-1■ shows the blocking mechanism of autoantibody binding to TSH receptors.

Clinical Presentation Graves' disease has a peak onset between 20 to 50 years of age and is seen in about a ratio of 10:1, women to men. Unlike diseases such as SLE, the incidence in blacks is lower than in Caucasians. There is not a strong link with HLA antigens but in the Caucasian population those with DRB1*0304, DRB1*0301, or HLA-DQA1*0501 are at increased risk for developing Graves' disease while presence of HLA-DRB1*07 may confer protection. The patient with Graves' disease generally has symptoms that include nervousness, palpitations, increased perspiration, fatigue, hyperkinetic behavior, weight loss, and tachycardia. (Table 8-3) About 50% have thyroid-associated ophthalmopathy (TAO) with characteristic eyelid retraction, periorbital edema, and in some patients, exophthalmia. Patients have diffuse goiter with enlargement of the gland up to 2 or 3 times normal size due to the overactivity. In a severe onset, referred to as thyroid storm, the patient may have fever, psychosis, weakness, and coma. Patients with Graves' disease may be treated with antithyroid drugs, surgery, and radioactive iodine ablation.

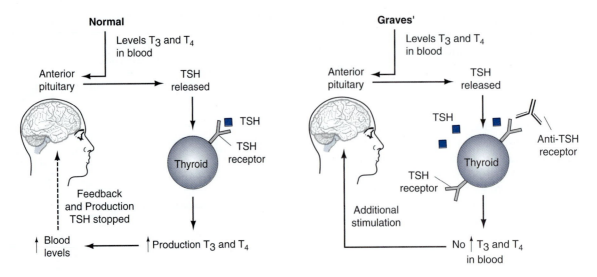

■ FIGURE 8-1 Mechanism of blocking antibodies in Graves' disease.

Laboratory Testing Diagnosis is often made on the basis of clinical symptoms alone. Laboratory tests show elevated T4 and T3 levels but low to undetectable TSH levels (Table 8-4). Over 50% of patients will have anti-TPO antibodies present and some patients may have elevated levels of antithyroglobulin. Table 8-4 shows a comparison of the laboratory results in patients with **Hashimoto's thyroiditis** and in those with Graves' disease.

Type 1 Diabetes Mellitus

Type 1 diabetes mellitus, formerly referred to as insulin dependent diabetes mellitus (IDDM) or juvenile diabetes, is recognized as a chronic disease in children and represents up to 10% of diagnosed cases of diabetes in the United States. It is characterized by abrupt onset in individuals younger than 20 years old with a peak onset between 10 and 14 years. Initially it was considered as a variation of adult onset diabetes (Type 2 diabetes mellitus) but is now recognized as an autoimmune disease characterized by the presence of antibodies specific for the beta cells (insulin-producing cells) in the islets of Langerhans in the pancreas. It is now recognized that cellular damage and production of autoantibodies may precede by years the appearance of clinical symptoms.

Initial cellular damage occurs as a result of a CD4+ and CD8+ lymphocytic infiltration of the pancreas which may be related to viral infection. It is believed that the virus initiates the autoimmune response by molecular mimicry with production of antibodies that cross react with epitopes on the pancreatic cells. Cox-

sackie B virus is most frequently associated with this type of autoantibody reaction, but rubella virus, rotavirus, and enteroviruses have also been linked. Macrophages and Th1 lymphocytes are activated during the viral infection and subsequently release cytokines such as IFN-γ, TNF-α, and IL-1 that contribute to the cellular destruction. Insulitis results in eventual atrophy and fibrosis of the pancreas.

Cellular antigens released into the circulation stimulate formation of autoantibodies to native insulin (IAA) or to islet cell antigen (ICA). Other antibodies that may be involved are autoantibodies to glutamic acid decarboxylase 1A-2 (GAD) and to tyrosine phosphatases IA-2B. Reaction of these autoantibodies with tissue antigens contributes to the eventual termination of insulin production and the consequent hyperglycemia.

Clinical Presentation HLA-D genes may contribute to genetic susceptibility to or protection from immune mediated diabetes, especially in patients of European origin. Increased susceptibility is associated with HLA-DR3 and -DR4, with up to 90% of patients having one or the other allele. Recently the beta chain of the DQ site has also been linked to a propensity to develop Type 1 diabetes. The majority of patients with IDDM have at least one of these alleles present. Individuals with HLA DQ1.2 appear to have a decreased risk for developing the disease. At this time, the routine testing for genetic markers is not of value for either diagnosis or management of Type 1 diabetes, but may be useful in screening nondiabetic family members who are considering donating a portion of their pancreas for transplant to the patient.

Patients with Type 1 diabetes mellitus suffer from hyperglycemia, ketoacidosis, and eventual absolute insulin deficiency. Ineffective cellular absorption and utilization of glucose results in the classic symptoms of extreme hunger, weight loss, tiredness, unusual thirst, nausea and vomiting, and frequent urination. Current treatment is lifelong insulin therapy, but research into the use of immune therapies including beta cell transplants is ongoing.

Laboratory Testing Patients have elevated serum and urine glucose, as well as increased ketone excretion. Plasma levels of insulin are decreased, and antibodies to native insulin may be detected.

Nervous System

Myasthenia Gravis **Myasthenia gravis** (MG) is a neuromuscular disease that affects more than 25,000 people in the United States. The underlying cause of MG is production of autoantibodies directed against specific subunit proteins on the acetylcholine receptor (AChR) at the neuromuscular junction. These autoantibodies block nerve transmission to the muscle. Normally acetylcholine is synthesized in the cytoplasm of terminal nerve endings and packed into vesicles that cross a cleft between the nerve ending and the AChR of the muscle. The interaction of acetylcholine with its receptor results in contraction of muscle fibers. The antibody interferes with signaling from nerve to muscle across the neuromuscular junction and may act via several mechanisms. First, the AChR site may be blocked by direct binding or by steric hindrance (Figure 8-2■). The AChR is thus unable to bind to sub-

unit sites which in turn prevents muscle contraction. An alternate mechanisms involves increased AChR degradation caused by cross-linking with the molecule. Yet another process involves activation of the complement cascade leading to damage of the postsynaptic membrane of the muscle.

Clinical Presentation Peak onset of MG in women is during the third decade of life (called early onset) and is linked to a different set of HLA alleles (B8 and Dr3) than those of late onset (B7 and DR2). Late onset usually occurs in males during the seventh decade of life. Overall, the incidence of the disease is slightly higher in women than in men. MG may be seen as a single autoimmune disease or may occur in association with other autoimmune diseases such as rheumatoid arthritis, systemic lupus erythematosus, or Sjogren's syndrome. MG has been linked with specific HLA types in the Caucasian population, the most common of which are HLA-A1, and HLA-B8. HLA-B8 is often linked to onset of disease in women under age 40.

Patients with MG have easily fatigued muscles and weakness that may cause temporary paralysis of specific muscle groups. Individuals often suffer from diplopia, drooping eyelids, and other facial weaknesses. Some experience chewing problems, difficulty in breathing, and inability to support the head or trunk. Weakness of the extremities will increase with use but recover normal action after rest. Therefore patients tend to have an increase in severity of symptoms during the course of the day. Some patients with MG also have hyperplasia of the thymus, and a few

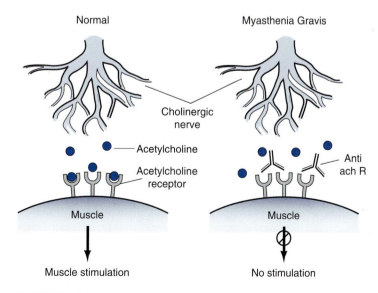

■ FIGURE 8-2 Mechanism of blocking antibody action in Myasthenia gravis.

develop thymoma (a tumor originating in the thymic epithelial cells).

Cholinesterase inhibitors have proved effective in slowing down the rate of degradation of acetylcholine. Steroids or immunosuppressive agents (such as azothiaprine or cyclosporine) that target T lymphocytes have also been used. Plasma exchange decreases the amount of circulating antibody and serves as short-term treatment to relieve acute symptoms. Intravenous immunoglobulins (IVIG) have also been used as adjunct therapy in combination with other agents. Thymectomy may be indicated in patients with a thymic mass, poor medical control, or generalized MG.

Laboratory Testing Either radioimmunoassay (RIA) or enzyme-linked immunosorbent assay (ELISA) may be used to detect anti-AChR antibodies. Antibody is present in almost 90% of MG patients. The titer of the antibody, however, is not related to the severity of the disease.

Multiple Sclerosis **Multiple sclerosis** (MS) is a progressive, relapsing inflammatory condition that affects the central nervous system (CNS), causing progressive neurological dysfunction. As with other autoimmune diseases, a combination of environmental and genetic factors triggers an autoimmune response. Viral agents such as Epstein-Barr virus and human herpes virus type 6 (HHV-6) have been suggested as causative agents and most likely initiate the reaction via molecular mimicry. In this disease, the interaction of myelin-reactive T cells and macrophages brings about formation of characteristic plaques or lesions within the white matter of the CNS, causing damage to the myelin sheath surrounding nerves. T_H1 lymphocytes secreting IFN-γ, initially activated during the viral infection, cross the blood-brain barrier. Multiple factors influence plaque formation, including a T cell reaction with myelin epitopes, an inflammatory reaction with an influx of cytokines (IL-1, TNF-α, IFN-γ) and chemokines, activation of the complement cascade by antibody-myelin binding, upregulation of adhesion molecules, and increased protease production. The resulting tissue damage includes demyelination and plaque formation in the brain and spinal cord, leading to interruption of nerve impulses. Plasma cells in the spinal fluid secrete oligoclonal IgG specific for myelin basic protein (MBP) or myelin glycoproteins. Binding of antibody to MBP further exacerbates the cycle of inflammation and plaque formation.

Clinical Presentation Peak incidence for the disease is in 20–50 year olds with approximately twice as many women affected as men. There is increased risk in people of Northern European heritage, and DRB1, DRB5, and DQB1 appear to be the risk-conferring MHC genes. The course of the disease is often a pattern of acute attacks alternating with periods of remission. Symptoms develop over a period of days, stabilize, and then the patient may improve. Symptoms are variable and include sensory loss, weakness in the limbs, clumsiness, spasticity, tremors, fatigue, vertigo, cognitive impairment, and memory loss. Treatment with steroids may help decrease immune reactions. Recently, routine injections with beta interferons and a synthetic protein similar to myelin protein have been used with success in some patients.

Laboratory Testing There is no single diagnostic test for MS. Clinical history, neurological exam, and appearance of a typical pattern of lesions or plaques seen on magnetic resonance imaging (MRI) are used most frequently in diagnosis. Total cerebrospinal fluid (CSF) protein levels are generally normal or slightly elevated. The IgG index, a nonspecific test for increased immunoglobulin (Ig), shows increased levels of IgG in the CSF as compared with serum IgG levels. Increased IgG levels accompanied by oligoclonal bands in the gamma region are attributed to localized intrathecal production of immunoglobulin. A comparison of serum IgG levels and bands to those found in the CSF is essential in determining whether the IgG is of CSF origin. Lack of oligoclonal bands in the plasma confirms the CNS origin of the IgG. Specific autoantibodies to myelin are not easily detected in CSF; it is suspected that they form immune complexes with myelin and are deposited in the CNS.

Goodpasture's Syndrome **Goodpasture's syndrome,** also known as anti-glomerular basement membrane (GBM) disease, presents with pulmonary hemorrhage and a progressive glomerulonephritis. Antiglomerular basement membrane antibodies (anti-GBM), which are characteristic of this disease, react with alpha-3 regions of type IV collagen, a collagen found primarily in the basement membranes of the alveoli and in the renal glomerulus. The exposure of a cryptic antigen on one of the chains appears to stimulate formation of this autoantibody. When the autoantibodies bind to collagen in the glomerulus, the immune deposits activate complement and trigger an inflammatory process. Subsequently, vascular functions are altered and glomerulonephritis occurs.

Clinical Presentation The disease is relatively uncommon and usually seen in Caucasians rather than African Americans. There is a strong HLA association with over 75% of patients with anti-GBM disease having either the HLA-DR15 or DR4 allele. Conversely, the presence of HLA-DR7 and -DR1 appear to offer some protection from the condition.

As a result of the renal damage, the patient's urine contains increased protein, elevated numbers of red blood cells, and red blood cell casts. Markers of impaired kidney function such as blood urea nitrogen (BUN) levels and creatinine levels are increased while creatinine clearance is decreased. Anti-GBM also reacts with antigens in the basement membrane of the alveoli. In this clinical presentation, symptoms include malaise, cough, dyspnea, and hemoptysis. Treatment includes immunosuppressive drugs such as corticosteroids or cyclophosphamide and use of plasma exchange to decrease antibody levels during an acute episode.

Laboratory Testing Immunoassay tests for anti-GBM show increased titers in patients with Goodpasture's syndrome. The specificity of these antibodies is confirmed using a Western blot technique. Direct immunofluorescence of biopsied renal tissue will demonstrate smooth linear deposits of IgG antibody and C3 on the basement membrane. This linear pattern (which shows the specificity of the antibody to the basement membrane) helps distinguish it from other immune-mediated diseases of the kidney such as acute poststreptococcal glomerulonephritis or SLE, which often show granular patterns typical of nonspecific immune complex deposits.

Hepatobiliary

This group of autoimmune diseases affects the liver and includes **autoimmune chronic hepatitis, primary biliary cirrhosis (PBC),** and **primary sclerosing cholangitis (PSC).** Hepatic damage is a result of the action of autoantibodies and/or inflammatory processes and may be confined to the bile ducts or may spread throughout the entire liver structure.

Autoimmune Hepatitis **Autoimmune hepatitis,** like all other types of hepatitis, is characterized by inflammation of the liver. In this disease all viral or toxin-related causes have been ruled out, and the cause is unknown. However, the condition has developed in a number of patients following acute hepatitis A infection. The condition may be seen in patients of all ages and has been reported to cause fulminant hepatitis or cirrhosis if untreated.

Type 1 and Type 2 autoimmune chronic hepatitis are characterized by age of onset and types of autoantibodies present. Type 1 is most common and is seen in all ages. The antibodies present are **antinuclear antibodies** (ANA) and anti-smooth muscle antibody (SMA). Type 2 is seen primarily in children up to about 14 years of age. The characteristic autoantibodies are directed against liver-kidney microsome type 1 antigens (anti-LKM). The target antigen is cytochrome monooxygenase (P-450), an enzyme involved in detoxification by hepatocytes.

The hepatocytes are destroyed either by cell-mediated cytotoxicity involving IL-2 and TNF-α or through antibody-dependent cytotoxicity (ADCC) involving IL-4 and IL-10. In ADCC, aggregates of antibody on the hepatocyte bind to the Fc receptors on the natural-killer cells which lyse the hepatocytes.

Clinical Presentation Both types of autoimmune hepatitis demonstrate a genetic predisposition and are linked to alleles of HLA-DRB1 genes, especially DRB1*0301. The ratio of persons affected is approximately 8:1, female to male. Individuals of northern European descent are most commonly afflicted, and the disease is rare in persons of African or Asian descent. Approximately one-half of those with Type 1 have other autoimmune conditions such as Graves' disease or **Sjogren's syndrome.** The patient may be asymptomatic or may present with fatigue, jaundice, anorexia, and abdominal pain. About 50% of patients have another autoimmune disease such as thyroiditis, rheumatoid arthritis, or Sjogren's syndrome. Although autoimmune hepatitis is responsive to treatment by corticosteroids, some patients may require several courses of treatment. Those patients nonresponsive to treatment may require a liver transplant.

Laboratory Testing Liver function tests show elevation of alanine aminotransferase (ALT), a liver enzyme, and bilirubin. Patients with Type 1 disease have an increased ANA titer, but no reaction pattern is characteristic of the disease. Anti-[SMA] directed against actin may also be detected in patients with Type 1 disease, while anti-LKM is found in those with Type 2. Titers of these antibodies are considered positive at levels of >1:80 in adults and 1:20 in children. Perinuclear anti-neutrophil cytoplasmic antibodies (pANCA) may also be present but are not specific for autoimmune hepatitis.

Primary Biliary Cirrhosis Destruction of the intrahepatic bile ducts caused by interaction of the mitochondrial antigens (usually enzymes) with anti-mitochondrial antibodies (MA) is the primary pathology evident in PBC.

Clinical Presentation This autoimmune disease primarily affects middle-aged individuals (50s and 60s), with almost 90% of them women. The disease has an insidious onset with symptoms that may include fatigue, increased skin pigmentation, dry eyes and/or mouth, jaundice, Raynaud's syndrome, and hepato- and/or splenomegaly.

Laboratory Testing Elevated levels of one or more of the following liver enzymes occur in PBC: alkaline phosphatase, gamma glutamyl transpeptidase, alanine aminotranferase, and aspartamine aminotransferase. Bilirubin is usually elevated. There may also be hypercholesterolemia, increased serum ceruloplasm, increased urinary excretion of copper, and elevated IgM levels. High titers of anti-MA are characteristically seen in over 90% of individuals with PBC; almost 50% of the patients also have increased ANA titers. The anti-MA is detected using indirect immunofluorescence with rat kidney cells containing increased concentrations of mitochondria as the substrate.

Primary Sclerosing Cholangitis **Primary sclerosing cholangitis** is the rarest of this group of autoimmune diseases and is characterized by inflammation of both the intrahepatic and extrahepatic bile ducts, leading to cirrhosis. It is frequently seen in patients with inflammatory bowel diseases such as ulcerative colitis. There is increased IgM and p-ANCA antibodies can be detected, but the presence of either of these antibodies is not specific for the disease.

Hematologic

The autoimmune hematologic conditions are usually fully covered in hematology texts, but the following section gives a brief overview of the most commonly encountered conditions.

Idiopathic Thrombocytopenia ITP, also known as immune thrombocytopenia purpura, is caused by immune destruction of platelets due to an autoantibody typically directed against a high-frequency platelet antigen. The antibody-coated platelets are destroyed in the spleen. ITP may have a chronic or acute course and may occur in either children or adults. In children, the disease tends to have an acute, postinfectious course that is self-limiting. Both sexes are almost equally affected. In adults, however, the course is usually chronic with almost 80% of the cases seen in women.

Clinical Presentation The primary presentation involves purpura, bruising, or excessive bleeding after minor cuts. Treatment involves use of intravenous immunoglobulin or steroids. Splenectomy is used in those cases refractory to other treatments.

Laboratory Testing Platelet counts are indicative of a severe thrombocytopenia. Special studies can be performed to identify the antiplatelet specificity.

Pernicious Anemia **Pernicious anemia** (PA) is the most common cause of vitamin B_{12} deficiency, a vitamin required for DNA synthesis and normal hematopoiesis. Intrinsic factor (IF), produced by parietal cells in the gastric mucosa, binds vitamin B_{12} in the duodenum. This complex is carried to the ileum where it is absorbed. Vitamin B_{12} cannot be absorbed without IF. In PA, an autoantibody directed against IF binds to the molecule and inhibits absorption of vitamin B_{12}. This blocking antibody is seen in the majority of patients. In addition, approximately 80% of patients develop autoantibodies to gastric parietal cells, resulting in chronic atrophic gastritis and the decreased production of IF.

Clinical Presentation The mean age at diagnosis for PA is about 60 years; slightly more women than men are diagnosed with the disease. PA may take as long as 20–30 years before development of clinical symptoms. The patient initially presents with symptoms of anemia, including fatigue and shortness of breath. In advanced cases the tongue is smooth and beefy red due to atrophic glossitis. Diarrhea and/or malabsorption are due to damage to the epithelial cells of the small intestine. In severe cases there may also be peripheral neuropathy or other neurological complications. Treatment involves monthly injections of vitamin B_{12}.

Laboratory Testing Laboratory diagnosis is often made from a peripheral blood smear. The red blood cells appear macrocytic and normochromic, and there are hypersegmented neutrophils due to the asynchonization of DNA synthesis and cell division. Pancytopenia is frequent. The mean corpuscular volume (MCV) and the mean corpuscular hemoglobin (MCH) are increased, but the mean corpuscular hemoglobin concentration (MCHC) is normal. Serum vitamin B_{12} levels are low, but folate levels are in the normal range. Definitive diagnosis is made with the Schilling's test. Immunofluorescent methods using mouse stomach can be also performed to detect patient antibodies to parietal cells.

Autoimmune Hemolytic Anemia **Autoimmune Hemolytic Anemia** (AIHA) is the result of IgG or IgM autoantibody directed against high-frequency antigens common to the membranes of most erythrocytes. In cold agglutinin disease (CAD), IgM antibodies that generally react optimally at 4°C may cause intravascular hemolysis by activating the complement cascade. These antibodies react with the I antigen on erythrocytes. In warm autoimmune hemolytic anemia (WAIHA), IgG antibodies to a high-frequency antigen belonging to the Rh system react optimally at 37°C and cause extravascular hemolysis when the immunoglobulin-coated cell binds to Fc receptors on splenic macrophages. Certain drugs may also stimulate immune mediated destruction of erythrocytes.

Clinical Presentation   The onset of WAIHA can be insidious or abrupt and may be a primary or secondary condition associated with hematologic abnormalities. In WAIHA, the initial symptoms, such as shortness of breath and tiredness, will often be generic. In CAD the patient often has agglutination or intravascular lysis of RBC in the extremities upon exposure to the cold.

Laboratory Testing   Laboratory testing will include hematologic tests to determine the extent of anemia. In addition, a direct antiglobulin test (DAT) will be performed to determine whether IgG or complement or both are attached to the patient's erythrocytes. An indirect antiglobulin test (antibody screen) will be performed to determine if there is also an alloantibody present. Identification of the antibody specificity in WAIHA is usually limited to reference laboratories.

SYSTEMIC AUTOIMMUNE DISEASES

Unlike the organ-specific diseases in which autoantibodies are directed against tissue specific antigens and the clinical symptoms are directly related to the site of damage, the systemic diseases are characterized by nonspecific symptoms and by antibodies that react with antigens found on or in multiple cells throughout the body. These diseases are characterized by damage directed against collagen in vascular or connective tissue. Deposits of immune complexes, presence of autoantibodies, and activation of an acute inflammatory response cause much of the damage, although a few diseases may be initiated by a T cell infiltration.

The most common systemic diseases are **rheumatoid arthritis** (RA) and systemic lupus erythematosus (SLE). Other less common diseases in this group are

listed in Table 8-1. The predisposing factors for the systemic diseases are the same as for single organ autoimmune diseases—genetic (including linkage with some HLA antigens), gender, and environmental factors.

Almost all of the systemic diseases have overlapping symptoms, especially in the initial stages of the disease. Patients must have specific clinical symptoms before the determination of a specific disease is made. Only a limited number of laboratory tests are usually used in clinical diagnosis of systemic autoimmune disease. Because few tests are specific for a single systemic disease, any given test may be positive for more than one disease, and each disease may result in positive reactions in several tests. The most common laboratory tests, their major uses, and diagnostic significance are described in this initial section.

Laboratory Testing   In the initial laboratory workup for a suspected autoimmune disease, a complete blood count (CBC), metabolic panel, urinalysis, and nonspecific tests for inflammation such as **C-reactive protein** (CRP) or erythrocyte sedimentation rate (ESR) will often be performed. In addition, two common tests, one for presence of **rheumatoid factor** (RF) and the other for the presence of antinuclear antibodies (ANA), will be ordered. In some instances complement levels will be measured. Specific follow-up tests for identification of the ANA may be performed in some diseases. In other cases, complement levels may be measured.

Nonspecific Tests for Inflammation   The ESR and the CRP tests are nonspecific indicators of inflammation and may be elevated during active autoimmune disease or in any number of conditions that are unrelated to autoimmune diseases. During an inflammatory episode, cytokines trigger physiological changes known as the acute phase response. This causes a number of changes in plasma proteins, including an increase in fibrinogen and other globulins and a decrease in albumin. Both the ESR and the CRP tests will be affected by these changes. The ESR may, however, be affected by incorrect handling of the specimen or by physiological factors (i.e., anemia) unrelated to inflammation. In addition, normal reference range values differ between men and women. CRP, on the other hand, is unaffected by underlying non-inflammatory conditions or gender. It generally rises within two hours of acute injury or infection and falls within 48 hours after resolution of the inflammation. In RA the CRP will remain elevated during periods of active disease.

Complement Levels Complement levels may be helpful in evaluating disease activity and in following the response to therapy in SLE or other diseases in which immune complexes are formed. CH_{50} (a measure of the total hemolytic activity of complement), C3, and C4 are commonly tested. If the total level of complement as measured by CH_{50} is decreased, then levels of individual components such as C3 and C4 may be evaluated. A high ANA titer and decreased complement levels are considered indicative of active SLE. On the other hand, increased production of complement may be found in some diseases such as RA.

Rheumatoid Factor (RF) The RF marker, an IgM antibody to the Fc fragment of an IgG molecule, is thought to be the result of damage to the Fc fragment of an IgG molecule. RF is seen in a variety of autoimmune conditions as well as in normal, healthy individuals, especially the elderly where a positive RF test may be found in 10%-25% of those individuals above the age of 70. It is elevated in about two-thirds of the patients with RA but may also be detected in SLE, Sjogren's syndrome, and scleroderma. It can also be seen in chronic hepatitis B, hepatitis C, or in malignancy. Titers of >1:80 are considered a positive result and usually correlated with a disease process, whereas titers of <1:40 are often seen in the elderly. A positive result supports a clinical diagnosis of RA but is not diagnostic, and a negative test does not rule out RA. Although the titer does not directly correlate with activity of the disease, a high titer is often indicative of a more severe clinical course. Latex agglutination, enzyme immunoassay (EIA), and nephelometry methods are available to detect RF. There are EIA methods that can be used to identify other immunoglobulin classes (Ig) of RF such as IgG or IgA, but these are not commonly used in routine diagnosis.

Antinuclear Antibodies The **anti-nuclear antibody (ANA) test** is probably the screening test used most often to diagnose collagen vascular diseases. While a positive test is not proof of an underlying disease, a negative test provides strong serological evidence against it. There are multiple antibody specificities that can be detected in this test, and a positive result indicates the need for follow-up tests to determine specificity of the antibody present. Results must be interpreted in light of clinical symptoms because the ANA may be positive not only in persons with collagen vascular diseases, but also in normal (nondiseased) individuals or in patients with nonautoimmune conditions. False positives may be due to increased age, thyroid conditions, chronic infections, or viral infections.

The most common method for detection is an indirect fluorescent antibody test using patient serum and cultured human epithelial cells (HEp-2). The initial screening is done by diluting patient serum 1:40 to avoid some false positives due to low titers of normal autoantibodies or to avoid non-specific binding of immunoglobulin to the cells. Titers of 1:40 are of questionable significance, especially if the patient does not have clinical symptoms. High titers of >1:160 usually indicate the presence of an autoimmune disease. There are multiple patterns of fluorescence and several are found in more than one disease. Table 8-5✪ lists the more common patterns and the diseases and antibodies associated with the pattern. There is also an EIA screening method that is less popular, but does not require a fluorescent microscope. The antibody patterns seen in this method are similar to those in the IFA method. EIA methods or immunodiffusion methods such as Ouchterlony double diffusion can be used to identify the specificity of the autoantibody responsible for the pattern.

Figures 8-3■ through 8-6■ show the common patterns seen in the fluorescent antinuclear antibody test. The homogenous pattern seen in Figure 8-3 shows fluorescence throughout the entire nucleus. The rim or peripheral pattern in which fluorescence is concentrated at the edge of the nucleus is shown in Figure 8-4. Figure 8-5 illustrates the nucleolar pattern which is characterized be a few large fluorescent dots. Figure 8-6 shows a speckled pattern characterized by small dots throughout the nucleus.

As noted in Table 8-5, the more commonly encountered antibodies include antinative or double stranded DNA (dsDNA), anti-Smith (SM), anti-SS-A/Ro, anti-SS-B/La, anti-SCL-70, and anti-RNP. Anti-dsDNA, which gives a peripheral or homogenous pattern, and anti-Sm which gives a speckled pattern are highly specific for SLE. The presence of anti-dsDNA is confirmed by an indirect immunofluorescent test using the hemoflagellate *Crithidia luciliae.* The kinetoplast of the organism contains a high concentration of dsDNA and fluoresces in the presence of anti-dsDNA in the patient's serum. Anti-histone antibodies, which react with histone, a component of chromatin, produce a homogenous pattern and are associated with drug-induced lupus. They are detected in approximately 90% of patients with drug-induced lupus due to anticonvulsant, anti-arrhythmic, or antihypertensive drugs. However, this type of antibody can also be found in SLE patients, RA patients, and in normal individuals.

The extractable nuclear antigens (ENAs) are a group of nuclear proteins associated with RNA that may stim-

✪ TABLE 8-5

Patterns of Positive ANA

Pattern	Antigen	Antibody	Disease
Homogenous	dsDNA	Anti-dsDNA	SLE
	DNA-histone	Anti-DNP	SLE
			Drug-induced lupus
	Histone	Anti-histone	Drug-induced lupus
Peripheral	dsDNA	Anti-ds-DNA	SLE
Speckled	Extractable nuclear antigen (RNA)	Anti-Sm	SLE
	RNA protein complex	Anti-SSA (Ro)	Sjogren's syndrome
			Scleroderma
			SLE (rare)
	RNA polymerase complex	Anti-SSB (la)	Sjogren's syndrome
			Scleroderma
			SLE (rare)
	DNA topoisomerase	Anti-Scl 70	Scleroderma
	Ribonucleoprotein	Anti-RNP	Mixed connective tissue disease
Centromere	Centromere	Anti-centromere	CREST
Nucleolar	Fibilarin	Anti-nucleolar	Scleroderma
	RNA polymerase		

ulate antibody formation in a number of different systemic autoimmune diseases, including Sjogren's syndrome and scleroderma. Anti-SS-A/Ro and anti-SS-B/La, which both give a speckled pattern, can be seen in Sjogren's syndrome or SLE. Antinucleolar antibodies are typically seen in patients with scleroderma.

Rheumatoid Arthritis

RA is a chronic disease characterized by inflammation of the peripheral joints and progressive destruction of the articular structures. The American College of Rheumatology has published a list of criteria for clinical diagnosis of RA. Patients must meet at least four of

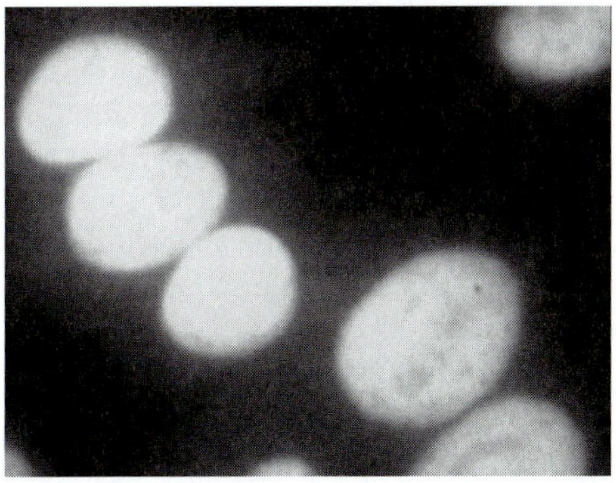

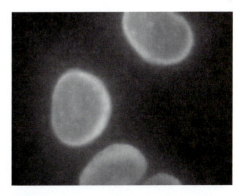

■ FIGURE 8-3 Fluorescent antinuclear antibody test showing homogenous pattern. Photo courtesy of E. Camellia St. John, MEd, MT(ASCP)SBB, Associate Professor, University of Texas School of Allied Health Sciences at Galveston.

■ FIGURE 8-4 Fluorescent antinuclear antibody test showing peripheral (rim) pattern. Photo courtesy of E. Camellia St. John, MEd, MT(ASCP)SBB, Associate Professor, University of Texas School of Allied Health Sciences at Galveston.

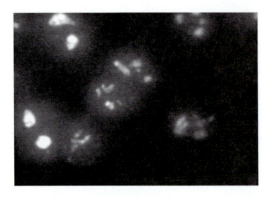

■ FIGURE 8-5 Fluorescent antinuclear antibody test showing nucleolar pattern. Photo courtesy of E. Camellia St. John, MEd, MT(ASCP)SBB, Associate Professor, University of Texas School of Allied Health Sciences at Galveston.

✪ TABLE 8-6

1987 Criteria for Classification of Rheumatoid Arthritis*

1	Morning stiffness of joints lasting 1 hour before improvement
2	Arthritis of 3 or more joint areas simultaneously have swelling or fluid
3	Arthritis of hand joints
4	Symmetric arthritis of same joint
5	Rheumatoid nodules
6	Serum rheumatoid factor
7	Radiographic changes typical of rheumatoid arthritis including erosions or bony calcifications

*A patient is said to have rheumatoid arthritis if the individual has at least 4 of the 7 criteria. Criteria 1–4 must be present for at least 6 weeks.

Adapted from the descriptions given on the website of the American College of Rheumatology. Originally published in Arnett, FC, Edworthy Sm, Bloch DA et al. The American Rheumatism Association 1987 revised criteria for the classification of rheumatoid arthritis. *Arthritis Rheum.* 1988;31:315–324.

these criteria to be considered for a diagnosis of RA (Table 8-6✪). Diseases such as SLE that have similar symptoms during the early stages of the disease may mimic or be confused with RA.

The underlying cause of the initial inflammation is believed to be related to molecular mimicry following infection by a virus or bacterium. The most common antigens involved are those of Epstein-Barr virus, but direct causation has not been proven. The response to this foreign antigen causes infiltration of the synovial area by T cells, B cells, segmented neutrophils, plasma cells, and macrophages. The cytokines released by the infiltration cells initiates an inflammatory reaction.

During the inflammatory process, an IgM antibody is directed against the IgG Fc region of antibodies present in the joint capsule. Immune complexes known as **rheumatoid factor** (RF), which consist of IgM anti-IgG bound to IgG, are deposited in the synovium of

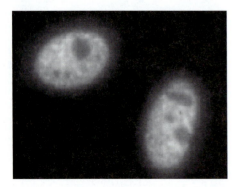

■ FIGURE 8-6 Fluorescent antinuclear antibody test showing speckled pattern. Photo courtesy of E. Camellia St. John, MEd, MT(ASCP)SBB, Associate Professor, University of Texas School of Allied Health Sciences at Galveston.

the joints and contribute to the inflammatory process. Complement binds to the immune complex, and the chemotactic factors C3a and C5a recruit additional macrophages to the area.

Cytokines such as IL-1 and TNF-α released by macrophages and lymphocytes also serve as chemoattractants that stimulate cellular infiltration and cartilage destruction. Collagenase, lysozymes, and other proteases released by neutrophils during phagocytosis of the immune complex cause further damage to cartilage. Activated B lymphocytes in the synovium secrete increased amounts of RF. IgG and IgA molecules that interact with the Fc region of IgG have also been identified. Figure 8-7■ shows a sketch of the comparison between a normal joint and one affected by RA, as well as some of the immune system components that promote inflammation and joint damage.

Clinical Presentation RA affects over 2 million Americans and is the most commonly encountered rheumatic disease. It affects women 2–3 times more frequently than men and usually has an onset starting during the third to fifth decade of life. The patient described in Case in Point #1 might well have RA. DRB1*0101, DRB1*0104, and DR4 genes are associated with an increased relative risk for developing RA, and

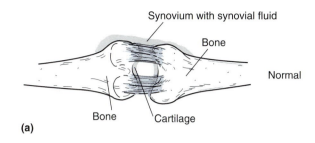

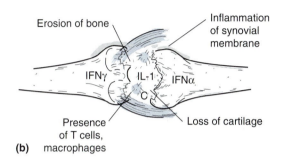

■ **FIGURE 8-7** (a) Normal joint; (b) rheumatoid arthritis.

at least one of these is seen in approximately 70% of patients with diagnosed RA. Patients with RA generally have higher rates of morbidity and mortality than individuals who are not affected with the disease.

Disease onset is insidious with nonspecific symptoms, including weight loss, low-grade fever, malaise, stiffness and tenderness of joints (especially upon arising in the morning), and progressive symmetrical joint inflammation. Small joints such as those in the wrist or ankles are affected first, followed by involvement of larger joints such as the knees and hips. Rheumatoid nodules may be seen on the joints of approximately 25% of patients with RA. These nodules are subcutaneous granulomas infiltrated with lymphocytes and plasma cells. Changes in the affected joints include inflammation of the synovial membrane, infiltration by mononuclear cells, and erosion of joint cartilage and bone. The ongoing process eventually leads to chronic pain, joint deformity, and limited range of motion. A few patients may develop Felty's syndrome which is characterized by the triad of RA, leukopenia, and splenomegaly.

There are several classes of drugs that may be used to treat RA. Treatment generally starts with non-steroidal anti-inflammatory drugs (NSAIDs) such as aspirin or ibuprofen to decrease pain and inflammation. The rate of damage to the joints may be decreased by the use of disease modifying antirheumatic drugs (DMARDs) such as methotrexate. Steroids may be given during periods of acute disease activity. Biologic disease modifier drugs, the newest group of drugs, serve to down regulate the biologic responses by interfering with the inflammatory responses created by TNF-α and IL-1. These drugs function like monoclonal antibodies and interfere with biological activity by binding to cytokines and preventing their interaction with cytokine receptors on the cells.

Laboratory Testing Patients with RA may have nonspecific findings such as a normocytic, normochromic anemia (anemia of chronic disease), decreased serum iron, elevated total protein, and an elevated ESR or positive CRP test. Synovial fluid is sterile, cloudy, and has an increased neutrophil count.

A major marker for RA is the presence of rheumatoid factor RF. Although RF is not specific for RA, approximately 80% of individuals with RA have elevated levels of RF, with levels of RF >60 U/ml (as determined by nephelometry) or a titer of >1:80 (by agglutination methods) considered significant. A small percentage of the normal population may be positive for RF. Patients with other systemic autoimmune disease such as SLE may also have elevated levels. Up to 25% of patients with RA may also show a positive ANA test.

Systemic Lupus Erythematosus SLE remains the classic example of a systemic autoimmune disease. It is characterized on a cellular level by inflammation and B cell activation. It is not known whether autoantibody production is due to nonspecific polyclonal B cell activation or to antigen specific activation. There have also been reports linking SLE with exposure to various viral agents, including the Epstein-Barr virus. Regardless of the initial activating event, the autoantibodies produced react with intracellular or extracellular antigens, including DNA, nucleoproteins, cytoplasmic proteins, or cell surface antigens. Complement activation results in increased chemotaxis of mononuclear cells such as macrophages that release cytokines such as IL-1. Circulating immune complexes of antigen and antibody are deposited in tissues and subsequently cause an inflammatory response, including complement-mediated destruction. The joints, skin, kidney, brain, and lungs are most often affected. Patients may also produce autoantibodies to erythrocytes, platelets, and clotting factors. Numbers of T suppressor cells are often decreased.

Clinical Presentation Prevalence of SLE in the United States is about 40/100,000 and is about three times more frequent in African Americans than in Caucasians. Hispanics and Asians also have a higher frequency of disease than Caucasians. About 90% of the patients with SLE are women and onset of symptoms generally occurs between the ages of 18–65, with most cases initially seen between 20–40 years of age. There is a strong link to the HLA system antigens including HLA DR2, HLA DR3, and to the HLA A1,B8, DR3 haplotype, as well as to environmental factors such as exposure to ultraviolet rays and to chemicals.

SLE has a variable course and progression with symptoms that range from mild to severe and with exacerbations alternating with periods of minimal symptoms or remission. There is a high morbidity usually due to cardiac, renal, or nervous system complications, and the mortality rate in those affected with SLE is about three times that of the general population.

Because of the multiple symptoms that overlap with other collagen vascular diseases, SLE is often initially difficult to diagnose. Patients with active SLE may present with alopecia, fatigue, fever, arthralgia, weight loss, joint swelling, arthritis, and myalgia. The patient presented in Case #1 has some of the nonspecific symptoms associated with SLE. Joints of the fingers, wrists, and knees are often affected, but there are no articular lesions such as those seen in RA. A skin rash aggravated by sunlight is another common symptom.

Less than 40% of patients, however, develop the characteristic butterfly rash that extends across the cheeks and nose. Other patients may develop Raynaud's phenomenon, pustular lesions, or urticaria. Diagnosis is based on criteria established by the American College of Rheumatology (Table 8-7✪). Four of the 11 classic symptoms must be present for SLE to be a probable diagnosis. SLE patients are often anemic due either to the anemia of chronic disease or to antibody-mediated destruction of the erythrocytes. A few patients have leukopenia or develop autoimmune thrombocytopenia. Patients with SLE have increased incidence of antiphospholipid syndrome with the presence of anticardiolipin antibodies and lupus anticoagulant.

Renal complications occur in about 50% of the SLE patients due to deposition of immune complexes in the glomerulus. Symptoms in patients with renal complications may resemble those of patients with acute glomerulonephritis. Other complications include myocarditis and damage to the vascular system of the CNS, leading to disorders such as memory loss, anxiety, and depression.

NSAIDs such as aspirin or ibuprofen are the first drugs used to control inflammation and pain. Patients

---

✪ TABLE 8-7

The 1982 Revised Criteria for Classification of Systemic Lupus Erythematosus*

1. Malar rash	
2. Discoid rash	Erythematosus scaling raised patches
3. Photosensitivity	Skin rash as a result of exposure to sunlight
4. Oral ulcers	
5. Arthritis	Nonerosive involving 2 or more peripheral joints
6. Serositis	Plueritis or pericarditis
7. Renal disorder	Persistent proteinuria >3+ or cellular cases
8. Neurologic disorder	Seizures or psychosis
9. Hematologic disorder	Hemolytic anemia with reticulocytosis or leukopenia (<4000/mL^3) on 2 or more occasions or thrombocytopenia (<100,000/mL^3) or lymphopenia (<1500/mL^3) on 2 or more occasions
10. Immunologic disorder	Anti-native DNA or anti-Sm or false positive serologic test for syphilis confirmed by treponemal test
11. Antinuclear antibody	Abnormal titer

*Adapted from the criteria published on the American College of Rheumatology website. Originally published in Tam EM, Cohen AS, Fries JF et al. The 1982 revised criteria for the classification of systemic lupus erythematosus. *Arthritis Rheum*. 1982;25:1271–1277.

Revision published in Hochberg MC. Updating the American College of Rheumatology revised criteria for the classification of systemic lupus erythematosus (Letter). *Arthritis Rheum*. 1997;40:1725.

may be given steroids or other immunosuppressive drugs to decrease inflammation during exacerbation of the disease. Other options include the use of anti-malarial drugs to control severe joint pain and the use of methotrexate or azothiaprine to suppress the immune system.

Laboratory Testing Patients with suspected SLE should have an ANA screen performed in addition to a routine CBC biochemical profile, and urinalysis. A positive ANA test is not a definitive diagnosis for SLE. As discussed earlier in this chapter, there are a number of other conditions, that give a positive ANA. In addition, a certain percentage of the normal population will have a positive ANA screen.

Patients with SLE most often show a positive ANA, decreased levels of complement (especially during flare-ups), increased levels of immunoglobulins or cryoglobulins, and deposits of immune complexes in organs , especially the skin and glomerulus. Deposits of these immune complexes can be seen in direct FA examination of tissue biopsies labeled with fluorescent tagged antihuman globulin. The pattern of deposits in the kidney biopsy may also provide a clue to the underlying disease. Deposits of immune complexes in SLE tend to be irregular and coarse, while those in Goodpasture's syndrome are smooth and linear.

As noted in Table 8-5, a number of different ANA patterns can be seen in SLE. However, the peripheral or homogenous patterns are the most common. Anti-dsDNA, which gives a peripheral pattern, and anti-Sm, which gives a coarsely speckled pattern, are autoantibodies specific to SLE. Anti-SS-A/Ro and anti-SS-B/La are found in SLE but also in Sjogren's syndrome. Patients with SLE often have biological false positive (BFP) results in non-treponemal syphilis tests (VDRL, RPR). Anticardiolipin antibodies are seen not only in SLE but also in other common connective tissue diseases. In patients with renal involvement, the urinalysis will demonstrate proteinuria, increased numbers of erythrocytes, white blood cells, and of casts.

In addition to classic SLE, there are other related conditions including discoid, drug-induced, and congenital (neonatal) lupus. A drug induced SLE, may present with symptoms similar to classic SLE but they are usually milder and limited to rash, fever, anemia, and arthritis-like joint pain. The most common drug to cause this is procainimide. Other drugs that are associated include isoniazid, phenytoin, and quinidine. The patient typically has anti-histone antibodies (homogenous pattern) and lacks the anti ds-DNA that is found

in classic SLE. In addition there are no immune complex deposits and complement levels are usually normal. The clinical symptoms subside within 4–6 weeks after the drug is stopped, although autoantibodies may be detected for up to 12 months.

Discoid or cutaneous lupus is limited to skin manifestations. It is characterized by photosensitive skin rashes with coin-shaped red lesions that scar upon healing. There may be ulcerations on the mucous membranes of the mouth and nose. Only about 10% of patients with discoid lupus will develop systemic SLE. The ANA screen is negative and diagnosis is made by biopsy of the affected area.

Congenital lupus is seen when autoantibodies cross the placenta and cause SLE-like symptoms, including photosensitive rash, thrombocytopenia, or other manifestations of lupus in the newborn. The autoantibody most frequently involved is anti-SS-A/Ro.

Antiphospholipid Syndrome **Antiphospholipid syndrome** (APS), a relatively uncommon hyper-co-agulability syndrome, is characterized by two different clinical presentations—either vascular thrombosis or complications of pregnancy. The underlying autoantibodies, which may be IgG, IgM or IgA class antibodies, are directed against plasma phospholipid proteins and are commonly known as anti-cardiolipin antibodies (ACA) or lupus anticoagulants (LA). These antibodies often require cofactors such as β2-glycoprotein I or prothrombin to demonstrate activity. LA is more commonly associated with thrombosis than ACA, despite the fact that LA causes deep vein thrombosis (DVT), acts to prolong in vitro clotting time and interferes with both procoagulant and anticoagulant pathways. The anti-β2 glycoprotein I binds to a β2 glycoprotein, which is a plasma phospholipid binding protein. The exact mechanism by which these antibodies cause thrombosis is unknown, although several mechanisms have been proposed. Activation of endothelial cells with resulting cytokine activation and expression of adhesion molecules is one possibility. Another possible mechanism is injury to vascular endothelium by an oxidant-mediated pathway. A third possibility is interference with regulation of coagulation. The phospholipid to which LA reacts may prevent activation of Protein C which in turn blocks inhibition of coagulation. Cardiolipin antibodies react with cardiolipin, a negatively charged phospholipid. These cardiolipin antibodies are similar to, but not the same as, those detected in syphilis tests such as the VDRL or RPR.

Clinical Presentation   APS may present either as a primary condition or as a secondary one often associated with SLE or a reaction to drugs or infection (especially viral agents). The prevalence of the syndrome as a primary disease is about 4 times more frequent in women than men but when it occurs as a secondary syndrome the prevalence is 7 to 9 times more frequent in women and the onset is primarily during the woman's reproductive years. Approximately 50% of patients with SLE may have APS as a secondary condition. The majority of patients with LA will also have ACA present. APS is diagnosed when the patient demonstrates typical clinical symptoms and the LA or ACA is positive on two separate occasions 8 to 12 weeks apart. Clinical symptoms include arterial or venous thromboses and miscarriage. The thromboses may be seen in small or large vessels and are commonly associated with painful leg swelling, stroke, myocardial infarction, pericarditis, renal proteinuria, and ulceration of the skin. The vascular thromboses most often present as a deep venous thrombosis of the leg although pulmonary vessels may be involved. If smaller vessels such as capillaries or venules are involved, the clinical presentation may resemble thrombotic thrombocytopenia purpura or hemolytic uremic syndrome. Some patients also develop thrombocytopenia or hemolytic anemia. Patients do not usually suffer from bleeding problems, despite prolonged coagulation tests. The clinical presentation in women is more frequently a complication of pregnancy with repeated loss of a fetus prior to birth due to placental thrombosis caused by LA.

Prophylactic aspirin does not appear to be effective prophylaxis against DVT, but may help women who have APS and recurrent fetal miscarriage. After a thrombotic event, patients may be treated initially with heparin and then switched to oral anticoagulants such as coumadin. Immunotherapies such as intravenous immunoglobulin (IVIG) or plasma exchange are under investigation.

Laboratory Testing   Diagnosis is based on the presence of either antiphospholipid or anti-lupus anticoagulant antibodies, or both, and either venous thrombosis or pregnancy complications. LA are identified when the activated partial thromboplastin time (APTT) is prolonged and not corrected by mixing with normal plasma. APTT tests using dilute Russell viper venom are also prolonged. The platelet neutralization procedure, considered a confirmatory test for the presence of LA, may also be performed. ACA antibodies are detected using an EIA test with cardiolipin-coated wells.

Sjogren's Syndrome   This autoimmune disease is characterized by pathological changes in the salivary and lacrimal glands. Patients present with decreased tear production, dry eyes (keratoconjunctivitis sicca), and dry mouth (xerostoma). Although it may develop as a primary disease, Sjogren's syndrome can also be secondary to other autoimmune diseases, including RA and SLE.

The disease is generally mild; however, it may become systemic, involving other exocrine glands including the pancreas and sweat glands. In addition, patients may be at increased risk of developing malignant B cell lymphoma.

After the initial triggering event, the salivary glands are infiltrated with T helper cells that recognize specific ribonuclear protein autoantigens of the cells. The immune reaction results in chronic inflammation.

Clinical Presentation   The disease generally begins in the fourth and fifth decade of life and affects women more frequently than men (9:1). Risk factors include a family history or the presence of specific HLA antigens. There appears to be a genetic predisposition to develop the disease in individuals with the HLA types of HLA B8, HLA-DR3, and HLA DRw52. Viruses may be a trigger, especially Epstein Barr virus (EBV) which can be latent in the salivary glands. Some studies have shown that patients with Sjogren's syndrome have a higher prevalence of antibodies to human herpesvirus 6 (HHV-6) or to lymphotropic viruses such as HTLV-1.

Symptoms commonly include the presence of dry eyes, often with a gritty feeling, burning, redness, and itching. The decrease in tears may lead to keratitis or ulcerative corneal lesions. Oral symptoms include insufficient saliva and difficulty in swallowing . The corresponding loss of antibacterial mucins in the oral secretions leads to increased risk of caries. A few patients may develop bilateral parotid swelling. The patient may also demonstrate drying of the mucous membranes of the gastrointestinal tract, respiratory tract, and urogenital tract. Skin may show erythema and ulcerations. Other less common systemic manifestations include arthritis and Raynaud's phenomenon. Treatment includes drugs to stimulate the flow of saliva and artificial tears to lubricate the eyes.

Laboratory Testing   Diagnosis is often primarily based on clinical symptoms. Ophthalmic tests include measuring the amount of tearing (Schirmer's test). A biopsy of the salivary glands demonstrating a classic inflammation with T and B lymphocytes and macrophages provides a differential diagnosis. Approximately 70% of patients show a positive ANA test with a speckled pattern typical of anti-SS-A/Ro or anti-SS-B/La. Studies have shown that patients with both autoantibodies have an increased risk of complications including non-Hodgkin's lymphoma. Patients may also exhibit a positive RF test or the presence of cryoglobulins.

Scleroderma (Systemic Sclerosis) **Scleroderma,** a nonorgan specific disease, is characterized by damage resulting from an active inflammatory process, as well as from the production of autoantibodies. The term scleroderma means hard skin, and the primary target tissue in this disease is the endothelium. Overproduction of collagen and other components of the extracellular matrix such as fibronectin characterize the condition. In a few persons, increased levels of fibrinogen, immunoglobulins, and C3 may also be found. There are variations of the disease including localized scleroderma, systemic sclerosis, and the **CREST syndrome** which is a limited form of the disease.

Clinical Presentation The etiology of scleroderma is unknown, but the presence of HLA antigens DR1, DR3, and DR5 appear to predispose individuals to the disease. Onset occurs most often in the fifth and sixth decades with women outnumbering men 15:1. African Americans are more frequently affected than Caucasians. The onset of the disease in men is more commonly associated with environmental or toxic exposures.

Clinical symptoms include a thickening of the skin, mild muscle weakness or atrophy, and stiffness. There are vascular lesions in almost all organs. Visceral complications include heartburn and dysphagia due to esophageal dysmotility and reflux. Pulmonary complications which are due to fibrosis include hypoxia and dyspnea. In the systemic form, damage may involve not only skin but also the heart, lung, and kidney. The CREST syndrome is characterized by calcinosis (calcium deposits under the skin), Raynaud's phenomenon, esophageal dysmotility, sclerodactyly (tightening of the skin on the fingers), and telangiectasia (spidery dilated capillaries on the face and hands).

Laboratory Testing Patients may have elevated creatinine kinase (CK) if muscles are involved and elevated BUN and creatinine if there is kidney involvement. Several autoantibodies may be found in patients with SS. Anti-centromere antibodies are characteristically seen in CREST. Anti-Scl 70, which is directed against the nuclear antigen topoisomerase, is commonly found in diffuse cutaneous presentations of the disease.

Other Systemic Autoimmune Diseases
Polymyositis/dermatomyositis is yet another systemic autoimmune disease. Polymyositis is an inflammatory myopathy characterized by muscle weakness and joint pain. In dermatomyositis, there is involvement of the skin, including a red to purple rash on face, neck, and chest. Both forms may be associated with other collagen vascular diseases. Up to 70% of patients show increased levels of serum creatine kinase and aldolase, as well as an elevated ESR. Approximately 25% will show increased lactic dehydrogenase. Severe cases will show increased myoglobin levels. Anti-Jo1 may be detected in the ANA test.

▶ PRIMARY IMMUNODEFICIENCY DISORDERS

DEFINITION AND DIAGNOSIS OF IMMUNODEFICIENCIES

The previous sections of this chapter focused on the potentially devastating consequences of an inappropriate immune response against self-autoimmunity. The remainder of this chapter is devoted to the consequences stemming from the inability of the immune system to respond to pathogens—immunodeficiency. This lack of response to pathogens, with infection as the result, is the most obvious consequence of an immunodeficiency disorder. However, defects in some arms of the immune response may result in an increased incidence of tumors, possibly due to a deficit in immunosurveillance, which is discussed in detail in Chapter 10.

Immunodeficiency disorders are conventionally divided into primary and secondary disorders. **Primary immunodeficiencies,** while the consequences may not be apparent for a number of years, are present at birth. They are genetic in nature, and may be the result of a spontaneous mutation or may be inherited. The immune system is so complex that it is estimated that about one in every 500 individuals in the United States has some sort of defect. However, because of the redundancy of many of the immune response pathways, most of the defects are minor or even subclinical. **Secondary immunodeficiencies** are due to some exogenous agent, such as human immunodeficiency virus (HIV) or severe nutritional defects. With the exception of intra-uterine infection with HIV, secondary immun-odeficiencies do not generally appear at birth.

Primary immunodeficiency disorders may be further subdivided on the basis of the cell type affected or the point at which maturation of the cell lineage is blocked. Virtually any point in maturation or in any immune mechanism is a potential target for a deleterious mutation. The most severe disorders, which may result in early death from overwhelming sepsis from viral, bacterial, or fungal organisms, are those that affect an immune pathway early in its ontogeny (Figure 8-7). Defects in the adaptive immune system tend, in general, to have more serious consequences than do defects in the innate immune system, although this does not hold true in all cases. **Severe combined immunodeficiency (SCID)** in its many forms is the subdivision occupied by the most severe disorders. Because cytokines produced by T cells participate in so many aspects of both the innate and adaptive immune response, pure T cell disorders may also be very severe. B cell deficiencies that result in an almost complete lack of immunoglobulin production are characterized by frequent serious infections, but lack of one class of immunoglobulin may not have any profound effect upon the immune system in general. Individuals with defects in the innate immune system, such as phagocytic or complement deficiencies, are generally plagued with pyogenic infections, but do not generally have an abnormal number of fungal or viral infections.

A great deal of progress has been made in recent years toward characterizing the exact molecular and genetic defects responsible for many of the primary immunodeficiencies. And lack of response to a particular class of pathogens combined with recognition of the missing portion of the immune response has led to further understanding of the pathways and mechanisms of the immune system.

Diagnosis of immunodeficiencies begins with an accurate history. The type of infection or other disease and a family history of similar disease will help in the selection of diagnostic laboratory tests, many of which were discussed in detail in Chapter 7. A CBC and differential count will point up abnormal numbers of a class of white blood cells. Quantitation of total immunoglobulin and subtypes may be performed. Incubation of cells followed by flow cytometry may be useful in determining a relative lack of cell subsets or proteins normally present on cells. Complement levels and function may be determined. Once the general type of immunodeficiency is established, genetic studies or molecular biological assays for specific gene products may be performed to determine the exact mutation involved. If the defect is inherited rather than spontaneous, genetic counseling may be in order.

SCID: SEVERE B AND T CELL DEFICIENCIES

Clinical Presentation of SCID

SCID is generally recognized during the neonatal period or shortly thereafter. The affected child generally shows failure to thrive due to diarrhea and persistent infections with *Candida, Pneumocystis jeroveci (carinii)*, varicella, adenovirus, respiratory syncytial virus (RSV), parainfluenza-3, cytomegalovirus (CMV), Epstein-Barr virus (EBV), and a host of other organisms. Skin lesions, such as eczema, rashes, and infections, are common. There is also an abnormal response to BCG vaccine if given at birth. Diagnosis is based upon clinical symptoms along with a small thymus, lack of tonsils or lymph nodes, hypogammaglobulinemia, and profound lymphopenia (<2,000).

Treatment of SCID

Until recently, most forms of SCID resulted in death in early childhood. Although increasingly potent antibiotic agents became available, children inevitably succumbed to infection. Replacement of immunoglobulins was also somewhat successful but not long lasting. However, modern transplantation and molecular biology hold the potential for cure rather than mere symptomatic relief. Bone marrow or hematopoietic stem cell transplantation now has a 95% cure rate if performed within the first three months of life. Although rejection of the transplant is not a problem in a child lacking a functional immune system, development of graft-versus-host disease from immunocompetent cells from a mismatched donor is a serious consideration. The most successful bone marrow or hematopoietic stem cell transplants have been those that were HLA-matched and depleted of T cells. The problems associated with transplantation are discussed in more detail in Chapter 9.

Molecular biology may eventually contribute the ideal therapy—replacement of the defective gene. Gene therapy not only requires purification of the stem cells to be transfected, but also identification and isolate of the appropriate gene. This approach was first attempted in a child with **adenosine deaminase** (ADA) deficiency, where the gene was inserted into the child's own lymphocytes. The approach was somewhat successful, but since lymphocytes eventually stop proliferating, the treatment was not permanent. Transfection of stem cells in 9 X-linked SCID patients was much more successful, but the Moloney tumor virus vector used in the transfection led to development of tumors in two of the children.

Selected Forms of SCID

The severity of SCID and the most common infectious organisms seen in patients with SCID depend on where the defect lies. **Reticular dysgenesis** is the most severe form. A stem cell defect before the lymphoid/myeloid progenitor split results in no cells from either lineage. The lack of B and T lymphocytes, NK cells, and myeloid cells (including phagocytes) results in a profound immunodeficiency characterized by bacterial, viral, and fungal infections, with death usually occurring in early infancy. Stem cell transplantation is currently the only cure for reticular dysgenesis.

ADA deficiency is one of the more common forms of SCID. It is inherited as an autosomal recessive disorder (and may be the immunodeficiency present in the child in Case in Point #2). ADA is an enzyme in the purine salvage pathway used by lymphocytes. A defect in or lack of the enzyme results in increased intracellular levels of adenosine and deoxyadenosine nucleotides, which would normally be salvaged by ADA. These nucleotides are toxic to cells that undergo rapid turnover, such as lymphocytes and thymocytes. Therefore, while individuals with ADA are capable of producing lymphocytes, they still exhibit profound lymphopenia (<500). These children may also have other abnormalities related to the effect of accumulating nucleotides in other rapidly dividing cells. Chondro-osseous dysplasia with skeletal abnormalities is not uncommon. Replacement of ADA has proven effective in relieving the symptoms, but bone marrow transplantation is more effective.

Toxic metabolites also build up in the autosomal recessive disorder purine nucleoside phosphorylase deficiency. Individuals lacking this enzyme had high intracellular concentrations of deoxyguanosine triphosphate. The result of this toxic accumulation may be the presence of nonfunctional immunoglobulins accompanied by autoimmunity and neurologic impairment.

A defect in the γ_c chain of IL2-R is the most common form of SCID. Because this receptor is used in signaling from IL2, IL4, IL7, IL9, and IL15, the defect is serious. T lymphocytes and NK cells are absent, while B lymphocytes are present but nonfunctional. These deficits can be traced to the need for IL7 in T-cell development and in B cell growth and maturation, and for IL15 in NK cell development. The defect is **X-linked.** Female carriers have skewed **X-inactivation** in lymphocytes so that all mature lymphocytes contain normal X chromosomes. However, X-inactivation is random in other cell types, including germ cells. Deficiency of JAK-3, a protein required for γ_c signaling, behaves phenotypically like the X-linked disorder. However, it is inherited as an autosomal recessive. Other signaling defects include a defect in the IL7-R alpha chain, which primarily affects T cells, and CD45 deficiency. In CD45 deficiency, T, B, and NK cells are all present. However, lack of CD45, a hematopoietic-cell transmembrane tyrosine phosphatase that regulates the *src* tyrosine kinases such as *lyk* involved in T and B cell receptor **signal transduction** results in lack of activation of these cell types. T, B, and NK cells are also all present but nonfunctional in p56*lck* deficiency where the tyrosine kinases necessary for the differentiation, activation, and proliferation of T cells are absent or defective.

An absence of T and B cells, but not NK cells, results from a deficiency of RAG1 and RAG2, which are required for B and T cell receptor gene arrangements. As explained in Chapter 3, B cells that fail to undergo productive rearrangement of immunoglobulin genes eventually die of apoptosis in the bone marrow. A similar fate awaits T cells that fail to rearrange their T cell receptor genes.

Nezelof syndrome may be classified as a form of SCID since there is a T cell defect with variable B cell abnormalities. The T cell defects result at least in part from thymic hypoplasia; T cell numbers are decreased but the CD4/CD8 ratio is normal. Immunoglobulin is produced but is nonfunctional. This syndrome is also associated with hemolytic anemia and thrombocytopenia.

T CELL ACTIVATION DEFICIENCIES

Because of the great impact T cell function has on the rest of the immune system, some T cell activation deficiencies behave clinically like SCID. However, unlike SCID, T cell activation deficiencies may be characterized by the presence of normal numbers of T cells. However, because the cells cannot be activated, they cannot proliferate. T cell activation deficiencies are rare, and have been identified through molecular techniques.

The **CD3 complex deficiency** has few to no CD3+ T cells. Since the CD3 complex is essential to T cell activation, absence of CD3 results in T cells that cannot be activated to perform effector functions or to proliferate. Autoimmunity or immunodeficiency may be the result of this particular disorder. Clinical behavior is variable, depending on the number of CD3+ T cells present.

A mutation in the gene for **ZAP-70,** a tyrosine kinase involved not only in T cell signaling but also in the positive/negative selection of T cells in the thymus, results in an immunodeficiency that resembles SCID in the type of infections common to individuals with the defect. There is a profound CD8+ lymphopenia. Numbers of CD4+ T cells are normal because these cells use *syk* tyrosine kinase while in the thymus. However, since this enzyme is present primarily in the thymus, the CD4+ cells in the periphery are not high functioning. NK cells and B cells are present in normal numbers, and immunoglobulin production does not appear to be affected.

MHC DEFICIENCIES

Although lack of MHC Class I or Class II expression affects all cells that normally have MHC on their surface, the greatest damage is done to the T cell arm of the adaptive immune response. Since T cells are only able to recognize antigens presented in the context of self-MHC, lack of MHC expression renders T cells unable to respond in the presence of antigen.

MHC Class II deficiency, also known as **bare lymphocyte syndrome,** is transmitted as an autosomal recessive. The genetic defect that has been identified so far is not in those genes encoding Class II proteins, but in the genes that regulate transcription of Class II genes. A number of mutations have been identified, most of which affect a multiprotein transcription factor that must bind to the MHC-Class II promoter to regulate transcription. Another mutation affects a transactivator involved in MHC Class II transcription. The consequences of an MHC Class II defect are severe and usually fatal without bone marrow transplantation. CD4+ T cells, which must express MHC Class II to remain viable, are few if present at all. CD8+ cells, which express MHC Class I, are present in normal or increased numbers. Because T cells provide help in the B cell response to many antigens and in class switching, B cells, while present, are not able to mount a response to T-dependent antigens. Clinical manifestations of MHC Class II defects include diarrhea, often due to *Cryptosporidia,* bacterial pneumonia, *Pneumocystis jeroveci* infections, septicemia, and viral infections. Therefore, these defects of expressed clinically in much the same was as the T cell activation deficiencies and SCID.

MHC Class I deficiencies have also been observed but are less severe than MHC Class II defects. Although an increased incidence in viral infections would be expected since CD8+ cells are active against virally infected host cells, most of the clinical disease seen is in the form of bacterial respiratory infections. CD8+ cells, which require MHC Class I for antigen recognition, and NK cells, which use MHC Class I pattern recognition as a means to avoid killing host tissues, are decreased in number. Hypothetically, an organ from an individual with an MHC Class I defect might be ideal for transplantation, since no cells in the body of that individual express MHC Class I. The genetic defects isolated to date have been mutations in TAP1 and TAP 2 proteins. These defects prevent loading of peptide into the MHC Class I molecule. Without peptide loading, MHC cannot be expressed on the cell surface.

DEFICIENT IMMUNOGLOBULIN PRODUCTION

There are many genetic defects underlying deficient immunoglobulin protection. Some of these defects affect all classes of immunoglobulin, leaving the individual susceptible to infection with the encapsulated organisms such as *Streptococcus pneumoniae, Haemophilus influenzae,* and *Staphylococcus* which require opsonization by immunoglobulin for effective clearance by the immune system. Infections with gram-negative organisms such as *Pseudomonas spp.* are also common, as are infections with echoviruses, Coxsackie viruses, adenoviruses, and *Ureaplasma.* Other defects only affect one class of immunoglobulin, and the clinical manifestations are limited in their severity.

X-Linked Agammaglobulinemia

This profound deficiency of all classes of immunoglobulins is also known as **Bruton's agammaglobulinemia.** It is the most common of the agammaglobulinemias and is manifested clinically by the absence of B lymphocytes, very small tonsils, lack of palpable lymph nodes, no germinal centers in lymph nodes, intermittent neutropenia, and frequent overwhelming infections as described earlier. There may also be defects in T cell activation, but these defects are most likely due to the lack of B cell antigen presentation to T cells. Autoimmune disorders are common although the mechanism leading to these disorders is unknown. The identified genetic defect is in the gene encoding B cell tyrosine kinase, one of the *src* family of cytoplasmic protein kinases. Since this enzyme is required for transduction of signals leading to B cell maturation, lack of the enzyme or presence of an abnormal enzyme leads to a halt in B cell maturation at the pro-B stage. Several different mutations in the gene have been reported, with the majority of mutations in the catalytic domain.

The multiple infections commonly seen in patients with X-linked agammaglobulinemia can be prevented with relative success by infusion of pooled gamma globulins. This provides immunoglobulins of all classes, but must be done periodically, taking into account the half-life of antibodies in the serum.

Autosomal Recessive B-Cell Negative Agammaglobulinemia

This form of agammaglobulinemia is not as common as the X-linked form. Although described as a single clinical syndrome, there have been mutations identified that affect different aspects of B cell maturation or activation. Some of the mutations, such as those affecting the μ heavy chain or in the λ 5/14 surrogate light chain, affect the ability of B cells to produce immunoglobulin. A defect in the gene encoding the Igα chain of the B cell receptor molecule affects antigen recognition and binding. Yet another mutation has been observed in the gene encoding BLNK, the B cell linker adapter protein involved in signal transduction.

Other Defects in Immunoglobulin Production

Common variable immunodeficiency (CVID) has not been identified so much by identification of a mutation or mechanism as by default. If an immunoglobulin deficiency is identified and the cause cannot be identified, CVID is considered as a diagnosis. It is likely that this immunodeficiency will eventually be split into subtypes as the various mutations and underlying mechanisms are identified.

Unlike the agammaglobulinemias, the disorder is not usually identified until the second or third decade of life. Patients commonly present with recurrent or chronic sinus or pulmonary infections caused by pyogenic organisms. Bronchiectasis is often present. B cell numbers are normal, but are defective in immunoglobulin production.

T cell function may be impaired as well. One subset of CVID is characterized by decreased IL2 production by CD4+ T cells, while another subset has low numbers of CD4+ T cells accompanied by an increased number of CD8+ T cells.

A variety of other clinical symptoms and disorders may also be present, lending weight to the possibility that several separate types of immunodeficiency are currently categorized as CVID. Lymphoproliferative disorders, including lymphadenopathy, splenomegaly,

and intestinal nodular lymphoid hyperplasia are not uncommon. A sarcoid-like lung disease characterized by noncaseating granulomas may be present. Individuals affected by CVID have an increased risk of malignancy, primarily lymphoma and gastric adenocarcinoma. Autoimmune disorders are also common, including HA, ITP, SLE, RA, and thyroid disease. Oligoarticular arthritis has been observed. Infections with *Giardia lamblia, Campylobacter, Salmonella,* and *Shigella* species frequently cause gastrointestinal problems, along with a malabsorption syndrome that resembles celiac disease but with no evidence of gluten sensitivity.

X-linked hyper-IgM disease is so named because of the normal to greatly elevated levels of IgM observed. Although this particular disorder is caused by a defect in CD40 ligand (CD154) carried on activated CD4+ T cells, the immunodeficiency is considered a B cell disorder. CD154 interacts with CD40 on B cells, an interaction that is required for B cell class switching. Therefore, the B cells are capable of producing IgM in response to a pathogen, but cannot make IgG, IgA, or IgE. This appears clinically as frequent pyogenic infections. Binding of CD40 on B cells to CD40 ligand also upregulates expression of CD80/86 on the B cells which serves as a costimulatory signal for T cell activation. Absence of this signal results in persistence of autoreactive T cells and inefficient immunosurveillance of tumors. Macrophages and monocytes are also affected since maximum activation of these cells is through CD40/CD40 ligand binding. Therefore, individuals with X-linked hyper-IgM have an increased incidence of autoimmune disease, malignancy, neutropenia, anemia, sclerosing cholangitis, and liver disease.

There is also an autosomal recessive form of hyper-IgM syndrome. This defect does not affect the T cells, but rather is an intrinsic defect in the B cells themselves. A deficiency of activation-induced cytidine deaminase, a mRNA-editing enzyme involved in the gene splicing required for class-switching, leads to impaired terminal differentiation of B cells. The laboratory picture of high levels of IgM accompanied by low or absent IgA, IgE, and IgG is similar to that of the X-linked form of the disease.

OTHER IMMUNODEFICIENCIES

Wiskott-Aldrich Syndrome

Wiskott-Aldrich syndrome, an X-linked disorder, was initially considered to be primarily a hematologic disorder rather than an immunodeficiency since thrombocytopenia is a feature of the disease. Platelets are generally small and defective, resulting in easy bruising and bleeding. However, although the immunologic features of the syndrome are variable, it is actually due to a mutation of the gene on the X chromosome encoding the Wiskott-Aldrich syndrome protein (WASP). This gene is preferentially expressed in both lymphocytes and in megakaryocytes, leading to disorders in these two seemingly unrelated cell types. Female carriers show nonrandom X-inactivation. The cytoskeletal glycoprotein (sialophorin, CD43) encoded by this gene binds signaling factors involved in the polymerization of actin molecules that is required for successful formation of microvesicles. Lack of WASP leaves the lymphocytes and megakaryocytes unable to undergo the cytoskeletal reorganization required for a response to stimuli.

Individuals with Wiskott-Aldrich syndrome may have in addition to thrombocytopenia, eczema, recurrent infections with encapsulated organisms, *P. jeroveci (P. carinii),* and herpes viruses, and autoimmune cytopenias. The disorder worsens with age, and is generally fatal with death commonly due to EBV lymphoma. Laboratory analysis commonly, but not invariably, shows IgE antibodies to common allergens, increased levels of IgA and IgE with normal levels of IgG and decreased IgM, decreased numbers of T cells, normal numbers of B cells that, however, lack CD21 (CR2), and a poor response to polysaccharide, isohemagglutinins, and some protein antigens.

Several different types of therapy have been used to treat this disorder. The most successful has been cure, rather than relief of symptoms, by bone marrow transplantation from an HLA-matched sibling. Intravenous immunoglobulin therapy can be used to supplement the immunoglobulins produced by the patient. Splenectomy may be required to alleviate severe thrombocytopenia.

Ataxia Telangiectasia

Ataxia telangiectasia is another syndrome with variable effects on the immune system. This autosomal disorder results from a mutation in a gene on chromosome 11 that encodes a phosphatidylinositol kinase required for DNA repair, cell division, and regulation of the cell cycle. The disease is so named because of the presence of an irregular gait (cerebellar ataxia) accompanied by oculocutaneous telangiectasias (spiderweb-like dilated capillaries). Bacterial infections in the sinuses and lungs are common, as are T lymphocyte malignancies. Many of the clinical symptoms may be attributed to sensitivity to ionizing radiation and increased chromosome breakage which is not repaired.

Both the humoral and cell-mediated immune response may be affected. IgA deficiency is very common, as is decreased IgG. A hypoplastic thymus may accompany a T cell deficiency.

Duncan's Disease

X-linked lymphoproliferative disorder, also known as Duncan's disease, becomes evident following a primary EBV infection. Instead of the usual self-limiting infection, individuals with the disorder develop an often fatal fulminant mononucleosis. If the primary EBV infection is not fatal, leukemia, lymphoma, aplastic anemia, cellular immune defects, or agammaglobulinemia may occur. The defect responsible for this disorder is in a gene encoding signaling lymphocyte activation molecule (SLAM)–associated adaptor protein (SAP). SLAM, present on T and B cells, forms a high affinity self-ligand which must be inhibited by SAP. If SAP is not present or is abnormal, EBV infection leads to uncontrolled T and B cell activation.

Omenn's Syndrome

Omenn's syndrome results from a RAG1 or RAG2 mutation that causes impaired rearrangement of B cell and T cell receptors. This is not to be confused with RAG1/RAG2 deficiencies, which are characterized by a complete lack of receptors. In Omenn's syndrome, there are no circulating B cells, and T cells in circulation are generally activated oligoclonal Th2 type cells that respond abnormally to antigen. The syndrome is characterized clinically by erythroderma and desquamation, diarrhea, hypereosinophilia, and elevated IgE levels. Currently, the only treatment for this fatal syndrome is bone marrow transplantation.

Job's Syndrome

Hyper IgE, aptly named **Job's syndrome** for Job of Hebrew Bible fame who was afflicted with boils, is characterized by high IgE levels (>2,000) accompanied by eosinophilia. Eczema is common, along with staphylococcal skin abcesses. Recurrent sinopulmonary infections with *H. influenzae* or *S. pneumoniae* occur along with lung cysts containing *Aspergillus* or *Pseudomonas.* As is characteristic of syndromes, the immune system is not the only body system affected. Defects in the skeletal system, including osteopenia, scoliosis, and pathologic fractures, are seen as well as delayed loss of primary teeth and facial abnormalities such as a broad nose, coarse features, and a triangular mandible.

DiGeorge Syndrome

DiGeorge syndrome, which occurs as a result of a deletion on chromosome 22 leading to abnormal development of organs originating from the third and fourth pharyngeal pouches in the embryo, has a variable phenotype. The variable immunodeficiency may be severe if the thymus is completely absent, but is often less severe if there is a partial thymus. Since the heart and the parathyroids are descendents of the same pharyngeal pouches, cardiac defects and hypocalcemia associated with hyperparathyroidism are often seen.

Some immunodeficiencies result from defects that are as yet undefined, and are part of syndromes that affect multiple organ systems. Biotin-decarboxylase deficiency, a metabolic disorder, is associated with convulsions, ataxia, alopecia, keratoconjunctivitis, and *Candida*-associated dermatitis in combination with IgA deficiency and a reduced number of T cells. Chromosomal abnormalities not directly affecting genes encoding proteins used in the immune response may also be associated with decreased immune function. Downs syndrome, Bloom's syndrome, xeroderma pigmentosum, and Fanconi's anemia are among these disorders. Cartilage-hair hypoplasia, which is characterized by skeletal dysplasia, dwarfism, and sparse, fine hair, may also present with a variable T cell immunodeficiency with or without a B cell deficiency or neutropenia. Individuals with this disorder have greatly enhanced susceptibility to varicella; exposure to the virus should be treated with acyclovir. Individuals with chronic mucocutaneous candidiasis have, in addition to persistent superficial candidial infections of the mucous membranes, skin, and nails, pyogenic sinopulmonary infections and viral infections, particularly with herpes simplex virus, varicella zoster virus, and respiratory syncytial virus. Polyendocrinopathies, including hypoparathyroidism, Addison's disease, autoimmune hepatitis, hypogonadism, hypothyroidism, pernicious anemia, and thymoma, are not uncommon. Diagnosis of this particular disorder is made by demonstration of selective anergy to *Candida* in a delayed type hypersensitivity test.

DISORDERS OF PHAGOCYTES

Since phagocytic disorders may affect either PMNs or monocytes, the major abnormalities are seen in the innate immune response. However, because of the interaction between macrophages and T cells, some disorders of monocytes or macrophages may ultimately affect the adaptive immune system as well. The disorders may be loosely characterized as those affecting the ability of phagocytes to kill ingested bacteria, disorders that alter chemotaxis and cell adhesion, those that cause an outright decrease in the number of phagocytes (particularly neutrophils), and defects affecting phagocyte activation.

Chronic Granulomatous Disease (CGD)

Chronic granulomatous disease (CGD) stems from a defect in NADPH oxidase, a compound enzyme that includes cytochrome b_{558} responsible for production of the reactive oxygen intermediates important to the killing of bacteria phagocytized by neutrophils. The disease may be inherited as an X-linked (70% of cases) or autosomal recessive disorder, with a number of mutations identified for each. In general, there is no cytochrome production in the X-linked form, while a defective protein is produced in the 30% of the individuals affected by the autosomal recessive form.

Persistent infections and tissue granulomas along with impaired wound healing characterize the disease. The infections are caused predominantly by catalase-positive bacteria such as *Staphylococcus, Nocardia,* and *Serratia,* and by *Aspergillus* and *Candida.* Many organisms produce hydrogen peroxide during metabolism, which kills them when contained in phagocytic vesicles. Therefore, the lack of reactive oxygen intermediates does not markedly affect killing of these hydrogen peroxide-producing organisms. However, those organisms that produce catalase are able to break down the hydrogen peroxide which they produce. In the absence of reactive oxygen intermediates, these organisms are able to survive in the phagocytic vesicles and to cause persistent infection. Osteomyelitis, liver abscesses, and severe gingivitis are not uncommon.

Diagnosis of CGD may be made through the nitroblue tetrazolium (NBT) test, or by dihydrorhodamine (DHR). In the NBT test, the PMNs are incubated with NBT and stimulated. If reactive oxygen intermediates are produced, the dye is reduced to formazan, a blue pigment that can be seen in the cells under the light microscope. CGD cells do not reduce the NBT. In the DHR test, the fluorescent dye DHR enters the cells to cause oxidation of NADPH if it is present. This can be detected through flow cytometry, which is of sufficient sensitivity to detect carriers of CGD as well as those with the disease. Treatment with IFN-γ is effective if a low level of cytochrome can be synthesized. Bactrim has been used with some success for prophylaxis and treatment of persistent infections.

Myeloperoxidase deficiency is the most common of the inherited disorders affecting neutrophils. Myeloperoxidase normally converts hydrogen peroxide. Since there are alternate pathways for destruction of phagocytized microorganisms, absent or defective myeloperoxidase does not generally cause disease with exception of occasional disseminated candidiasis in diabetics.

Chediak-Higashi Syndrome

Chediak-Higashi syndrome, inherited as an autosomal recessive mutation in the gene encoding LYST, a cytoplasmic protein involved in vacuole formation and function, results in abnormal lysosomal granules. Both hematologic and neurologic systems are affected in this disorder. Giant granules are seen in neutrophils as a result of abnormal fusion of primary and secondary granules. Both chemotaxis and degranulation are impaired. The granules themselves lack elastase and cathepsin G. In addition to the predictable recurrent infections caused by *Staphylococcus aureus* or beta-hemolytic streptococci, individuals with the syndrome often have nystagmus, neuropathy, mental retardation, and partial oculocutaneous albinism. Abnormal granules in the platelets lead to platelet dysfunction accompanied by easy bruising.

Leukocyte Adhesion Deficiency (LAD)

Leukocyte adhesion deficiency (LAD) Type 1 is inherited as an autosomal recessive. The lack of the β2 subunit of CD18 leads to an integrin-mediated adhesion defect. Although neutrophils, macrophages, and lymphocytes all use integrins for adhesion following chemotaxis, only neutrophils, which lack the VCAM-1/VLA-4 pathway, are affected. Because adhesion is of neutrophils is affected but not production, leukocytosis is present. A delayed separation of the umbilical cord is the first indication of this form of immunodeficiency. Throughout life, recurrent infections with *Staphylococcus spp., Candida,* gram-negative bacteria such as *Pseudomonas* and *Klebsiella spp.,* and *Aspergillus* are common. Because the integrins are required for T-B cell interactions, some defects in the adaptive immune system may be seen as well. Diagnosis of this rare defect may be made by flow cytometry, which, with the appropriate antibody and positive control, can confirm the absence of CD18 and CD11, which requires CD18 for expression.

An even rarer immunodeficiency is caused by a defect in carbohydrate fucosylation. Individuals with LAD Type 2 lack sialyl-Lewis[x], which is the ligand for P- and E-selectins present on endothelial cells. Presumably because these selectins are involved in migration of cells other than lymphocytes during ontogeny, these individuals may have dysmorphic features, growth retardation, and neurologic deficits. In addi-

tion, because carbohydrate fucosylation is required for expression of blood group antigens, the Bombay blood group phenotype, which lacks not only A and B blood group antigens but also the H substance present on blood group O cells, may be present.

Rac2 (*ras*-related C3 botulinum toxin) deficiency disturbs the normal migration of neutrophils. This substance is the main GTPase for neutrophils and is integral to the function of the actin skeleton. A deficiency or abnormal protein disrupts the ability of the neutrophil cytoskeleton to undergo the necessary changes in conformation required for migration.

Cyclic Neutropenia

Cyclic neutropenia results from a mutation in neutrophil elastase (ELA2). This autosomal dominant disorder, which may improve over time, is characterized by extremely low numbers of neutrophils for every 3–6 days occurring every 21 days. During this time, there might also be a decrease in the numbers of monocytes, lymphocytes, and platelets. As might be expected, persistent bacterial infections, including cellulitis caused by *Clostridium,* occur during times of neutropenia. Bone marrow biopsies show a lack of granulocyte precursor maturation which improves during the normal portions of the cycle.

In contrast to the production of normal numbers of neutrophils during some periods in cyclic neutropenia, severe congenital neutropenia results from the failure of myeloid cells to mature past the promyelocytic stage. Monocytes and eosinophils are unaffected by this defect in myeloid maturation and may be present in increased numbers. Children with this disorder may have a number of organ systems affected by persistent infection with organisms such as *Staphylococcus aureus* and *Pseudomonas aeruginosa*. Treatment with granulocyte-colony stimulating factor (G-CSF) may improve the outlook for these children.

A number of mutations have been observed in the IFN-γ receptor or in the IL12 receptor. IL12, made by macrophages, stimulates T lymphocytes and NK cells to make IFN-γ which is in turn required for activation of macrophages and neutrophils. Failure to produce these cytokines have resulted the development of systemic mycobacterial infections, *Salmonella* and *Listeria* infections, histoplasmosis, disseminated disease following BCG vaccination, and infection by a variety of viruses including cytomegalovirus, respiratory syncytial virus, and Varicella zoster. One mutation has been identified in the IL12 receptor beta chain. The lack of this receptor renders T cells and NK cells unable to respond to IL12, which in turn limits the secretion by

SECONDARY IMMUNODIFICIENCIES

163

these cells of IFN-γ. An alternate mutation produces a defect in the p40 subunit of the cytokine itself. IFN-γ receptor mutations may also occur in either the ligand-binding (R1) or signaling (R2) chains.

COMPLEMENT DEFICIENCIES

Deficiencies may occur in virtually any component of the complement system. Pyogenic infections are common, since these organisms are usually phagocytized following opsonization. Immune complex formation is also another common manifestation of some of the complement deficiencies. The complement deficiencies may be divided into frank deficiencies of factors C1-9, deficiencies of regulatory proteins, deficiencies of binding proteins, and deficiencies of inhibitors. A review of the complement system, covered in Chapter 5, will help increase your understanding of the importance to the immune system of the complement components.

Both pyogenic infections and autoimmune disease are associated with C1q deficiency. The appearance of systemic lupus erythematosus or glomerulonephritis may be due to the presence of microorganisms that may trigger an autoimmune response, or may be the result of an ineffective clearance of antigen-antibody complexes. This scenario recurs occasionally as the result of C2 deficiencies, which are the most common complement deficiencies in Caucasians and are generally asymptomatic. Deficiencies of C3 and C4 show a similar pattern. Infections with *Neisseria* are the hallmark of deficiencies of complement components 5-9. Although a deficiency of C9 is generally asymptomatic, disseminated infections and recurrent meningitis may occur with lack of the other components.

An autoimmune response to the Bb portion of C3 convertase is associated with Type II membranoproliferative glomerulonephritis and partial lipodystrophy. The autoantibody produced, C3 nephritic factor, binds to Bb and stabilizes it to activate the alternate pathway. The end result is a deficiency of both C3 and B as the result of constant activation and consumption. Consumptive C3 deficiencies are also result from a lack of Factor H, the regulatory protein for C3bBb which competes with Bb, or Factor I, a regulatory protein that cleaves both C3b and C4b. An X-linked lack of properdin, which stabilizes C3bBb, leads to increased pyogenic infections and severe infections with *Neisseria*.

Deficiencies of other inhibitory and regulatory components do not generally result in development of bacterial infections or immune complex disease. Absence of C4 binding protein, which binds to C4b

to facilitate Factor I cleavage, is manifested clinically as angioedema.

Paroxysmal Nocturnal Hemoglobinuria (PNH)

Paroxysmal nocturnal hemoglobinuria (PNH) is the result of a deficiency of decay-accelerating factor (DAF). In normal red blood cells, DAF, homologous restriction factor (HRF), and protectin (CD59) all bind to the cell membrane via glycosyl phosphatidylinositol anchors. These proteins protect the red blood cells from lysis caused by constant activation of the alternate pathway. CD59 is accompanied by sialic acid in mammalian cells, and is able to inhibit formation of the membrane attack complex. DAF causes dissociation of C3/C5 convertases. If either of these proteins is not present, the red blood cells become much more susceptible to complement-mediated lysis, particularly at times of lower oxygen tension such as seen during sleep. Lack of C1 inhibitor results in hereditary angioedema, where a vasoactive C2 fragment causes a noninflammatory edema.

▶ SECONDARY IMMUNODEFICIENCIES

IMMUNODEFICIENCIES DUE TO NUTRITIONAL DEFICITS, TUMOR, OR IMMUNOSUPPRESSION

Secondary immunodeficiencies occur, by definition, as a result of some underlying cause other than a genetic mutation present at birth. There are multiple causes of these secondary immunodeficiencies. Virtually all infants have a brief period of immunodeficiency after maternal immunity has waned, but the infant immune system is not totally competent. Many viruses briefly down regulate at least some aspect of the immune system. For example, measles virus may occasionally suppress IL12 production, which in turn decreases cell-mediated immunity. In general, these brief periods of immunodeficiency only result in mild, if any, clinical disease.

Nutritional defects, tumors, and immunosuppression can cause a longer lasting immunodeficiency with more serious consequences. Marasmus, the end stage of malnutrition, is characterized by insufficient production of proteins of all types, while less severe protein-calorie malnutrition suppresses all aspects of the immune system. Selective mineral deficiencies, particularly iron, zinc, and selenium, may also result in a decreased immune response.

Replacement of hematopoietic cells in the bone marrow by tumor cells also decreases the immune response, not by immunosuppression but because of a lack of stem cells capable of providing the need replacement immune cells. Since tumor cells are often proliferating, the radiation and chemotherapeutic drugs used to treat cancer usually target rapidly dividing cells. Unfortunately, these treatments are equally as toxic to the frequently dividing hematopoietic cells in the bone marrow.

Individuals who have had their spleen removed also have a mild secondary immunodeficiency. The resident macrophages of the spleen, or the Kupffer cells, play a prominent role in phagocytosis and destruction of bacteria, particularly *Haemophilus influenzae*. Splenectomized individuals, particularly children who have had their spleens removed because of sickle-cell crisis, are at a moderately increase risk of pneumonia.

The current generation of immunosuppressive drugs available has made transplantation of many solid organs highly successful. Some of these pharmarcologic agents, along with steroids, are also used to treat active autoimmune disease. However, the effectiveness of these drugs at decreasing the immune response to the allograft in transplantation or to self in autoimmune disease also results in an inability of the immune system to respond to pathogens as well. This form of secondary immunodeficiency is a major cause of morbidity and mortality in allograft recipients.

HIV-INDUCED IMMUNODEFICIENCY

The clinical manifestation of HIV infection was first reported in 1981 in San Francisco, Los Angeles, and New York City. Physicians had noticed an unexplained increase in opportunistic infections with rare organisms such as *P. carinii* and in the incidence of Kaposi's sarcoma in young men. These individuals had greatly decreased cell-mediated immune responses and almost absent CD4+ T cells. Patient histories showed some common elements—virtually every patient seen with this new syndrome was homosexual or the partner of a homosexual, an intravenous drug user, or had received a blood transfusion before 1985. The syndrome was termed **acquired immunodeficiency syndrome (AIDS).**

The number of cases of HIV infection and of AIDS has escalated over the past 20 years, although public education about the risk and effective prevention have slowed the increase in the United States. Current estimates suggest that as many as one million Americans are infected with HIV. This number pales before the estimate of worldwide infection—36.1 million.

Although HIV was originally identified in the homosexual population, heterosexual contact is now believed to be the major mode of transmission in about 75% of the new cases. Maternal-fetal transmission is also escalating, particularly in sub-Saharan Africa. The most effective means of viral transmission is passage of infected cells (lymphocytes or monocytes) from one individual to another. Contact with infected blood, either incidental, by reuse of an infected needle, by transfusion or organ transplant, or through sexual contact has been the most common mode of transmission. It is also believed that infectious particles may be transmitted by contact with saliva or through semen.

HIV was identified as the organism responsible for AIDS by Luc Montagnier of France and Robert Gallo of the United States. The virus is a classic retrovirus. As such, it is comprised by two identical strands of RNA along with a core containing viral proteins surrounded by a phospholipid bilayer of host cell membrane and viral proteins. The RNA has a series of genes coding for elements essential to the virus. The long terminal repeat (LTR) is used to integrate viral DNA into the host and to bind to host transcription factors. *gag* genes encode nucleocapsids core and matrix proteins, while *pol* genes encode **reverse transcriptase,** protease, integrase, and ribonuclease. The coat proteins gp120 and gp41, which are required for binding to CD4 on the surface of T cells and to chemokines and which mediate cell fusion, are encoded in the *env* genes. Infectivity of the virus is enhance by *vif*, while *vpr* increases the nuclear import of viral DNA and arrests the host cell cycle in G_2. *tat* aids in elongation of the viral transcriptase. Increased nuclear export of unspliced or incompletely spliced viral RNA is accomplished by *rev* proteins. Proteins encoded by *vpu* and *nef* affect the host cells. *vpu* decreases host expression of CD4 and increases release of viral particles from the infected cells, and *nef* does the same while also decreasing host MHC Class I expression.

HIV preferentially infects CD4+ T lymphocytes and monocytes/macrophages. These cells are targeted through binding of the gp120 *env* protein to CD4 on the T cell surface. This binding is necessary but not sufficient for entry and production infection of the virus. Different strains of the virus, termed T-tropic or M-tropic (for T lymphocytes or monocytes), interact also with molecules that normally function as receptors for chemokines on the host cells. T cells express the

CXCR4 (fusin) coreceptor, while monocytes and macrophages express CCR5.

Once the virus has entered the host cell, it must be intercalated with host DNA in order to be expressed. Since the viral RNA cannot be integrated into DNA, reverse transcriptase encoded by the *pol* genes is used to make a DNA copy of the viral RNA genome, or a provirus. Other enzymes are used to integrate this DNA into the host cell genome, where it is may be replicated. The viral DNA may remain latent for long periods of time or may be expressed.

Expression generally results in the death of the infected cell. There are several mechanisms by which HIV is believed to cause cell death. The most prominent mechanism is through osmotic or calcium-influx mediated lysis caused by increased permeability of the host plasma membrane after viral budding. Interaction of gp120 with CD4 may also cause formation of multinucleated giant cells, which will kill any uninfected cells that form a syncytium with infected cells. This is probably a rare event in vivo, and has mostly been observed in vitro. Unintegrated viral DNA and large quantities of nonfunctional viral RNA are toxic to the infected cells, and production of the virus may interfere enough with synthesis of proteins vital to the host cell to cause cell death. Finally, some of the infected cells are killed by the host's own CD8+ T cells.

HIV does not begin as AIDS. The acute primary infection may cause fever and lymphadenopathy for a few weeks, but is rarely recognized clinically unless suspected exposure to HIV can be documented. The infection then becomes chronic, often for a long period of time. Full-blown AIDS may not appear for months to many years. The average time from viral infection to death of the individual is about 9–12 years.

Initially, there is a strong immune response to the virus. Although antibody is not present during the acute infection, HIV-specific antibody and cytotoxic T cells decrease the amount of virus present in the blood to a stable level after the initial viremia. However, the virus continues to replicate, particularly in the lymph nodes, which serve as a major replication site. The virus, like any other pathogen in the blood, is filtered through the lymph nodes and spleen to be captured by the follicular dendritic cells present in the follicles of these organs. By the time AIDS is diagnosed, the normal architecture of the lymph nodes is often destroyed.

During the chronic phase of the infection, the virus remains latent. Since there is enough of an immune response to control the infection early in the course of the disease, it becomes obvious that the virus is able to evade the immune system. There are a number of ways by which this may happen. First, the viral reverse transcriptase is extremely error prone. This results in an extremely high mutation rate, with some investigators estimating the occurrence of a mutation during every tenth replication. Most individuals who have longstanding HIV infection show evidence of multiple subtypes. Therefore, cells and antibodies generated during the initial strong immune response may not recognize subtypes produced later in the course of the illness. HIV is also capable of down regulating host expression of MHC Class I. The decreased expression or lack of MHC Class I protein on infected cells decreases lysis of these cells by CD8+ T cells, which recognize infected cells by antigen presentation in the context of self MHC Class I. Finally, T_H^1 CD4+ T cells appear to be eliminated to a greater extent than are T_H^2 cells. This means that there is a preferential decrease in cells making cytokines that enhance the immune response, while cells that may inhibit the immune response survive. Therefore, there is a preferential inhibition of cell-mediated immunity.

Inevitably, the viral load gradually increases, while the number of CD4+ T cells decreases. Once infected, a CD4+ T cell dies rapidly—the half-life of an infected cell is about 1.5 days. Immunodeficiency is not apparent early in the course of the disease, but is apparent once enough T cells have been killed. The diagnosis of AIDS is based on the presence of either antibodies to HIV or the presence of virus in the blood, <200 CD4+ T cells/mm^3 blood, impaired or absent delayed type hypersensitivity reactions, and the presence of opportunistic infections.

Laboratory tests show the increase in viral load accompanied by a loss of immune response. PCR assays for viral RNA quantitate the number of copies of the genome present in the plasma and provide an estimate of the viral load. This is particularly useful in assessing the status of the disease and the prognosis for the patient if performed shortly after the acute stage. Antibody specific for HIV can be identified, and Western blot analysis can confirm the presence of viral protein. Flow cytometry is useful in estimating the number of CD4+ T cells. As the disease progresses, IgG and IgA levels decrease along with a concomitant increase in B cells expression low levels of CD21. The ability of both T and B cells to proliferate in vitro decreases, first as a response to specific antigens such as influenza, then to alloantigens, and finally to mitogens.

The clinical aspects of AIDS include opportunistic infections, including *P. carinii* pneumonia and disseminated candidiasis. Other opportunistic infections may cause intractable diarrhea. Kaposi's sarcoma, normally a rare and indolent cancer arising late in life, may be extremely aggressive. Viral replication in the brain may result in the AIDS dementia complex of decreased cognition, poor motor performance, and altered behavior.

The development of antiviral drugs has led to increased survival of HIV-positive individuals and lengthened the time between infection and development of AIDS. Different classes of these drugs are directed toward various points in the viral life cycle. The major classes are either nucleoside analogs such as zidovudine (AZT), which block the action of reverse transcriptase or are protease inhibitors that block the viral protease responsible for cleavage of precursor proteins into subunit need for production of a new virion. **Highly active anti-retroviral therapy (HAART)** is currently the most commonly used approach and involves a combination of drugs, generally two different nucleoside analogs along with one protease inhibitor. However, these drugs may have serious side effects, are extremely expensive, and eventual treatment failure is not uncommon.

In a world where smallpox has been eliminated since 1979 and where vaccines to many other viruses are in common use, development of a vaccine to HIV seems logical and appropriate. However, failure by individual investigators and by pharmaceutical companies to develop such a vaccine is not due to lack of trying. HIV poses some unique challenges to vaccine development. First, the rapid mutation that confounds the immune system also makes it difficult to produce a vaccine that is effective against enough subtypes to be protective. The long latent period of the virus may mean that the virus will be protected from any host immune response boosted by a vaccine, since most vaccines target the disease rather than prevent infection. Furthermore, most vaccines are derived from either attenuated or killed virus. HIV is not antigenic when killed, and the use of an attenuated virus is not currently acceptable. The route of delivery is also a concern, since most HIV infections occur through sexual transmission rather than through a respiratory or gastrointestinal route. Should a vaccine be developed, testing that vaccine would also be a concern. Vaccines are commonly tested first in animal models to determine safety and efficacy. Unfortunately, dependable and affordable animal models are not available. Therefore, public education as to the routes of transmission of HIV, risk factors, and preventive measures such as condoms and a closely monitored blood supply is currently the major weapon in the global attempt to contain the HIV epidemic.

SUMMARY

An imbalance in the immune system's tolerance for and recognition of self-antigen and foreign antigen is responsible for the onset of autoimmune disease. Genetic and environmental factors, as well as gender, contribute to the relative risk of developing one or more of these conditions. Viral and/or bacterial agents may play a role in the process by mechanisms such as polyclonal activation of B cells, molecular mimicry and development of cross-reactive antibodies, epitope spreading, and production of superantigens.

The classification of autoimmune diseases is generally divided into organ-specific diseases in which the damage is limited to a single organ/organ system or systemic diseases in which the damage affects multiple organ systems. The autoantibodies produced in organ-specific disease react with an antigen unique to that organ whereas they are directed against antigens common to cells throughout the body in systemic disease. The mechanisms of damage within the organs may be mediated by invasion of T lymphocytes, reactions of autoantibodies to surface receptors or cellular antigens, or deposits of immune complexes that instigate inflammatory reactions.

Treatments for autoimmune diseases have often included drugs that affect the entire immune system. As a greater understanding of the balance in cellular interactions, the role of cytokines in the disease process, and the role played by HLA alleles in determining relative risk unfolds, treatments may become more focused and may eventually become preventative.

Immunodeficiencies are not uncommon; however, many do not cause any clinical symptoms. Primary immunodeficiency disorders are the result of a genetic mutation, and are present at birth, although the clinical symptoms may not yet be apparent. Secondary immunodeficiencies occur because of some external factor—malnutrition, cancer, or infection, particularly by HIV.

Immunodeficiency disorders are generally first identified as the result of recurrent or persisting infections in the affected individual. Diagnosis of immunodeficiencies begins with an accurate individual and family history, which will help in the selection of diagnostic laboratory tests. Diagnostic tests of most of these disorders may include a CBC and differential count, quantitation of total immunoglobulin and subtypes, FACS analysis of cell subtypes and surface proteins, and analysis of complement. Additional genetic studies or molecular biological assays for specific gene products may be performed to determine the exact mutation involved.

Although the symptoms of immunodeficiency diseases may be controlled through replacement therapy of cells or factor or by prophylactic use of antibiotics and aggressive treatment of infection, the definitive treatment for many of these disorders is bone marrow or stem cell transplantation. This therapy is not without difficulty, and graft-versus-host disease remains a serious concern. The ideal therapy would be transfection of a normal gene into the patient's own stem cells, which could then be reinfused. Some progress has been made toward this end, but the process is still in its infancy and is not yet even remotely possible for those disorders for which no specific mutation has been found.

POINTS TO REMEMBER

▶ An imbalance in the immune system's tolerance to and recognition of self-antigen and foreign antigen is responsible for the onset of autoimmune disease.

▶ Environmental and genetic factors play a role in the development of autoimmune disease.

▶ Autoimmune disease is more common in women than in men, and occurrence of multiple autoimmune diseases is not uncommon.

▶ Autoimmune diseases may be categorized into organ-specific or systemic subclasses.

▶ Damage in autoimmune disease may be caused by a self-directed cell-mediated immune response, by autoantibody, or by immune complex deposition.

▶ Autoimmune disease is currently treated by immunosuppressive drugs that target the entire immune response rather than solely the autoimmune response.

▶ Categorization of immunodeficiency disorders is purely artificial. The interaction between the innate and adaptive immune systems and humoral and cell-mediated immunity means that a defect in one arm of the immune system will inevitably affect other parts of the immune response.

▶ Immunodeficiency disorders may be asymptomatic or may result in recurrent or persistent life-threatening infections, cancers, or autoimmune disease.

▶ Primary immunodeficiency disorders are the result of a genetic mutation and are present at birth. Secondary immunodeficiencies are the result of some external factor.

▶ Autoimmune diseases are the result of an overvigorous and inappropriate immune response, while immunodeficiency diseases represent the failure of some (or all) portion(s) of the immune response.

LEARNING ASSESSMENT QUESTIONS

1. About _____ of the population has at least one autoimmune disease.
   a. 0–10%
   b. 10–20%
   c. 20–30%
   d. 30–50%

2. When antibodies are made to antigens on a microorganism that are also able to cross-react with host antigenic determinants that closely resemble that organism's antigens, the mechanism leading to development of autoimmune disease is called
   a. exposure of sequestered antigens.
   b. molecular mimicry.
   c. epitope spreading.
   d. sequestration of antigen.

3. One of the strongest links between presence of a particular MHC gene and development of an autoimmune disease has been made between HLA B27 and
   a. insulin-dependent diabetes mellitus.
   b. systemic lupus erythematosus.

   c. Graves' disease.
   d. ankylosing spondylitis.

4. Myasthenia gravis is an example of a(n) _____ autoimmune disease.
   a. organ-specific
   b. systemic
   c. immune complex-mediated
   d. cell-mediated

5. Patients with _____ commonly have a positive ANA screen and decreased levels of complement, particularly during periods of active disease.
   a. Hashimoto's thyroiditis
   b. rheumatoid arthritis
   c. systemic lupus erythematosus
   d. systemic sclerosis

6. Which of the following is not an example of a primary immunodeficiency disorder?
   a. LAD type I
   b. Nezelof's syndrome
   c. AIDS
   d. SCID

7. True or false: Some primary immunodeficiency disorders may also be associated with one or more autoimmune diseases.

8. Increased infections caused by _____ are associated with deficiencies in immunoglobulins.
   a. viruses
   b. bacteria
   c. fungi
   d. protozoa

9. The most severe form of SCID is caused by
   a. X-linked immunodeficiency.
   b. ADA deficiency.
   c. reticular dysgenesis.
   d. JAK-3 deficiency.

10. HIV binds to and enters CD4+ T cells via an interaction between
    a. HIV gp120 and T cell CD3.
    b. HIV gp41 and T cell CD3.
    c. HIV gp120 and T cell CD4.
    d. HIV gp41 and T cell CD4.

REFERENCES

Bach, J. F. 1995. Organ-specific autoimmunity. *Immunol Today* 16:353.

Benoist, C. and D. Matis. 2001. Autoimmunity provoked by infection: How good is the case for T cell epitope mimicry. *Nat Immunol* 2:797.

Berger, E. A, P. M. Murphy, and J. M. Farber. 1999. Chemokine receptors as HIV-1 coreceptors: Roles in viral entry, tropism, and disease. *Ann Rev Immunol* 18:657.

Buckley, R. H. 2000. Primary immunodeficiency diseases due to defects in lymphocytes. *N Eng J Med* 343:1313.

Candotti, F. and R. M. Blaese. 1998. Gene therapy of primary immunodeficiencies. *Springer Semin Immunopathol* 19:493.

Chapel, H., R. Geha, and F. Rosen. 2003. Primary immunodeficiency diseases: An update. *Clin Exp Immunol* 132:9.

Cohen, O. J. and A. S. Fauci. 2001. Current strategies in the treatment of HIV infection. *Adv Int Med* 46:207.

Fischer, A. 2001. Primary immunodeficiency diseases: An experimental model for molecular medicine. *Lancet* 357:1863.

Fischer, A., M. Cavazzana-Calvo, G. De-Saint-Basile, et al. 1997. Naturally occurring primary deficiencies of the immune system. *Ann Rev Immunol* 15:93.

Haase, A. T. 1999. Population biology of HIV-1 infections: Viral and CD4+ T cell demographics and dynamics in lymphoid tissues. *Ann Rev Immunol* 17:625.

Hausmanns, S. and K. W. Wucherpfennig. 1997. Activation of autoreactive T cells by peptides form human pathogens. *Curr Opin Immunol* 9:831.

Hacein-Bey-Abinas, S., F. Le Deist, F. Carlier, et al. 2002. Sustained correction of X-linked severe combined immunodeficiency by ex vivo gene therapy. *N Engl J Med* 356:1185.

Hacein-Bey-Abina, S., Von Kalle, C., Schmidt, M. et al. 2003. LMO2-associated clonal T cell proliferation in two patients after gene therapy for SCID-X1. *Science* 302:415.

King C. and N. Sarvetnick. 1997. Organ specific autoimmunity. *Curr Opin Immunol* 9:863.

Kohn, D. B. 2001. Gene therapy for genetic haematological disorders and immunodeficiencies. *J Int Med* 249:379.

Mascola, J. R. and G. J. Nabel. 2001. Vaccines for the prevention of HIV-1 disease. *Current Opin Immunol* 13:489.

McDevitt, H. O. 2000. Discovering the role of the major histocompatibility complex in the immune response. *Ann Rev Immunol* 18:1.

Rocken, M. and E. M. Shevach. 1996. Immune deviation—the third dimension of nondeletional T cell tolerance. *Immunol Rev* 149:175.

Rose, N. R. 1998. The role of infection in the pathogenesis of autoimmune disease. *Semin Immunol* 10:5.

Shiomchik, M. J., J. Craft, and M. J. Mamula. 2001. From T to B and back again: Positive feedback in systemic autoimmune disease. *Nat Rev Immunol* 1:147.

Smart, B. A., H. D. Ochs. 1997. The molecular basis and treatment of primary immunodeficiency disorders. *Curr Opin Pediatr* 9:570.

Theofilopoulos, A. N. 1995. The basis of autoimmunity. Part I: Mechanisms of aberrant self-recognition. *Immunol Today* 16:90.

Theofilopoulos, A. N. 1995. The basis of autoimmunity. Part II: Genetic predisposition. *Immunol Today* 16:150.

9

Transplant Immunology

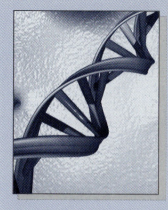

■ CHAPTER CHECKLIST

After reading and studying this chapter, the reader should be able to:

1. Identify the genetic components of the major histocompatibility complex.
2. Describe how these components (identified in objective #1 above) interact to present antigens at the protein level.
3. Describe the acceptable clinical and laboratory parameters for solid organ/bone marrow transplant.
4. Relate the elements involved in transplant rejection.
5. Discuss the relevance of HLA and disease association.
6. Identify the most common HLA associated diseases.

⊚ CASE IN POINT

A 13-year-old girl born with one diseased kidney requires an organ transplant. Laboratory tests show her father to be an acceptable donor. After the transplant, she did well for 2 years although she often skipped her medicine. When her kidney started to fail, her father offered to donate his only remaining kidney. In lieu of this, the search was widened to other family members who might be compatible. Her uncle was determined to be a suitable candidate. She was transplanted, with the stipulation that she would take her medicine to guard against rejection.

ISSUES TO CONSIDER

After reading the patient's case history, consider

- Reasons why the patient's father and uncle were considered to be suitable donors
- Laboratory tests that led to this conclusion
- Reasons why you would expect siblings to be suitable donors
- Factors that led to relatively early graft failure
- Prevention of future graft rejection

IMPORTANT TERMS

Allele
Alloepitope
Allogeneic
Ankylosing spondylitis (AS)
Autologous
CD4 T lymphocyte (T⁻ helper cell)
CD8 T lymphocyte (T⁺ suppressor cell)
Codominant
Crossing over
Cytokines
Dendritic cells
Endocytosis
Endogenous
Exogenous
Gene

Graft versus host disease (GVHD)
Haplotype
Heterodimer
Heterozygous
Homologous
Homozygous
Human leukocyte antigen (HLA)
Immunocompetent
Immunoglobulin superfamily
Interferon
Law of Independent Assortment
Law of Segregation
Linkage disequilibrium
Linked

Major histocompatibility complex (MHC)
MHC restriction
Narcolepsy
Natural-killer (NK) cell
Odds ratio
Polymorphic
Private epitopes
Progenitor cell
Pseudogene
Public epitopes
Recombination
Split
Spondyloarathropathies
Tolerance
Tumor necrosis factor-α (TNF-α)

▶ INTRODUCTION

Opportunities for clinical laboratory scientists/medical technologists to expand their knowledge are not restricted to the "traditional" laboratory areas of chemistry, hematology, microbiology, and blood banking. The field of transplant immunology or histocompatibility introduces the technologist to a new set of theoretical concepts and technical skills. To ensure compatibility between an organ donor and a potential recipient, this laboratory performs procedures generally not available in most clinical labs. These tests tend to be manual and time consuming (usually 3–6 hours per test), expensive, and low volume. Since they are performed on purified cell populations (as opposed to serum), the primary reagents are cells and sera, which require complex quality control. In the past, most of these reagents had to be obtained locally through extensive screening. As the clinical lab as evolved, so has histocompatibility testing, from cellular and serological procedures to those that can be accomplished by DNA methods. This chapter and Chapter 15 serve as an introduction to this challenging and fast-paced corner of laboratory medicine.

▶ THE MAJOR HISTOCOMPATIBILITY COMPLEX

The human **major histocompatibility complex (MHC)** is a cluster of **genes** found on the short arm of chromosome 6 at band 21 (6p21). These genes code for proteins that have a role in immune recognition. The proteins complex with peptide fragments from degraded viral and bacterial antigens and "present" them to T lymphocytes. The interaction between the degraded fragment and the T cell receptors stimulates the T cell to produce molecules aimed at destruction of the cell and the foreign antigen it carries. Transplanted tissue may trigger a similar destructive mechanism (termed rejection) if the recipient's cells recognize the MHC protein products on the surface of the transplanted tissue as "foreign" or if **immunocompetent** cells transplanted on the donor tissue target the "foreign" cells of the recipient for elimination. Testing performed in the histocompatibility laboratory prior to transplant is just one of a series of steps taken to minimize the chances of rejection by ensuring compatibility between a donor and the potential recipient.

HISTORICAL BACKGROUND

A successful blood transfusion depends upon ABO compatibility between the donor and the recipient. In the 1920s, Landsteiner was the first to suggest that a successful transplant may employ a similar mechanism. Gorer noted that recipient mice usually rejected tumors transplanted among unrelated mice. This led to the description of a complex of mouse antigens, termed H-2, which when matched between donor and recipient, markedly improved the ability of the graft to survive. These were called the major histocompatibility antigens (MHC). In the 1950s, the human MHC, termed **human leukocyte antigen (HLA),** was identified after studying antibody responses to white blood cells. Cytogenetic studies later localized the human MHC genes to the short arm of chromosome 6 (6p21). Today we know that the protein products of these genes are involved in all aspects of immune recognition. In utero, the HLA system plays a role in thymic T-cell receptor (TCR) selection and in the maturation of antigen-specific T cells. The presence of this system is critical to the ability of the individual's immune system to distinguish "self" from "not self." T cells in the fetal thymus are eliminated by apoptosis if they do not have TCRs that bind to self antigen or if they have TCRs, that bind too strongly to self antigens. There is also a well-documented association between the presence of certain HLA antigens and disease. Table 9-1✪ outlines significant events in the definition of the human MHC.

ORGANIZATION OF THE HUMAN MHC ON CHROMOSOME 6

The HLA genes code for molecules that play a role in the immune response. The human MHC encompasses a 3.6 million base pair region. Within this area, 224 gene loci have been identified. Approximately 128 of these genes are believed to be actively expressed with about 40% having some type of immune system function. The region is subdivided into three regions (Class I, Class III, and Class II, in that order). The map order

---

✪ TABLE 9-1

Significant Events in the Definition of Human MHC

Date	Event
1920s	Leukocyte antigens observed in humans
1950s	Existence of leukocyte antibodies (leukoagglutinins) demonstrated in sera of patients immunized by blood transfusion or pregnancy.
	These leukoagglutinins defined a series of polymorphic, genetically determined antigens.
	The first human HLA alloantigen shown to be genetically determined was "MAC." This was later named HLA-A2 plus HLA-A28.
	This system was analogous to the MHC of mice.
1960s	Association between human leukoagglutinating antibodies and tissue transplantation inferred from studies of skin graft recipients preimmunized with peripheral blood leukocytes from the prospective donor.
	Leukoagglutinins causing leukopenia shown to be induced by alloimmunization. Allospecificity demonstrated.
	Microlymphocytotoxicity (CDC) test introduced.
	Computer technology defined clusters of antisera reactive to discrete antigens later shown to correspond to Bw4 and Bw6.
	First World Health Organization workshop convened in Durham, NC, to compare and evaluate techniques and exchange ideas, reagents, concepts.
	Miniaturization of the CDC enabled use on a routine basis.
	Amos modification of the CDC enhanced test sensitivity.
	A two-locus model for HLA was proposed based on family studies. Each locus was believed to have multiple alleles. The two loci were later identified as HLA-A and HLA-B. Together they composed the Class I HLA.
1970s	Another HLA locus, distinct from the previous serology defined HLA loci was proposed; named HLA-Dw.
	The mixed lymphocyte culture (MLC) test allowed definition of Class II antigens through their ability to stimulate allogeneic T cells; the 7-day MLC test used to define HLA-D series.
	Cellular techniques used to identify antibodies in alloantisera that were reactive with HLA-D molecules.
	Using B lymphocytes as the target cell, serologically defined determinants were correlated with HLA Dw.
	International histocompatibility workshop uses MLC to define the HLA-D series; serologic specificities for HLA-D termed DR for D-related.
	The existence of a third Class 1 HLA locus, HLA-C, was confirmed.
	Serologic testing and immunochemical studies identified additional Class II antigens, DR52, DR53, DR51, and DQ.
	Role of HLA genes in immune response and MHC restriction defined.
1980s	Class II DP locus identified.
1990s	Initial studies began characterizing DNA coding sequences and locations of genes on MHC by molecular biology.

and position of genes within these regions has been determined by meiotic linkage studies and molecular techniques such as DNA cloning, DNA sequencing, and pulsed field gel electrophoresis. The HLA system is the most **polymorphic** in man. The resulting variability in the amino acid sequence of the proteins coded for by these loci allows the body to adapt to a wide variety of invading pathogens, a characteristic believed essential to species survival and that is thought to be maintained in the population by selection. The proteins coded by the HLA region are members of the **immunoglobulin superfamily** (e.g., having an antibody-like structure with constant and variable regions).

INHERITANCE/HAPLOTYPES

The MHC genes are **linked.** Because of their close proximity, they segregate as a group or **haplotype** during meiosis. Since one copy of chromosome 6 is inherited from each parent, each individual inherits two haplotypes and, thus, two sets of HLA genes. The gene **alleles** can be **homozygous** or **heterozygous,** and gene expression is **codominant.** By convention, the paternal haplotypes are designated a and b, and the maternal haplotypes are designated c and d. For any given mating, inheritance of a particular haplotype follows Mendel's **Law of Segregation** and **Law of Independent Assortment.** The chance of inheriting a particular haplotype is 1 in 4 or 25%. The probability of two sibs being HLA identical is 25% (Figure 9-1■). The patient in the case study has an HLA type that is a one haplotype match with that of her father. Testing in the HLA laboratory distinguishes the alleles present on a particular haplotype.

Occasionally, a physical exchange of genetic material can occur between haplotypes during parental meiosis. The probability of **crossing over** or **recombination** occurring between linked genes is proportional to the distance separating the two loci. Molecular data suggest that certain regions along the chromosome may be prone to recombination. The presence of these "hot spots" within the HLA region may also affect the likelihood of recombination. Approximately 2% of offspring may demonstrate a recombinant genotype.

INHERITANCE/DISEQUILIBRIUM

Statistics predict that two alleles will occur together on the same haplotype at a specified incidence in the population with the expected frequency being a product of the frequencies of the individual alleles ($f_1 \times f_2 = f_{expected}$). Actual observations, however, demonstrate that these rates are higher than would be expected on the basis of chance alone. This effect, termed **linkage disequilibrium,** appears to be related to ethnicity and nationality. For example, the expected frequency of the HLA-A1 and HLA-B8 alleles occurring together would be 1.6% ($f_{HLA-A1} \times f_{HLA-B8}$ or 0.16×0.1). However, in certain Caucasian populations in Northern Europe, the frequency is as high as 8%. In specific populations, certain combinations of HLA alleles may provide a selective survival advantage.

CLASS I MHC

Organization of the Class I Region

Within the Class I region of the human MHC, there are over 20 genes. Many are nonfunctional (**pseudogenes**). The Class I region can be subdivided into six subregions, designated HLA-A, HLA-B, HLA-C, HLA-E, HLA-F, HLA-G, and HLA-J (Figure 9-2■). The "classical" Class I molecules (HLA-A, HLA-B, HLA-C), those directly involved in immune recognition, are transmembrane **heterodimers** consisting of an α-chain and a β-chain. The genes in the Class I-MHC region on chromosome 6 code for the α-chain protein, which has a structure resembling the heavy chain of an immunoglobulin molecule. The other half of the heterodimer, the β-chain, is a 12-kilodalton protein called β2-microglobulin. This protein has a structure similar to an immunoglobulin light chain and is coded for by a gene on chromosome 15. The β2-microglobulin gene sequence is highly conserved and not variable.

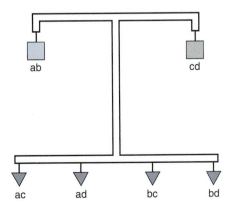

■ **FIGURE 9-1** Possible genotypes when paternal and maternal haplotypes are combined (ab = paternal; cd = maternal).

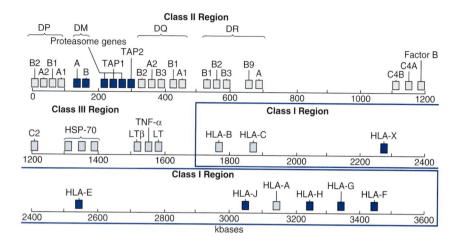

■ FIGURE 9-2 Map highlighting the Class I region of the human MHC. The products coded by each subregion are shown. Not all genes are included.

After translation, while still in the cytoplasm, the α-chain bonds noncovalently with β2-microglobulin to form the Class I molecule. On the cell surface, β2-microglobulin remains attached to the α-chain and does not come in contact with the cell surface. This association must be intact in order for Class I molecule to function (Figure 9-3■).

Each "classical" transplantation gene has eight exons. On the translated protein, three domains, each having 90 amino acid residues, are located extracellu-

larly (α1, α2, α3). The α3 domain is highly conserved. The α1 and α2 domains, located at the top of the protein, interact with each other through a series of β-pleated sheets to form a unique groove whose shape is determined by the structure of the amino acids lining it. This genetic polymorphism serves to produce a groove with a unique conformation.

Endogenous peptide antigens derived from proteins synthesized in the cell de novo (e.g., viral peptides) have shapes allowing them to fit within the Class I groove if they are conformationally similar, analogous to the fitting together of two pieces of a puzzle. The size of the typical fragment fitting in the groove is 6–10 amino acids. Proteins coded for within the Class II MHC region assist in antigen degradation (e.g., LMP 2, LMP 7) and transportation of the degraded fragments from the cytoplasm to the endoplasmic reticulum (e.g., TAP1, TAP2). Once the Class I–fragment binding occurs, the complex is transported to the cell surface, where the Class I protein "positions" itself such that the peptide antigen fragment lying within the groove is accessible for binding with the T cell receptor on a circulating **CD8 T lymphocyte (T-suppressor cell).** This will occur only if the Class I molecule and the CD8 T lymphocyte share a class I allele product (**MHC restriction**). Other amino acid residues within the α1-α2 groove interact with the T-cell receptor assist in the recognition process (Figure 9-4■).

If the T lymphocyte becomes activated, it will release molecules (e.g., **cytokines**) that will initiate immune destruction of the antigen and the presenting cell. The T lymph also serves to protect the cell presenting the

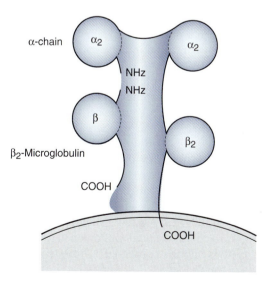

■ FIGURE 9-3 Structure of the HLA Class I molecule. Adapted from: KuKuruga D and Eisenberry AB. Used by permission American Society of Clinical Pathologists.

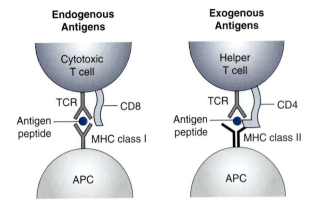

Endogenous Antigens
Exogenous Antigens

■ **FIGURE 9-4** The cell surface interactions between T lymphocytes and antigen presenting cells (APC). The T cell receptor on the T suppressor/CD8 and T helper/CD4 lymphocytes recognizes antigen presented by either the MHC Class I or Class II molecules, respectively. Adapted from: KuKuruga D and Eisenberry AB. Used by permission American Society of Clinical Pathologists.

antigen from the actions other cells (e.g., **natural killer** or **NK cells**) that may directly lyse and destroy it. The serological tests performed in the HLA laboratory use alloantisera and monoclonal antibodies to define the alleles coding for the amino acids within the α1 and α2 region of the Class I MHC molecule.

Cell Surface Expression

Class I proteins are expressed on the cell surface of almost all nucleated cells and platelets and to a limited extent on reticulocytes. The level of expression is highest on lymphoid cells and lowest in brain, muscle, and sperm cells. Atypical RBC may also express Class I antigens on young cells (Bg^a, Bg^b, Bg^c). On any given cell surface, there are thousands of Class I proteins. The number can be increased or decreased by molecules released from stimulated T helper cells (e.g., cytokines such as **interferon** γ and **tumor necrosis factor-α** or **TNF-α**). These molecules bind to DNA sequences upstream from the start of the Class I gene sequence and serve to increase the rate of transcription. Tumors and certain viruses (e.g., HIV) have been shown to suppress Class I gene transcription. Other molecules can act to increase the affinity of cellular interactions and to transmit costimulatory signals.

Other Class I Genes

Gene cloning has identified approximately 20 "nonclassical" or Class 1b genes. Many are pseudogenes. The Class 1b genes are indirectly involved in the immune recognition and may serve as mediators in the adaptive immune response. They are homologous to the "classical" transplantation antigens in structure and need to be associated with β2-microglobulin for expression. However, unlike their classical cousins, these genes have a low level of allelic polymorphism, low cell surface expression, and a variable distribution pattern. HLA-E and HLA-G may protect cells against the actions of NK cells. The function of HLA-F is not known.

CLASS II MHC

Organization of the Class II Region

A comparison of the DNA sequences of the Class I and Class II genes suggests that these MHC genes arose by a series of successive gene duplications with the original gene duplication giving rise to the Class I HLA-A and HLA-B genes and more recent duplications generating the Class II genes. The Class II region of the human MHC spans 1100 kilobases of DNA (Figure 9-5■). Many of the genes within this region are pseudogenes. Like the Class I protein, the Class II molecule is a heterodimer with an α and β chain. However, unlike the Class I MHC, both the α- and β-chain genes are coded for within the Class II region. There are several Class II MHC subregions (DR, DQ, DP, DM, DO) and each contains at least one expressed and β gene. The five-exon α-chain gene codes for a 28,000 MW transmembrane polypeptide similar in structure to an immunoglobulin heavy chain. The six-exon β-chain gene codes for a 33,000 MW transmembrane polypeptide similar in structure to an immunoglobulin light chain. Like the Class I polypeptide, the newly transcribed Class II α and β proteins bind noncovalently in the cytoplasm of the cell to form a protein heterodimer that will associate with any conformationally suitable **exogenous** antigen of 12–30 amino acids in length. These fragments are degraded, soluble, and particulate peptide antigens (e.g., from bacteria) taken up in cells by **endocytosis**. This Class II complex is transported to the cell surface where, similar to the Class I protein, the Class II heterodimer "positions" the antigen fragment for presentation to a circulating **CD4 + T lymphocyte (T-helper cell)** (see Figure 9-4). The extracellular region of the protein can be separated into two domains (α1β1 and α2β2) with each α and β segment having 90 amino acid residues. The α2β2 region is homologous to the immunoglobulin constant region domain and is highly conserved. The α1β1 region is similar to the Class I α1α2 domains and is highly polymorphic. Like the α1α2 domains of the Class I MHC protein, the α1β1 domains interact at the top of the molecule to form a groove that accommodates peptide

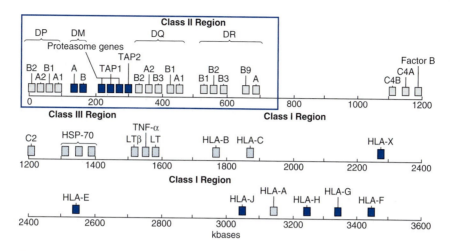

■ **FIGURE 9-5** The Class II region of the human MHC. The products coded by each subregion are shown. Not all products are included. From: Henry JB, 2001. Used by permission.

fragments of specific conformations (Figure 9-6■). The recognition of the peptide antigen by the T-cell receptor stimulates the CD4 lymphocyte and initiates the immune response (Table 9-2✪).

Subregions of the Class II MHC

There are three main subregions of the Class II MHC: DR, DQ, and DP (see Figure 9-5). In the DR region, there is one *DRA* gene (α-chain) that produces a DRA protein that is similar in all haplotypes. Nine *DRB* genes (β-chain) have been identified. The DRB1 pro-

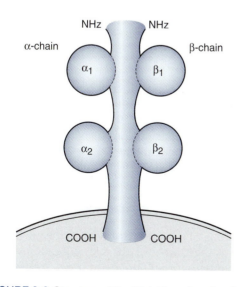

■ **FIGURE 9-6** Structure of the HLA Class II molecule. Adapted from: KuKuruga D and Eisenberry AB. Used by permission American Society of Clinical Pathologists.

tein (*DRA* gene plus *DRB1* gene) makes up over 50% of the total number of Class II proteins present on the surface of the cell and is the predominant Class II protein present. The *DRB1* gene is highly polymorphic, with sequence differences giving rise to 18 different *DRB1* alleles with over 306 sub-alleles (Table 9-3✪).

The presence of certain DRB1 alleles impacts the expression of other β-chain genes. All alleles except DRB1*01 (the first allele identified), DRB1*08 (the eighth allele identified), and DRB1*10 (the tenth allele identified) are associated with the expression of a second β-chain gene. These genes are *DRB3*, *DRB4* or *DRB5*. The DRB1 alleles associated with the expression of *DRB3* are DRB1*03, *11, *12, *13, and *14. The resulting protein, DR52 (*DRA* plus *DRB3*), is present on the surface of the cell at a concentration 10 times less that that of DRB1. The DRB1 alleles associated with the expression of *DRB4* are DRB1*04, *07, and *09. The protein is DR53 (*DRA* plus *DR4*). The DRB1 alleles associated with the expression of *DRB5* are DRB1*15 and *16. The protein is DR51 (*DRA* plus *DR5*). *DRB2* is a pseudogene and is not expressed.

The DQ subregion contains two *DQA* and two *DQB* genes. The *DQB1*-gene loci are polymorphic. Serologic testing has identified nine DQ heterodimers of which there are 39 alleles (Table 9-3). The *DQA2* and *DQB2* genes are similar to *DQA1* and *DQB1*, but no functional products are produced. DQ molecules represent 15–20% of the total Class II molecules on the cell surface.

The DP subregion contains two *DPA* and two *DPB* genes. The *DP*-gene loci are polymorphic. Seventy-seven gene products and 84 alleles (DwP1 through

---

✪ TABLE 9-2

How the CD4+ Helper T Cells Affects the Immune Response.

- Help B lymphs to differentiate into antibody producing cells
- Help other T lymphs to differentiate into cytotoxic cells or cells with a suppressor function
- Act as a cytotoxic cell, directly killing cells with the appropriate target (cells expressing Class II MHC complex with specific antigen)
- Function as a cell with suppressor functions causing a dampening of the immune response
- Produce a number of biologically important molecules (e.g., INF gamma) that augment the immune response and increase expression of MHC molecules on target cells
- Produce growth factors (e.g., IL2) that effect a wide range of cells from hematopoietic progenitor cells to mature lymphs

From: Henry, 2001.

DwP4) have been identified (see Table 9-3). *DPA2* and *DPB2* are pseudogenes. The level of DP expressed in the cell is very low and is associated primarily with platelets.

Cell Surface Expression

Class II molecules are present on the surface of B lymphocytes, activated T lymphocytes, antigen presenting cells (APC) such as monocytes and macrophages and **dendritic cells.** Gene expression may be affected by the binding of upstream regulatory sequences by molecules released from activated cells (e.g., interferon-γ and cytokines).

Other Class II Genes

The DO and DM gene products form heterodimers that are expressed inside of the cell. Located in specialized intracellular compartments, they assist the binding of newly synthesized Class II molecules to a peptide antigen. DM may regulate and stabilize peptide binding to DR, DQ, and DP. DO is believed to negatively regulates the function of DM. Other genes from the Class II region encode components of proteosome complex, a macromolecular structure that degrades proteins in the cytoplasm. This complex is also associated with a peptide transporter that is involved in moving peptides from the cytoplasm to the endoplasmic reticulum.

CLASS III MHC

The Class III MHC region encodes complement components (e.g., C2, C4, Bf) that are involved in cleaving C3, critical to initiating an inflammatory response. Other genes in this region such as 21-hydroxylase (Cyp21), heat shock protein 70 (Hsp70), and TNF-α are not involved in the immune response.

THE IMMUNE RESPONSE

The binding of a peptide fragment in the polymorphic groove of the Class I or Class II molecule is the first step in initiating the immune response. The ability of a fragment to fit within this space is dependent on the shape of the groove as configured by the amino acids lining it. Variability of the amino acid sequence, as de-

---

✪ TABLE 9-3

Numbers of Alleles with Official Names at Each Locus by December 1998

Locus	Number of Alleles	Locus	Number of Alleles
HLA-A	239	HLA-DQA1	19
HLA-B	475	HLA-DQB1	39
HLA-C	74	HLA-DPA1	15
HLA-E	5	HLA-DPB1	84
HLA-G	14	HLA-DOA	8
HLA-DRB1	306	HLA-DMA	4
HLA-DRB3	19	HLA-DMB	5
HLA-DRB4	9	TAP1	6
HLA-DRB5	14	TAP2	
HLA-DRB6	3	MICA	15
HLA-DRB7	2		

From: Bodmer et al., 1999.

termined by the DNA allele present on the individual's haplotype, results in different shaped grooves, and thus the ability to accommodate different peptide fragments produced from proteins manufactured within the cell (endogenous or viral antigens) or phagocytized proteins (exogenous or bacterial antigens). The Class I and Class II molecules can also bind to self antigens that are produced in the normal process of cellular protein degradation. Generally, these are not recognized by the TCR (**tolerance**). Cells with TCR that do bind strongly to self antigens are generally eliminated in the thymus by apoptosis. If these self reactive cells should be released into the peripheral circulation, they may trigger a self-destructive process that could lead to autoimmunity.

In transplant patients, most immune responses are generated not from bacterial, viral antigens or self antigens, but from presentation of **alloepitopes** derived from the transplanted tissue to circulating T lymphocytes. There are two types of alloepitopes present on the transplanted tissue. **Private epitopes** are unique to a single gene product. **Public epitopes** are present on more than one gene product. They can reside on the same HLA molecule as a private epitope but at a different site (e.g., HLA-B). Some public epitopes may be widely distributed (e.g., Bw4 and Bw6). Cross-reactive groups (CREGS) have been defined that categorize the cross-reactive alleles of HLA-A and HLA-B (Table 9-4✪). The identification of CREGS is important for

patients who await transplantation or who require repetitive platelet transfusions.

NOMENCLATURE

The numerical designation of HLA Class I and Class II alleles is determined at international workshops sponsored by the World Heath Organization (WHO) Committee for HLA nomenclature. Here, serological and cellular defined specificities are compared and defined. These collaborative forums also serve as a platform to exchange ideas and typing reagents among participating laboratories.

In 1968, the HLA nomenclature committee designated two series for the MHC: HL-A and HL-B. Specificities were numbered sequentially according to the order of their discovery (e.g., HL-A2) with the letter "w" indicating provisional acceptance of a particular type (e.g., HL-Aw2). When the allele was formally accepted, the "w" was dropped. In 1975, new nomenclature was developed to accommodate the increasing number of loci that had been identified. Serology had defined a third Class I locus (HLA-C) and a specificity present only on B cells (HLA-D) and HL- was replaced by HLA- (e.g., HL-A2 was now HLA-A2). The numerical designation of HLA alleles started with 1 except for B. The "w" designation was retained. In 1984, the nomenclature was modified to include the HLA-D subregions of DR, DQ, and DP. To avoid confusion between HLA-C locus alleles and complement components, the "w" prefix was permanently retained for HLA-C locus alleles. Further nomenclature revisions were made with the development of DNA technology to determine the nucleotide sequences of allelic genes (Table 9-5✪).

Initially, HLA nomenclature involved the name of the HLA molecule followed by a number that reflected the sequential order in which the serological specificity was defined. Over time, as typing sera got more discriminating, serologic specificities were **split.** For example, HLA-B44 and B45 were initially thought to be private epitopes. They were later shown to share specificity with HLA-B12, which was identified first. Thus, HLA-B44 and HLA-B45 are splits of previously identified HLA-B12. Because of this, HLA-A and HLA-B specificities may not be numbered consecutively. With the progression of typing from serological and cellular methods to DNA based methods, a single serologically defined specificity may include as many as 50 different allele products (Table 9-3). New alleles are described in regular reports of the WHO nomenclature committee

✪ TABLE 9-4

Summary of Some of the Major Public Epitopes or Cross-Reactive Groups (CREG) of HLA-A and HLA-B Gene Products.

CREG	Associated HLA Gene Product	Approximate Antigen Frequency (%)
1C	A1,3,9,10,11,28,29,30,31,32,33	80
2C	A2,9,28,B17	66
5C	B5,15,17,18,35,53,70,49	59
7C	B7,13,22,27,40,41,47,48	64
8C	B8,14,16,18	37
12C	B12,13,21,40,41	45
4C	A24,25,32,34,Bw4	85
6C	Bw6, Cw1,3,7	87

From: American Society for Histocompatibility and Immunogenetics.

✪ TABLE 9-5

How HLA Alleles are Named

Description	Example
HLA designates MHC	HLA
HLA is followed by a capital letter indicating a specific MHC gene locus	HLA-A or HLA-B or HLA-C or HLA-D
All genes in D region followed by a second capital letter indicating a specific subregion	HLA-DR, HLA-DQ or HLA-DP
Loci coding for specific alleles based on serologic typing	HLA-A2
Gene locus followed by "*" and then a two-digit number indicating the specific allele most closely associated with the serologic specificity; DNA methods are numbered in the order in which they are described.	HLA-A*02
Allele specificity can be narrowed using high-resolution DNA methods.	HLA-A*0201 → 0210

(Figure 9-7■). All nucleotide sequences are deposited in Gen Bank.

▶ CLINICAL APPLICATIONS

HLA AND TRANSPLANTATION

The challenge of transplantation is to achieve long-term survival of the transplanted tissue. The major barrier to accomplishing this is the MHC. Transplanted tissues are rejected when the recipient's T cells are directly stimulated by a donor (foreign) MHC peptide or they are indirectly stimulated by the presentation of fragments from ingested donor-grafted tissue by recipient (self) MHC molecules to recipient T cells. The humoral and cell-mediated immune responses generated by recognition of these alloepitopes lead to graft rejection and are inevitable unless the patient receives adequate immunosuppression. The most common cause of graft rejection, particularly in teenagers, is the failure to take the immunosuppressive drugs regularly. This was the case with the patient in the case study. During rejection episodes, the induction of the Class I and Class II antigen expression in certain cells that do not normally express these molecules contributes to allograft rejection. Finding an HLA-compatible donor is critical but does not always ensure a successful transplant. Acute allograft rejection remains a major block

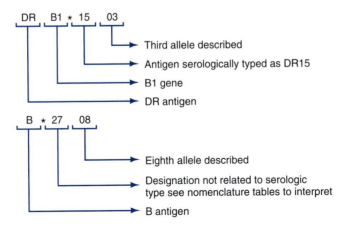

■ FIGURE 9-7 Pictorial description of HLA-DR nomenclature.
From: Hurley and Ng, 1994. Used with permission.

to long-term graft survival. Chronic allograft rejection is also a problem—the average life span of a solid organ allograft is about 10 years. Also important is achieving tolerance to donor alloantigens without suppression or obliteration of the protective functions of the immune system.

SOLID ORGAN TRANSPLANTATION

Kidney transplantation is the therapy of choice for patients with end stage renal disease. HLA-matching is part of the donor selection process and is performed pretransplant. Donors and recipients should be ABO and HLA compatible and must have a negative T cell and B cell donor specific cross-match when tested with the appropriate sera. (See Chapter 15 for a description of laboratory techniques.) Nonrenal solid organ transplants involve heart, lung, liver, pancreas, and small intestine. These are now accepted therapeutic procedures with approximately 58–67% of transplanted patients still living 5 years posttransplant. Depending on the type of nonrenal transplant, HLA compatibility testing and pretransplant donor crossmatching may not be necessary prior to transplant. However, because serum antibody screens of the recipient showing the presence of antibodies against the tissues of the prospective donor are an immunologic risk factor, these are recommended before transplant to identify the state of sensitization. Patients identified for heart, lung, pancreas, and small intestine transplant generally get pretransplant HLA typing and an antibody screen (termed PRA or panel reactive antibody). If the PRA is negative, the heart and lung recipients do not need pre-transplant crossmatching. All liver workups are done post-transplant.

The procurement and allocation of organs within the United States is arranged through the United Network of Organ Sharing (UNOS). Congress chartered this organization in 1964. In the UNOS system, organ distribution is based on a point system incorporating medical need, patient's time on the waiting list, PRA status, HLA-type, and age. To accomplish this, the continental United States has been divided into 11 UNOS regions that contain approximately 63 organ procurement organizations (OPO). When an organ becomes available, it is offered to transplant patients within that OPO region first. It is offered outside the region if a 6-antigen match is found or if the transplant surgeons refuse the organ. The ultimate decision to transplant or not to transplant always rests with the transplant surgeon.

The organ procurement process is initiated when a potential donor is identified (Figure 9-8■). Individuals

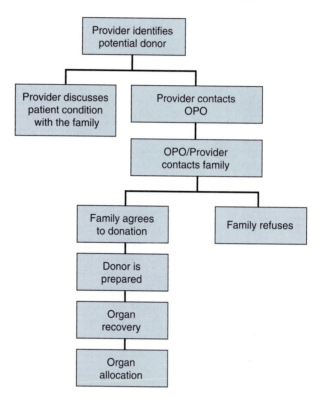

■ FIGURE 9-8 Typical scheme for organ procurement when a donor becomes available.

can donate either tissues or tissues and organs. Donors eligible to donate tissue and organs are those having cardiac function but no neurological activity. These include drowning, shooting and car accident victims, and patients with brain tumors and cerebral hemorrhage. Donors with neurological but no cardiac function are not eligible to donate organs because of the lack of blood perfusion (circulation) through the organs but may donate tissues (e.g., skin). Two conditions are contraindicative to organ donation. These are potential donors who are HIV positive or who have metastatic carcinoma.

When a potential donor is identified, the health care provider contacts the local OPO, who reviews the medical records to determine if the patient would be a suitable donor. Meanwhile, the provider approaches the patient's family to tell them the patient's condition. It is recommended that the subject of organ donation not be broached until the OPO has determined if the patient is an acceptable donor. Studies have shown that successful organ procurement is affected by (1) where the family is asked (not at the bedside), (2) who asks them (known/trusted provider), and (3) if a period of time has elapsed between the news that their loved one will not survive and the request for donation. If the family agrees to organ donation, the cost of medical care from that point on is paid for by the OPO. The patient is then prepared for donation, and the organs are harvested.

The first step in the allocation process is sending donor blood or tissue, usually lymph nodes, to HLA laboratories within that procurement region. Each laboratory has their own list of potential recipients who have been previously ABO typed, HLA typed, and tested for HLA antibodies. The information from each location is entered into the UNOS computer system by the local OPO for each potential recipient. When each laboratory receives the donor specimen, they HLA type the donor and perform crossmatches with each patient on their waiting list. The OPO confirms that all laboratories in their region obtained the same HLA type for the donor and enter the crossmatch results for each patient into the UNOS computer system. For kidney transplants, organ allocation is based on a point system. Points are awarded for (1) time on the waiting list, (2) degree of mismatch (with a complete match or 0-antigen mismatch getting the most points), (3) PRA ≥ 80% (patient has an antibody and shows potential compatibility with this donor), (4) medical urgency, (5) age (with pediatric patients less than 11 years old getting priority), and (6) donation status (if they ever donated an organ in the U.S.). The UNOS computer system ranks the patients based on these criteria. The patient with the most points, who is crossmatch negative, is the most likely candidate for that organ. However, the decision to transplant lies with the transplant surgeon, who can accept or refuse the organ. If the surgeon refuses the organ for that patient, it is offered to the transplant surgeon of the next patient on the list, and so on. If no one accepts the organ locally, it goes outside of the region and then nationally. This system favors local distribution and small transplant centers. The UNOS system has recently been challenged by the Department of Health and Human Services, which favors national distribution with the sickest person in the most need getting priority.

PROGENITOR CELL TRANSPLANTATION

Since 1997, the ease of **progenitor cell** collection has made it the transplant method of choice for patients with hematopoietic cell malignancies, bone marrow failure, certain inherited metabolic disorders, and congenital immunodeficiency syndromes. Sources of progenitor cells include bone marrow, growth factor

mobilized peripheral blood, and umbilical cord. Progenitor cell transplantation is the most difficult of all clinical transplants because it involves the transfer of an entire immune system. At the time of transplant, the recipients are totally immunodeficient, due to either inherited deficiencies (SCID) or pretransplant conditioning (chemotherapy or irradiation). Preconditioning serves to eliminate malignant cells and to prevent the recipient's immune system from rejecting the infused donor progenitor cells. The best donor is the recipient himself. **Autologous** transplants are performed if the malignancy is one that does not involve the bone marrow, is not genetic, or involves an identical twin. The next best is an identical twin or an HLA-matched brother or sister. However, since over 70% of patients requiring a transplant do not have an HLA-matched sibling, they are forced to turn to a national registry to find a compatible donor (**allogeneic** transplants). Following transplant, the greatest danger to the recipient is **graft versus host disease (GVHD)** where the lymphocytes present in the progenitor cell transplant respond to the foreign MHC of the recipient. GVHD is a risk whenever immunocompetent cells are transplanted, either intentionally or as a component of a solid organ graft. The survival rate following progenitor cell transplant varies with the disease and the transplant facility. Survival of patients with chronic myelomonocytic leukemia after hematopoietic cell transplantation with cells from an unrelated donor is 40% to 60% while patients with aplastic anemia have survival rates ranging from 30% to 50%, but as high as 90% depending on patient age.

Prior to progenitor cell transplant, members of the patient's immediate family are typed for HLA-A, HLA-B, and HLA-DR to determine if there is a match with the recipient and to establish inheritance of the haplotypes. HLA typing can be performed using serological or DNA procedures. Most DR typing is DNA-based and performed at high resolution to ensure a complete allelic match with the patient. Some degree of mismatching may be beneficial in stimulating an immune response against tumor cells. Some studies show that single HLA-mismatches may be tolerated and that the chance of relapse is greater for patients receiving an HLA-matched graft.

HLA AND DISEASE ASSOCIATION

The first connection between HLA and disease in humans was proposed in 1967. The HLA-antigenic cluster designated "4c" (now called the 5-CREG, a group of HLA-antigens that includes B5, B35, B18) was shown to be present more frequently in patients with Hodgkin's disease (51%) as compared to healthy individuals (27%). Although it was a weak association (**odds ratio** = 2.8), the findings were significant enough to begin the quest for more HLA-associated diseases. By the early 1970s two research groups independently reported the very strong association of HL-A27 or HL-A w27 (now known as HLA-B27) with **ankylosing spondylitis (AS).**

Current Issues

Today, there are hundreds of diseases that have been suggested to have HLA associations of varying degrees (Table 9-6✪). The clinical value of an HLA association

depends on whether HLA typing can be used to aid in the diagnosis of a disease or to predict the likelihood that an individual will develop a disease. Since the HLA association in most diseases is incomplete, HLA typing for disease diagnosis is requested in very few circumstances. The low predictive value, however, should not diminish the significant observations that HLA genetic factors do contribute to disease susceptibility and prompt a need for continued investigation into the MHC's role in disease etiology.

The case-control study is the simplest way to accumulate data for a disease association study. Once completed, the data are analyzed using a 2X2 contingency table. Table 9-7✪ shows a study of 63 African American

✪ TABLE 9-6

Some HLA-Associated Diseases

Disease	HLA[a]	Frequency in % Pts[b]	Cts	RR[c]
Celiac disease	DQ2	99	28	>250
Ankylosing spondylitis	B27	>95	9	>150
Reiter's disease	B27	>80	9	>40
Narcolepsy	DQ6	>95	33	>38
Acute anterior uveitis	B27	68	9	>20
Subacute thyroiditis	B35	70	14	14
Type I diabetes	DQ8	81	23	14
Type I diabetes	DQ6	<1	33	0.02
Multiple sclerosis	DR2,DQ6	86	33	12
Rheumatoid arthritis[d]	DR4	81	33	9
Juvenile RA[e]	DR8	38	7	8
Behcet's disease	B51	57	14	8
Psoriasis vulgaris	Cw6	87	33	7
Addison's disease	DR3	69	27	5
Graves' disease	DR3	65	27	4
Myasthenia gravis	DR3	50	27	2

[a]Serologically defined HLA molecules: many diseases are associated with only one or some of their subtypes.

[b]Data mainly from Norwegian patients and controls. Behcet's from Japanese study.

[c]Relative risk, that is, how much more frequently the disease occurs in individuals carrying versus those not carrying the given HLA molecule.

[d]Seropositive RA.

[e]Early onset pauciarticular JRA.

From: Thorsby, 1997.

✪ TABLE 9-7

A 2 × 2 Contingency Table Analyzing Disease Association Data for RA in African American Patients

Subjects	DR4+	DR4-	Total
Patients	14 (22%) (a)	49 (b)	63
Controls	12 (7.4%) (c)	150 (d)	162
Total	26	199	225

$X^2(1dt) = 9.74$; $p = 0.002$, Odds ratio = ad/cb = 3.6

From: Acton, 1993.

subjects with seropositive rheumatoid arthritis (RA) that showed 14 of the 63 possessed DR4 compared with 12 of the 162 matched controls. The chi-square (9.74) and p-value (0.002) are both significant, indicating that seropositive RA in African Americans is associated with DR4. Once the frequency of an HLA type is shown to be significant in the patient population, the strength of the association can also be assessed. Woolf's Odds Ratio (OR) calculates the odds that an individual with a given HLA type will develop a given disease. For RA, the OR is 3.6. Thus, the odds of an African American with DR4 having seropositive RA are 3.6 fold greater than someone who does not have DR4.

Relative Risk and Its Relevance to HLA-Disease Association

What are some ways HLA-disease association information can be used? Many diseases can be stratified based on their association with MHC genes. MHC association studies can help in (1) differential diagnosis (e.g., **narcolepsy**), (2) defining clinical subgroups in diseases (e.g., insulin-dependent diabetes mellitus,

IDDM), (3) revealing clusters of diseases such as the seronegative **spondyloarthropathies,** (4) predicting pathogenesis and natural history of infectious diseases, and (5) predicting response to therapy.

Narcolepsy is a sleep disorder characterized by excessive daytime sleepiness (hypersomnolence), sleep attacks, cataplexy, sleep paralysis, and hypnogogic hallucinations. If a physician has a patient who initially demonstrates some symptoms of hypersomnolence, but does not quite fit the classic narcolepsy picture, an HLA-DR/DQ typing could be useful. DR2 and DQ1 are strongly associated with narcolepsy in Japanese and Caucasians. The association is not as strong in African Americans. Molecular studies have shown that the true association in all races, with few exceptions, appears to be DQB1*0602. If the patient is DR2+ and/or DQ1+, then they are likely to have latent narcolepsy that will manifest in time. This information aids the physician in the diagnosis and treatment of the patient.

One of the strongest disease associations ever observed is that of HLA-B27 with ankylosing spondylitis (AS). B27 is also associated with a group of conditions called the seronegative spondyloarthropathies (Table 9-8✪). The common feature of the spondyloarthropathies is inflammation. The site of the inflammation generally determines the disease subset. Not only is B27 associated with all these diseases, but also there is considerable clinical overlap between them. A patient diagnosed with one of spondyloarthropathies may subsequently develop another in the group. Interestingly, a number of gram-negative enteric organisms are thought to be possible causative agents of some of these diseases (e.g., *Yersinia, Klebsiella, Shigella, E. coli,* and *Salmonella*).

A number of HLA phenotypes are associated with the natural history of infectious diseases. Many studies have looked at the differences between reduced and in-

✪ TABLE 9-8

Association of HLA-B27 with Seronegative Spondyloarthropathies in the Caucasian Population.

Disease	Odds Ratio	Disease	Odds Ratio
Ankylosing spondylitis (AS)	117	Acute anterior uveitis	15
Reiter's disease	48	Juvenile chronic arthritis	15
Lone aortic regurgitation	39	Psoriatic arthritis	4
Reactive arthritis	26	Whipple's disease	4
Crohn's disease+AS	23	Ulcerative colitis	2

From: Acton, 1993.

creased rates of progression to AIDS in HIV-1 positive individuals. Some HLA associations have been found. DRB1*0702 has been associated with a reduced rate of progression. B27 has been associated with a slower loss of both square root CD4 count and loss of CD4 percentage. The A1, B8, DR3 haplotype is associated with rapid loss of both markers. B35 may not only be a risk factor for a more rapid progression to AIDS, but also may predict the likelihood that opportunistic infections and Kaposi's sarcoma will occur. Several studies have shown that HLA is related to side effects and detrimental responses to some drugs. In other cases, there are either good responders or resistant or nonre-

sponders; for example, the lack of response to the hepatitis vaccine that is seen in some people with the A1, B8, DR3 haplotype. Although HLA-DR appears to mediate HBsAg presentation, it is unclear why certain HLA alleles are more frequent among the nonresponders.

DNA technology has defined MHC genes at the nucleotide sequence level. This higher technology does not change the way disease association studies are designed or how the data are collected and analyzed but does provide more precise information. This may allow better definition of the exact gene involved in the disease state and provide insight into possible etiological mechanisms.

SUMMARY

Realization that while tissues could be successfully transplanted between identical twins but not between any other individuals and identification of the proteins on the cell surface responsible for the resulting immune response has led to the development of transplant immunology and the field of histocompatibility. Patients who are prospective recipients of either a solid organ allograft or of a stem cell transplant are

routinely "tissue typed" for Class I and Class II MHC antigens and for the presence in their plasma of antibodies to MHC antigens. In general, a higher degree of matching for these antigens has led to improved graft survival. Certain haplotypes of MHC antigens are also strongly linked to the development of some diseases, particularly ankylosing spondylitis and autoimmune disorders.

POINTS TO REMEMBER

▶ The HLA field began following the discovery that some human leukocyte antigens turned out to be histocompatibility antigens.

▶ The major barrier to organ transplantation is the response of immunocompetent cells to foreign HLA antigen. Currently, this barrier can only be overcome by the use of immunosuppressive drugs.

▶ HLA matching improves short- and long-term graft survival, as well as avoiding serious graft versus host disease.

▶ As a genetic marker, HLA typing has been useful in paternity and forensic areas, disease predisposition, and prediction of a patient's response to therapy (Figure 9-9■).

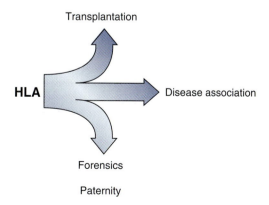

■ FIGURE 9-9 Schematic relationships involving the MHC in humans.

LEARNING ASSESSMENT QUESTIONS

1. Which of the following is an accurate descriptor of the class II MHC molecule?
   a. Associated with β-2 microglobulin on the surface of the cell
   b. Coded for by a gene on chromosme 15
   c. Transmembrane protein present on the surface of B lymphocytes
   d. Binds with the CD8 receptor on T lymphocytes

2. Which of the following statements is *not* true?
   a. Because of close linkage, the MHC alleles are always inherited as a haplotype.
   b. Homozygosity for a HLA allele indicates two identical copies have been inherited.
   c. HLA Class I molecules present endogenous antigens to circulating CD8+ lymphocytes.
   d. GVHD occurs when transplanted donor cells attack incompatible recipient antigens.

3. In solid organ transplants,
   a. liver transplant patients are HLA typed and cross-matched prior to transplant to insure compatibility.
   b. the decision to transplant an organ always lies with the transplant surgeon.
   c. a point system is used to determine who is the best candidate for a heart transplant.
   d. organ allocation is determined by the sickest patient.

4. Nomenclature HLA-A*0201 → 0210 indicates that
   a. there are 10 HLA-A2 genes.
   b. HLA-A2 is polymorphic at locus 0201.
   c. there are 10 identical alleles for HLA-A2.
   d. the HLA-A2 locus codes for one of 10 possible alleles.

5. Which change would increase Relative Risk for disease Y with HLA type X?
   a. Fewer patients with the disease Y observed in the sampled population.
   b. Fewer total individuals with HLA type X in the sampled population.
   c. Fewer controls with HLA type X in the sampled population.
   d. Fewer patients with disease Y but without HLA type X in the sampled population.

REFERENCES

Acton, R. P. 1993. Relationship of genes within the major histocompatibility complex to disease states. In: *Tissue Typing Reference Manual,* 3rd ed., ed. G. N. Tardif and J. M. MacQueen, SEOPF, Richmond, VA.

Beck, S. and J. Trowsdale. 1999. Sequence organization of the Class II region of the major MHC. *Immunol Rev* 167:201–10.

Bennington, J. L. 1984. *Dictionary of Laboratory Medicine and Technology.* W. B. Saunders Company, Philadelphia.

Billingham, R. E. and E. S. Silvers. 1971. *The Immunobiology of Transplantation.* Prentice Hall, Upper Saddle River, New Jersey.

Bjorkman, P. J., M. A. Saper, B. Samraoui et al. 1987. Structure of the human class I histocompatibility antigen, HLA-A2. *Nature* 329:506–12.

Bjorkman, P. J. and P. Parham. 1990. Structure, function and diversity of class I major histocompatibility complex molecules. *Annu Rev Biochem* 59:253–58.

Bodmer, J. G., S. G. E. Marsh, E. D. Albert, et al. 1997. Nomenclature for factors of the HLA system, 1996. *Vox Sang* 73:105–30.

Bodmer, J. G., S. G. E. Marsh, E. D. Albert, et al. 1999. Nomenclature for factors of the HLA system, 1998. *Vox Sang* 77:164–91.

Brodsky, F. M., L. Lem, A. Solache, and E. M. Bennett. 1999. Human pathogen subversion of antigen presentation. *Immunol Rev* 168:199–215.

Dausset, J. 1981. The major histocompatibility complex in man. *Science* 213:1469–74.

Dausset, J. and J. Colombani, eds. 1972. *Histocompatibility Testing.* Munksgaard, Copenhagen.

Dupont, B. 1989. Antigen Society #5 Report (B5, B51, Bw52, B18, B35, Bw53). In: *Immunobiology of HLA,* vol. I: *Histocompatibility Testing 1987,* ed. B. Dupont. Springer-Verlag, New York.

Gorga, J. C. 1992. Structural analysis of class II major histocompatibility complex proteins. *Crit Rev Immunol* 11:305–35.

Henry, J. B., ed. 2001. *Clinical Diagnosis and Management by Laboratory Methods.* W. B. Saunders, Philadelphia, pp. 927–48.

Hurley, C. K., G. Ng, and G. Hegland. 1994. *Interpretation of DNA-based typing of HLA and correlation with serologic types for Bone Marrow Transplantation: A guide for Transplant Coordinators.* Georgetown University.

Klein, J. 1987. *Natural History of the Major Histocompatibility Complex.* John Wiley and Sons, New York.

KuKuruga, D. and A. B. Eisenberry. 1993. Roles of molecular tools in tissue transplantation. *Lab Med* 24:589–95.

Momberg, F. and G. J. Hammerling. 1998. Generation and TAP-mediated transport of peptides for major histocompatibility complex class I molecules. *Adv Immunol* 68:191–56.

Morris, P., J. Shaman, M. Attaya, et al. 1994. An essential role for HLA-DM in antigen presentation by class II major histocompatibility molecules. *Nature* 368:551–54.

Parham, P., E. J. Adams, and K. L. Arnett. 1995. The origins of HLA-A,B,C polymorphisms. *Immunol Rev* 143:141–80.

Perkins, H. A. 1997. HLA typing for transplantation of stem cells from unrelated donors. *Lab Med* 28:451–55.

Rodey, G. E. 1991. *HLA beyond Tears.* De Novo, Inc., Atlanta, GA.

Rodey, G. E. and T. C. Fuller. 1987. Public epitopes and the antigenic structure of the HLA molecules. *Crit Rev Immunol* 7:229–67.

Roitt, I., J. Brostoff, and D. Male. 1989. *Immunology,* 2nd ed. C. V. Mosley Company, St. Louis, MD.

Singer, D. S. and J. Maguire. 1990. Regulation of expression of Class I MHC genes. *Crit Rev Immunol* 10:235–57.

Terasaki, P. I. 1991. Histocompatibility testing in transplantation. *Arch Pathol Lab Med* 115:250–54.

Thorsby, E. 1997. Invited anniversary review: HLA associated diseases. *Hum Immunol* 53:1–11.

Walker, R. H. 1993. HLA and disease. In: *AABB Technical Manual,* 11th ed.

10

Tumor Immunology

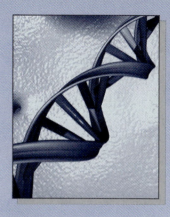

■ **CHAPTER CHECKLIST**

After reading and studying this chapter, the reader should be able to:

1. Differentiate between benign and malignant tumors.
2. Identify metastatic spread as the major impediment to cancer treatment.
3. List environmental, physical, genetic, hormonal, and viral factors as agents responsible for cellular transformation leading to the development of tumors.
4. Describe the detection and importance of tumor-specific transplantation antigens.
5. Distinguish between tumor-specific (TSA) and tumor-associated antigens (TAA).
6. Explain how technological developments have made it possible to examine TAA within individual patient tumors.
7. List the five specific categories of TAA recognized by CD8+ cells.
8. Discuss the potential for use of monoclonal antibodies against TAA as a passive immunotherapeutic strategy.
9. Explain the hypothesis of immunosurveillance and why it is actively debated currently.
10. Discuss evidence showing an immune response to TAA.
11. Explain the utility and the drawbacks of the CA-125II assay.
12. Discuss possible reasons why patients do not always reject a tumor even if they have mounted humoral and cellular responses against the tumor.
13. Using specific examples, differentiate between active and passive immunotherapeutic strategies.

 CASE IN POINT

A 42-year-old woman referred to a gynecologic oncologist after experiencing abdominal bloating/fluid retention was diagnosed with late stage (Stage IIIC) ovarian cancer with CA-125 levels >20,000 U/ml (Normal Range = 0–35 U/mL). She underwent extensive debulking surgery to remove the majority of the tumor, followed by six rounds of postoperative chemotherapy consisting of monthly doses of carboplatin and paclitaxol. Four weeks after her last round of chemotherapy, CA-125 levels dropped to 10 U/mL, but her oncologist cautioned her that ovarian cancer carries a high likelihood for recurrence and that recurrent tumors are usually resistant to the original chemotherapy regimen.

ⓒ CASE IN POINT (continued)

Because of this, her oncologist recommended that she consider enrollment in an experimental immunotherapy protocol.

ISSUES TO CONSIDER
After reading the patient's case history, consider

- ⓐ The type of immunotherapy (humoral vs. cellular, active vs. passive) that should be considered for this patient.

- ⓐ How the immunotherapy can be individualized to this patient's tumor.

- ⓐ Why this patient is a better candidate for experimental immunotherapy than someone with late stage disease.

- ⓐ The principles of the CA-125 assay and its value in screening, diagnosis, monitoring, and disease prognosis.

- ⓐ The success rate for experimental immunotherapy of cancer.

- ⓐ Why immunotherapy is not used as a front line treatment instead of surgery and/or chemotherapy

- ⓐ The inherent danger in immunotherapeutic strategies targeting single TAAs and how to avoid this danger.

IMPORTANT TERMS

Autologous
Benign
Carcinogen
Carcinoma
Cellular transformation
Clinical staging
Concomitant immunity
Cytotoxic T lymphocyte (CTL)

Homologous
Immunoselection
Immune surveillance
Immunotherapy
Malignant
Metastatic
Neoplasm
Oncogene

Sarcoma
Tumor suppressor gene
Tumor-associated antigen (TAA)
Tumor-specific antigen (TSA)
Tumor-specific transplantation antigen (TSTA)

▶ INTRODUCTION

The discipline of tumor immunology had its modest beginnings during the latter part of the nineteenth and early part of the twentieth century. Earlier demonstrations that immunization as well as passive serum therapy might protect against certain infectious diseases sparked interest as to whether similar approaches might be useful in the treatment of human cancers. Very early efforts to apply the lessons learned from the immunologic treatment of infectious diseases to naturally occurring tumors in man and animals were largely failures. It was not until the development of transplantable tumor lines in the context of experimental animal models that important insights began to unfurl. In 1912, Georg Schone published a book summarizing nearly a decade of experimental investi-

gations in the new field of tumor immunology. In this work, he summarized a set of rules that governs the acceptance and rejection of tumor transplants and coined the phrase transplantation immunity. These rules are remarkably similar to the present day laws of transplantation that apply to skin and solid organ grafts. Paul Ehrlich, one of the founding fathers of modern immunology, made the fundamental observation in 1906 that transplantation of a tumor into an animal host in which an identical tumor had become previously established would invariably result in the failure of the second tumor to grow. He interpreted this result, which he termed athrepsie, as reflecting the depletion of an essential nutrient by the established tumor, thus starving the secondary transplant and preventing its outgrowth. Today, we know that the basis of Ehrlich's observations is a phenomenon known as

concomitant immunity in which the initial tumor stimulates an immune response incapable of having an impact on a large, established primary tumor, but fully capable of rejecting the relatively small secondary tumor inoculum at a distant site.

Most of the tenets of modern human tumor immunology have their roots in the elegant studies in animal model systems that began with Ehrlich and Schone in the early part of this century and continue to the present day. Although this chapter focuses on those elements of tumor immunology germane to human neoplasms, it is important to maintain a perspective for the vast information base that was established in conjunction with experimental animal models, without which our present day understanding of human tumor immunology and continued advances in cancer immunotherapy would not be possible.

▶ CAUSES OF TUMOR FORMATION

NEOPLASM, CARCINOMA, AND SARCOMA

Cancer cells are generally defined as abnormal cells that proliferate in a highly unrestrained manner leading to the formation of a **neoplasm** or tumor. If the neoplastic cells remain clustered together in a localized mass, the tumor is classified as **benign.** On the other hand, if the cells have the ability to invade surrounding tissue and spread, then the tumor is classified as **malignant.** If these invasive tumors spread to other parts of the body and form secondary tumors, they are classified as **metastatic.** Metastatic spread is the major impediment to successful cancer treatment. Cancers are generally named according to their tissue or cell of origin. For example, cancers arising from epithelial cells are termed **carcinomas,** while those arising from muscle or connective tissue are termed **sarcomas.** Glandular tumors are called adenomas if they are benign and adenocarcinomas if they are malignant. Cancers of the hematopoietic and immune systems are termed leukemias, lymphomas, and myelomas, and cancers of the nervous system are generally named according to their cell of origin, such as astrocytoma, glioma, neuroblastoma, and retinoblastoma.

Once again, very elegant studies in animal model systems throughout the first half of the twentieth century firmly established that environmental, physical, and viral factors could each be responsible for **cellular transformation** leading to the development of tumors. Among the more significant findings from such studies was the identification of the multiple steps involved in carcinogenesis and the firm establishment of viral etiologies for many different animal tumors. Subsequent investigations during the last decade of the century also identified genetic elements that can predispose the host to tumor development.

ENVIRONMENTAL FACTORS

The precise etiology of many human tumors can often be less clear. In a high proportion of cases, the exact cause of a particular tumor can only be inferred, such as unusually high incidences of certain types of tumors in a population occupationally exposed to toxic and potentially carcinogenic chemicals. Potent carcinogens such as methylcholanthrene (MCA) and benzanthracene were used extensively in animal model systems to induce tumor formation. It is assumed that these and related compounds have similar activities in the formation of human tumors. Since populations in the developed world are constantly exposed to low levels of potential carcinogens in the environment through pollution and chemical contamination of water and food sources, it is often difficult to pinpoint a specific environmental exposure that ultimately leads to a transformation event and tumor development.

PHYSICAL FACTORS

Physical factors can also be directly responsible for initiating certain tumors. Perhaps the best example of this is the association between increased exposure to ultraviolet radiation from the sun and the subsequent development of certain skin cancers such as malignant melanoma. Other forms of radiation, such as that associated with exposure to nuclear weapons, are causally linked with the increased incidence of leukemias and lymphomas. Cells of bone marrow origin, with their high turnover rate, are particularly vulnerable to radiation-related neoplasms.

GENETIC PREDISPOSITION

The possible genetic predisposition to certain types of cancer has been recognized for some time. The pattern of familial occurrence of breast and ovarian cancers, for example, strongly suggested a genetic influence on the development of these human cancers. In fact, a family history of ovarian cancer is the single most important risk factor for the development of this disease, although the great majority of ovarian cancers are sporadic in nature and less than 10% can be clearly defined as hereditary. The identification in 1994 of

BRCA1 and BRCA2, two **tumor suppressor genes,** has further solidified the concept of genetic predisposition to certain cancers. If a patient is found to have mutations in either of these genes, her lifetime risk for developing breast or ovarian cancer is greatly increased. To date, well over 100 mutations have been mapped in BRCA1. Both BRCA1 and BRCA2 genes are inherited in an autosomal dominant manner and can, therefore, be passed on from either parent.

HORMONAL FACTORS

In addition to environmental, physical, and genetic factors that may affect the development of certain tumors, hormonal factors can also play a role. This is perhaps most evident in breast cancer where epidemiologic studies over the past 20 to 30 years have revealed a number of significant breast cancer risk factors that are linked to hormonal changes in the population. These include (1) nulliparity or increased age (>35 y/o) at first full-term pregnancy, (2) early age of first menstruation, and (3) late onset of menopause. Studies also suggest an increased risk of breast cancer among postmenopausal women who have received hormone replacement therapy, although there is no convincing data indicating a similar increased risk among women who used oral contraceptives. Breast tumors can be classified as either estrogen receptor (ER) positive or negative based on their expression of this hormone receptor. Likewise, prostate tumors can be grouped as either testosterone receptor positive or negative. In many cases, the therapy for hormone receptor positive and negative tumors can be vastly different.

VIRAL ORIGIN

Although viruses were clearly identified as the agents responsible for a number of animal leukemias and sarcomas, it was only within the past 30 years that a viral etiology for human cancers was clearly established. According to several current estimates, viruses presently are the cause of approximately 20% of all cancers that occur worldwide. Only a handful of viruses are responsible for these tumors in immunocompetent hosts, including (1) hepatitis B and C viruses (HBV and HCV; primary hepatocellular carcinomas), (2) Epstein-Barr virus (EBV; Burkitt's lymphoma and nasopharyngeal carcinomas), (3) human T cell leukemia virus I (HTLV-I; certain adult T cell leukemias), and (4) human papilloma viruses (HPV; cervical carcinomas). For most of these, the mechanism of cellular transformation has not been precisely defined. For example, while EBV ex-

presses two proteins of known oncogenic potential (i.e., LMP and EBNA-2) it is unclear how these and other viral genes bring about cellular transformation. Hepatitis viruses as well as HTLV-1 carry no known **oncogenes,** and only certain genetic strains of HPV (e.g., HPV-16 and HPV-18) are associated with cervical carcinomas. One feature that unites these widely differing viruses is their capacity to establish latent infections, a basis for viral persistence. Persistence, in turn, can produce a state of chronic immune stimulation that can lead to hyperplasia and, eventually, neoplasia. It has been proposed for viruses lacking a viral oncogene that chronic stimulation can lead to activation of cellular oncogenes. This is thought to be the case in HBV infection. Primary HBV replication takes place in the liver and, in over 95% of infected individuals, HBV replication ends with the development of neutralizing antibodies and immunity to reinfection. The remaining 5% of infected individuals exhibit persistent infection and, when symptomatic, chronic hepatitis B. Worldwide, there are thought to be >300 million chronic carriers of HBV. Chronic HBV infection is causally linked to 80% to 90% of primary hepatocellular carcinomas (PHC), accounting for over 500,000 cancer deaths annually.

► IDENTIFICATION OF TUMORS

Extensive research conducted in the context of animal models during the 1970s and 1980s revealed striking differences among different experimental tumors of the same histologic type based on the initiator of tumor formation. Two different tumors (e.g., tumor A and tumor B) induced by the same chemical **carcinogen** in the same inbred strain of mice and resulting in the same histologic type of tumor (e.g., sarcomas) express individually unique tumor antigens. In these studies, tumor antigens were defined in the context of transplantation resistance. For example, when mice representing the strain of tumor origin were immunized with killed tumor A cells, they resisted subsequent challenges with live tumor A cells, while nonimmunized mice succumbed to rapid tumor growth. However, mice immunized with tumor A cells were not protected from tumor growth when challenged with live tumor B cells. Likewise. Tumor B-immunized mice are not protected from challenges with live tumor A cells. Thus, tumor A and tumor B express individually unique **tumor-specific transplantation antigens (TSTA).** In fact, if one were to examine a panel of 12-15 different tumors, all of which were derived from the identical mouse strain with the same carcinogen, one would likely find transplantation immunity only in the context of **homologous** tumor cell immunization and challenge. This most likely represents the highly random processes involved in chemical carcinogenesis, although the same rules apply to spontaneous tumors with no identifiable etiology. Since it is estimated that most human tumors fall into the "spontaneous" category, the issue of individually unique tumor antigens would appear to require that any immunotherapeutic strategy take this into account. Fortunately, responses to other tumor antigens obviate the need for such individualized approaches.

In contrast to chemically induced and spontaneous tumors, cells transformed by oncogenic viruses express common or highly conserved TSTA. For example, virtually all erythroleukemias induced in a single strain of mice by Friend leukemia virus (FLV) express common TSTA and, therefore, can cross-protect another strain of mice in transplantation/challenge experiments such as those discussed earlier. Even cells of different histologic type that are transformed by the same virus tend to share common TSTA. Similarly, cells from different strains of mice transformed by a common oncogenic virus also share common TSTA, although true transplantation resistance cannot be assessed in allogeneic recipients where tumor rejection can be based on differences in histocompatibility antigens.

Obviously, determinations of unique versus common TSTA can only be made in conjunction with animal models and not in the context of human tumors. Therefore, there is a need to characterize antigens associated with human tumors in a manner exclusive of transplantation resistance. The two general terms that have been used to describe human tumor antigens are **tumor-specific antigens (TSA)** and **tumor-associated antigens (TAA).** Tumor specific antigens are those antigens found only on transformed cells and not expressed by any normal tissues. Tumor associated antigens, on the other hand, are those antigens expressed in a native or mutated form by tumor cells that are also found in association with normal tissues. With the realization that the majority of tumor antigens are not expressed exclusively by tumor cells, but are present on normal cells, the term tumor specific antigen has largely fallen out of use; in favor is the more precise descriptive term—tumor-associated antigen.

IDENTIFICATION AND CHARACTERIZATION OF HUMAN TAA

The major technologic advances of the late 1980s and early 1990s, particularly molecular-based strategies, have greatly facilitated the identification and charac-

terization of human TAA. The clear emphasis of most of these studies over the past 15 years has been focused on TAA recognized by T lymphocytes, particularly **cytotoxic T lymphocytes (CTL),** from patients with various types of tumors. These CTL are largely CD8$^+$ lymphocytes that recognize TAA epitopes in association with MHC class I molecules (see next section). Much of this work involved studies of antigens expressed by human melanomas. The reason for this focus is the ease with which a stable cell line can be derived from most primary melanomas and propagated indefinitely in vitro. This is in clear distinction to the great difficulty that investigators continue to have in establishing stable cell lines from most other primary human tumors, such as breast, lung, and gastrointestinal tumors, to name but a few.

The first identification of a human TAA recognized by a patient's own CTL was reported in 1991 by Dr. Thierry Boon in Belgium. As depicted in Figure 10-1■, the feasibility of this elegant study was made possible by the successful derivation of a stable melanoma cell line from the patient's tumor that expressed multiple TAA, including antigen E. Boon's group then isolated and propagated a clone of the patient's CTL, with specificity for antigen E that could recognize and lyse his or her own (i.e., **autologous**) melanoma cell line. By co-culturing the CTL and the autologous melanoma cell line, the group was able to select an antigen loss variant cell line that lost expression of the putative target TAA (antigen E) such that these cells were no longer recognized or lysed by the patient's Ag E-specific CTL. Boon's group then constructed a cosmid library consisting of DNA fragments from the original (i.e., E$^+$) melanoma cell line. These were subsequently transfected into the E$^-$ antigen loss variant, and the stable transfectants were cloned and tested for recognition by autologous CTL in the form of TNF-α production. Once a susceptible tranfectant was identified, fragments of the DNA that conferred CTL recognition (i.e., TAA expression) were transfected into the antigen loss variant until a relatively small segment of the DNA encoding the target TAA (i.e., antigen E) was identified. The gene encoding this TAA was designated MAGE-1. Using overlapping peptides representing the coding regions of the DNA segment, the actual 9 amino acid epitope that served as the target for the CTL was eventually identified. This overall approach and its subsequent molecular refinements have served as prototypes for strategies aimed at identification of new TAA epitopes in the context of human tumors.

Importantly, Boon's group took these observations one step further by investigating the expression of the MAGE-1 gene in normal tissues and tumors belonging

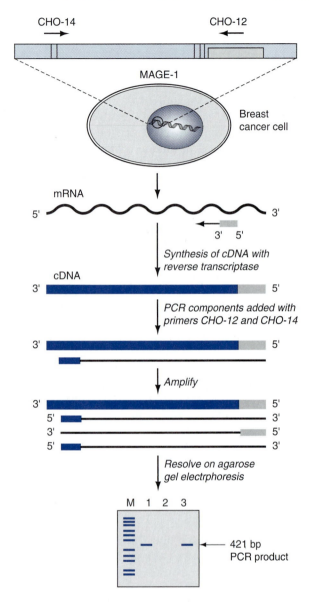

■ **FIGURE 10-1** Detection of MAGE-1 gene expression by reverse transcriptase-PCR.

With the development and refinement of the polymerase chain reaction (PCR) technology in the early 1990s, it became possible to examine the expression of TAA within individual patient tumors. Once the nucleotide sequence of the TAA gene was delineated, a specific molecular probe could be constructed that could measure gene expression at the level of mRNA using a technique called reverse transcriptase PCR (RT-PCR). The schema for performing such analyses is depicted in Figure 10-2■, using MAGE-1 gene expression as an example.

Although molecular approaches have proven valuable in the identification of human TAA, other strate-

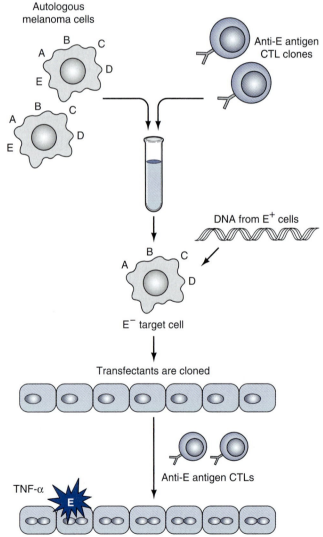

■ **FIGURE 10-2** MAGE-1: Human melanoma antigen-encoding gene.

to other tissue types. They found that no normal tissues except testicular tissue expressed MAGE-1. Additionally, they found that MAGE-1 expression was not restricted to melanomas, but could be found in association with a broad range of tumor types including lung, breast, and colon tumors. These latter findings were particularly significant since it clearly established that human TAA that serve as targets for CTL are not individually unique, but are shared among a variety of histologically diverse tumors.

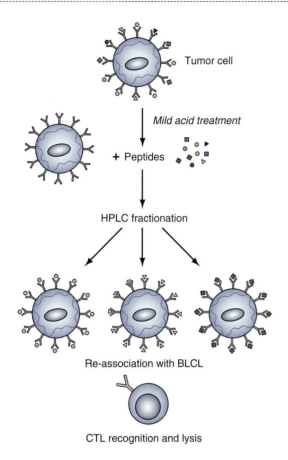

FIGURE 10-3 Identification of CTL target peptides.

| Tumor cell |
| Mild acid treatment |
| + Peptides |
| HPLC fractionation |
| Re-association with BLCL |
| CTL recognition and lysis |

⊗ TABLE 10-1

Human Tumor-Associated Antigens

Melanoma-Melanocyte Differentiation Antigens	Cancer-Testes Antigens
	MAGE-1
MART-1 (Melan-A)	MAGE-3
Gp100	BAGE
Tyrosinase	GAGE
Mutated antigens	NY-ESO-1
k-ras	**Nonmutated shared**
P53	**overexpressed antigens**
Tumor Viral Antigen	a-fetoprotein
HPV16 E7	MUC-1
	CEA
	HER-2/neu

MHC class I-restricted, recognized by CD8+ cells

gies have also had great utility. One such strategy, involving a more biochemical approach, is depicted in Figure 10-3■. This takes advantage of the fact that tumor cells express the subset of TAA recognized by CD8+ cells as 9–10 amino acid peptides presented in the context of MHC class I molecules. These TAA peptides can be easily eluted from tumor cells by mild acid treatment, and the isolated peptides can be further purified and sequenced. Those TAA that serve as target antigens for CTL can be easily identified by coating autologous B lymphocyte cell lines (BLCL) with purified peptides and measuring their susceptibility to in vitro lysis by patient effector cells. Once again, this technique has been most successful in defining TAA expressed by melanomas since cell lines can be easily established and the large numbers of cells required for these analyses can be readily grown in vitro.

The various technologies discussed earlier, in addition to others not mentioned, have permitted tumor immunologists to further subdivide human TAA recognized by CD8+ cells into five specific categories based on the pattern of expression relative to normal host tissues. These categories (listed in Table 10-1⊗) include (1) melanoma-melanocyte differentiation antigens, (2) mutated antigens, (3) tumor virus antigens, (4) cancer-testes antigens, and (5) nonmutated, shared, overexpressed antigens. Under each of these categories in Table 10-1, a partial listing of representative TAA is included. With the exception of tumor virus antigens, most of these TAA bear a striking similarity, if not identity, to normal self antigens. This may be the underlying basis for their relatively weak immunogenicity.

MART

MART is an acronym for melanoma antigen recognized by T cells and serves as a representative TAA belonging to the melanoma-melanocyte differentiation group. MART-1 is expressed by melanomas, melanocyte cell lines, and human retinal tissue. Anti-MART CTL are restricted by the HLA A*0201 allele and recognize an epitopic peptide with the amino acid sequence AAGIGILTV. Patients receiving MART-stimulated T cells sometimes develop a depigmentation condition known as vitiligo, most likely due to the reactivity of MART-specific CTL with normal melanocytes in the skin.

Among the mutated human TAA, p53 mutations are the most common, with base substitutions occurring in over 90 different codons. Codon 12 and 61 mutations in k-ras occur at high frequencies in certain tumors, with up to 85% of human pancreatic tumors expressing a codon 12 (glycine to valine) mutation. HPV 16 encodes the E7 TAA that is found in association with a high frequency of cervical carcinomas. The MAGE family is composed of at least 12 closely related genes, all of which are silent in all normal adult tissues except testes, hence the classification as "cancer-testes" antigens. In contrast to MART-1, the MAGE-1 gene encodes a TAA restricted by HLA A*0101, with the epitopic sequence EADPTGHSY. HER-2/*neu* is an interesting representative of the final group of TAA. This TAA has homology with epidermal growth factor (EGF) and is expressed by normal tissues. In malignant tumors, HER-2/*neu* is overexpressed in a nonmutated form. Therefore, this class of TAA is fully expressed on a variety of normal tissues, but when overexpressed, is recognized by host T cells as non-self. Despite this sequence identity with normal tissue components, there have been no reports of autoimmune phenomenon accompanying anti-HER-2/*neu* cellular reactivities in cancer patients.

Although a wide range of TAA have been identified in the context of recognition by CD8+ T cells, there are an increasing number of TAA that have been shown to interact with monoclonal antibodies, thus opening the door for potential targeting of human tumors in passive immunotherapeutic strategies. These monoclonal anti-TAA antibodies, manufactured in the laboratory, can be used alone or as conjugates coupled to cytotoxic or radiotoxic agents. Finally, it should be noted that several of these antibodies react with determinants of the TAA that were defined by T cell recognition. Herceptin (trastuzumab), for example, is a humanized monoclonal antibody that recognizes a portion of the HER-2/*neu* molecule in metastatic breast cancer, and is presently in Phase III clinical trials.

Although individual TAA were discussed earlier, it is important to recognize that a single tumor cell is likely to express a mosaic of different TAA and that a single cancer patient can potentially develop immune responses to each of them.

▶ IMMUNE RESPONSE TO HUMAN TUMORS

In 1970, Macfarlane Burnet proposed the concept of **immune surveillance** as a normal homeostatic process by which the immune system recognizes and eliminates cells that are a "result of somatic mutation or some other inheritable change represent potential dangers to life." Burnet went on to propose this as a

mechanism by which the host immune system detects and destroys tumor cells. According to this concept, transformation events occur spontaneously on a frequent and regular basis. Host T cells eliminate the resulting small numbers of tumor cells before they can expand into a clinically apparent tumor. In addition, it was proposed that the immune system played a critical role in the control of tumor growth and regression of established tumors. Several lines of evidence appeared to support these ideas. First, analysis of an extensive human autopsy database suggested that the actual incidence of human tumors was more than clinically apparent. Histologic examination revealed that many tumors contained lymphocytic infiltrates. Additionally, spontaneous regression of certain tumors, particularly melanomas, had been observed. Last, the occurrence of human tumors is greatest in young children and in older adults, both periods when the immune system is not functioning optimally. However, Burnet's hypothesis, although quite attractive, is still actively debated by the present community of tumor immunologists. It has been difficult to demonstrate that human tumors are subject to immune surveillance. Both mice and humans deficient in T cells have relatively similar incidences of common tumors to those with fully intact immune systems. Most of the increased tumor incidences seen in immunodeficient or chronically immunosuppressed patients are virally associated cancers. Thus, immune surveillance appears to be important in the control of virus-associated tumors, but it is unclear what role, if any, it may play in conjunction with spontaneous tumors that account for most human cancers.

Beyond the concept of immune surveillance, the more operative question to be addressed is whether patients mount a humoral and/or cellular immune response against their own tumors. We have partially addressed this in our previous discussion of TAA recognized by CD8+ T cells. But even studies predating Boon's identification of MAGE-1 began to address this question. In these in vitro experiments, patient lymphocytes and inactivated autologous tumor cells were co-cultured, and the resulting cellular responses were delineated. Again, many of these studies were focused on malignant melanoma because of the ease in deriving stable tumor cell lines. The sources of patient lymphocytes included peripheral blood, draining lymph nodes, or even lymphocytes that had infiltrated the actively growing tumor itself. These latter cell are termed tumor infiltrating lymphocytes or TIL. The results of studies in many laboratories revealed that these mixed cultures could generate both CD4+ helper T cells and

CD8$^+$ CTL capable of recognizing the autologous tumor. The characteristics of these immune responses suggested that the patient lymphocytes had been "primed" in vivo in response to the growing tumor. Therefore, patients apparently do mount a demonstrable cellular immune response against certain tumors. It is presently uncertain whether this is true for most human tumors.

Early attempts to use patient sera to measure reactivity against a variety of human tumors largely failed to confirm humoral antitumor reactivities. A more recent approach termed SEREX (serologic analysis of recombinant cDNA expression libraries), however, has proven extremely useful in defining TAA that are recognized by patient antibodies. In this assay strategy, sera from cancer patients are utilized to screen cDNA expression libraries prepared from fresh tumor material. Proteins recognized by patient antibodies, but not antibodies from normal, healthy individuals, are characterized and included in a comprehensive database. This technique has been used to identify nearly 100 gene sequences, some representing previously described TAA, but many that represent a large group of previously unknown TAA genes. Therefore, it appears that, in addition to cellular anti-TAA responses, patients also elicit TAA-specific antibodies.

Antibodies other than those derived from patient sera have also been used to identify TAA. Monoclonal antibody technologies, most of which involve immunization of mice with human tumor cells followed by derivation and extensive screening of hybridomas secreting TAA-specific antibodies, have proven instrumental in the identification of oncofetal TAA such as carcinoembryonic antigen (CEA) and α-fetoprotein (AFP), differentiation TAA such as common acute lymphoblastic leukemia antigen (CALLA), MUC-1, CA-125, and prostate-specific antigen (PSA). These monoclonal antibodies were not only valuable in the identification of specific TAA, but also have been incorporated into assay strategies that measure the relative quantity of these antigens in the circulation of patients being screened or treated for certain cancers. Levels of these TAA are highly reliable indicators of the remaining tumor burden following surgery or chemotherapy, and are also very early indicators of tumor recurrences. Some of these monoclonal antibodies are also being evaluated as potential therapies in ongoing clinical trials that are further discussed in this chapter.

The present generation of CA-125 test referred to in our opening Case in Point is known as the CA-125II assay. This is a radioimmunoassay in which a monoclonal capture antibody bound to polystyrene beads is used to bind CA-125 antigen present in a patient's serum. A second monoclonal antibody, coupled to a radioactive tag (^{125}I), is used as a tracer to detect the CA-125 complexed to the antibody-coated beads. By constructing a standard curve with each run of the assay, the amount of CA-125 present in a sample can be calculated. This amount is expressed in arbitrary units per milliliter (U/mL). This is, therefore, an indirect means of measuring residual tumor burden in a patient. A value of 35U/mL or greater is generally considered indicative of residual tumor in a patient who has completed front-line therapy. Although the CA-125II assay is an extraordinarily helpful monitoring tool for the clinician, there are a number of potential drawbacks. First, elevated CA-125 levels are only detected in approximately 80% of women with ovarian cancer, thus rendering the assay useless to the 20% of patients with CA-125 negative tumors. There is also a variable, and sometimes high, "false positive" rate among high-risk or healthy women. These two caveats illustrate the limitations of the CA-125II assay as a single modality diagnostic test for the presence of ovarian cancer. When used for screening, the assay results must be evaluated in the context of a pelvic exam and additional testing such as transvaginal sonography. The assay has greatest utility as a prognostic tool in monitoring the levels of CA-125 in association with surgical and chemotherapeutic interventions and in identifying relapses resulting from therapeutic failures as depicted for our Case in Point in Figure 10-4■. Because of the potential risks and disposal concerns of working with radioisotopes, efforts are presently underway to convert this radioimmunoassay into a luciferase-based assay with read-out on a luminometer.

▶ MECHANISMS OF TUMOR ESCAPE

If patients do mount humoral and cellular responses against their own tumor, why then is it not rejected? There are a number of reasons for this, the first of which may be the simple kinetics of tumor growth versus the ontogeny of a TAA-specific immune response. Simply stated, the time required to initiate an effective immune response may be significantly longer than the time required for a primary tumor to become established. The immune response is notoriously ineffective in handling excessively large tumor burdens. But it is not always the primary tumor that causes the most problems since it can often be removed by the surgeon

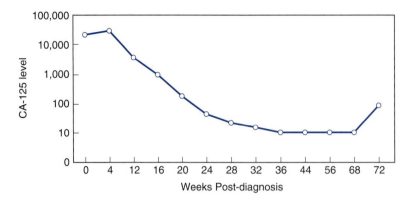

■ **FIGURE 10-4** CA-125 Levels following diagnosis and treatment of ovarian cancer.

or greatly reduced by chemotherapy and/or radiation. The major problem in clinical oncology is the metastatic spread of small tumor cell foci and establishment of metastases at sites distant to the site of the primary tumor. Since these are much smaller numbers of tumor cells than found in the primary tumor, why then doesn't the immune response, in a manner similar to Ehrlich's observation of concomitant immunity, prevent their metastatic spread?

There are a number of mechanisms whereby tumors can evade the immune response. Tumor cells tend to be genetically unstable and routinely generate genetic variants as a consequence of this instability. Under an immune pressure, variants capable of avoiding immune destruction would have an overall increased "fitness" or survival advantage. **Immunoselection** of resistant variants, perhaps with even greater metastatic or growth potential, could be a consequence of the anti-TAA immune response. This process could be envisioned as an in vivo analogue to Boon's in vitro selection of an antigen loss variant as part of his MAGE-1 identification process. Other possible mechanisms of tumor escape are listed in Table 10-2✪. Some tumors, particularly melanomas, have been shown to effectively down-regulate their MHC class I molecules in the setting of immune pressure. This, in turn, greatly decreases the overall frequency of cell surface TAA epitopes, presented in the context of class I molecules, at the cell surface where they can be recognized by immune effector cells. In the presence of anti-TAA antibodies, tumor cells have been shown to modulate their surface antigens, internalizing them and removing them from immune recognition. Tumor cells are also capable of producing immunosuppressive molecules such as TGF-β and IL-10. Fas ligand (Fas-L) present on

certain tumor cells has been shown to effectively mediate apoptosis of antitumor effector CTL. Tumors cells can also express TNF-α–related apoptosis-inducing ligand (TRAIL) as another means of eliminating anti-TAA effectors. A tumor cell is akin to an antigen-presenting cell (APC) since it displays processed epitopes in conjunction with MHC class I and II molecules. Engagement of the T cell receptor (TCR) in the absence of the costimulatory molecule CD28 or engagement of CD40 ligand (CD40L) can lead to a state of T cell unresponsiveness or anergy. Antitumor effectors can be actively eliminated through activation-induced cell death (AICD), fratracide, and clonal exhaustion, all under the control of the growing tumor. Last, dendritic cells are an essential component of the antitumor response. Proinflammatory cytokines are needed in order to optimally activate DC and induce their maturation. Tumor cells have been shown to compromise the production

---

✪ TABLE 10-2

Possible Mechanisms of Tumor Escape

- MHC down regulation
- Antigenic modulation
- Production of immunosuppressive molecules (e.g., TGF-β, IL-10)
- Expression of Fas-L on tumor cells
- Expression of TNF-α-related apoptosis-inducing ligand (TRAIL)
- TCR engagement in absence of CD28, CD154 (CD40L) ligation leading to T cell anergy
- Activation-induced cell death (AICD), fratracide, clonal exhaustion
- Absence of proinflammatory cytokines that induce DC maturation

of these critical cytokines in a number of settings. In summary, in the same fashion as have certain viruses (e.g., cytomegalovirus [CMV]) evolved mechanisms to evade or compromise immune recognition, tumor cells have likewise developed a set of processes aimed at self-preservation in the face of an immune response.

▶ IMMUNOTHERAPY AND TUMOR VACCINES

The seemingly unending listing of possible tumor escape mechanisms would predict that attempting to facilitate or augment the immune response of the patient through immunotherapeutic strategies would be an insurmountable task. It is certainly true that the **immunotherapy** of cancer has held great promise for over a decade, yet that promise is yet to be realized in the form of highly efficacious immunotherapy regimens. Although there are a number of reasons for this, perhaps the most important is the manner in which such trials were initially conducted. As illustrated in Figure 10-5■, up until the mid-1990s, experimental immunotherapeutic trials were structured after trials of new experimental chemotherapeutic compounds. Because of toxicity concerns, these modalities were first evaluated in patients with late-stage disease who had failed all conventional treatments. While this may have relatively minor effect on chemotherapy evaluations, these patients had overwhelming tumor burdens and very little remaining immune function. It is not surprising, therefore, that very few of the initial immunotherapeutic strategies made it beyond this first phase of testing. With the realization that the real promise of immunotherapies was not the elimination of large primary tumor burdens, but rather control of residual tumor following initial surgical, radiologic, or chemotherapeutic intervention, the overall setting for testing new immunotherapeutic strategies dramatically changed. Now the testing occurs in a setting that would be most like the setting for intended use of a particular immunotherapeutic strategy, namely, the setting of minimal residual disease. Cancers that are most amenable to this type of strategy are those at high to moderate risk of recurrence. In the Case in Point, the patient's tumor responded well to the combined debulking surgery and repeated chemotherapy regimen (see Figure 10-4), but the patient was at high risk for recurrence, having been diagnosed at a late stage (IIIC) of disease. In this manner, a patient can first receive "standard of care" primary treatment for their cancer and then participate in a rational immunotherapy trial during their period of remission.

CLINICAL STAGING IN THE STANDARD CARE OF TREATMENT

The standard of care treatment for most human cancers very much depends on the process of clinical "staging." Specific treatment strategies are inherently linked to discrete stages of clinical disease. Each type of cancer (i.e., lung vs. breast vs. colorectal versus ovarian, etc.) is subject to a unique **clinical staging** system. As an example, ovarian cancer is a surgically staged disease, meaning that the exact stage of disease cannot be determined until a thorough surgical examination is performed. The International Federation of Gynecologists and Obstetricians developed the standard staging system in use for primary carcinoma of the ovary. This system consists of four major stages and three subcategories within each of the first three major stages. Stage I is defined as growth limited to the ovaries while Stage II involves growth in one or both ovaries with pelvic extension. Stage III is defined as tumor involving one or both ovaries with peritoneal implants or metastases, and Stage IV involves tumor on one or both ovaries as well as intra- and extra-peritoneal metastases. In most cases, a specific prognosis is linked to the specific clinical stage at the time of diagnosis. The higher the stage at diagnosis, the poorer is the overall clinical prognosis. The overall success or failure of a specific therapy (including potential immunotherapies) must be considered in conjunction with the stage of the cancer at the time of diagnosis.

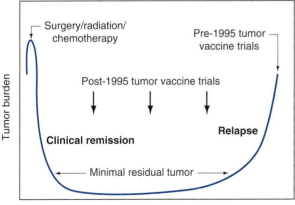

■ **FIGURE 10-5** Experimental immunotherapeutic trials.

IMMUNOTHERAPEUTIC STRATEGIES

All immunotherapeutic strategies fall into one of two categories—active or passive. Active therapies are those in which some form of tumor cell immunogen (e.g., killed tumor cells, peptides, peptide-pulsed dendritic cells, recombinant DNA, recombinant vector expressing TAA genes, etc.) is administered to the cancer patient who then actively mounts an immune response (either humoral, cellular, or both). Passive immunotherapies are those in which immune components, either antibodies or antigen-activated and expanded effector cells, are administered to the patient and are expected to "traffic" into the sites of tumor growth and exert their antitumor effects. For either of these strategies to be effective, the target tumor tissue must have a well-established blood supply. Necrotic areas of the tumor would not be accessible to immune cells or antibodies.

PASSIVE CELLULAR IMMUNOTHERAPY

A large body of clinical research has been devoted to evaluating the feasibility and potential efficacy of passive cellular immunotherapy, with mixed results. By far the most promising of these strategies is the ex vivo activation and expansion of patient effector cell population using a variety of dendritic cell stimulation platforms. Dendritic cells pulsed with tumor RNA, DNA, and peptides are all currently under active investigation. Perhaps the greatest progress has been made recently with application of monoclonal antibodies (MoAb) as therapeutic modalities. As mentioned earlier, Herceptin has produced interesting benefits to a subgroup of breast cancer patients enrolled in early trials. There are also ongoing trials using MoAb against TAA such as MUC-1, HER-2/*neu,* and CA-125, some with equally promising early results. These antibody strategies often involve MoAb conjugated directly to radiotoxins such as ^{90}yttrium and ^{131}iodine. There are presently a number of ongoing clinical trials in various phases of investigating the potential efficacy of anti-TAA antibody therapy.

The number of potential forms of active TAA immunogens (i.e., cancer vaccines) under consideration for clinical trials continues to increase. At the forefront of many of these strategies are the DC-based immunogens. Although vaccines against individual TAA are under initial evaluation, the ultimate goal would be to have a vaccine containing multiple TAA matched to those expressed by the individual patient's tumor. By stimulating a broad array of anti-TAA reactivities, the possibility for selection of a more highly tumorigenic or metastatic variant could be avoided. Recombinant viral vectors are also receiving close scrutiny, especially adenovirus-based strategies that include molecules to facilitate in situ DC activation. One of the very real challenges for the tumor immunologist is the development of highly sensitive and specific immunoassays to evaluate in a quantitative manner the immune responses elicited by these different immunotherapeutic agents.

Finally, with the completion of the Human Genome Project, and the continued identification of human genes that put individuals at risk for developing certain types of cancer, the move toward a preventive cancer vaccine for such tumors may be in the realm of possibility. Again, the rationale would be to immunize a person at risk prior to the expression of a clinically apparent tumor, in hopes that an accelerated immune response, primed by immunization, would be better able to prevent the establishment of the primary tumor.

SUMMARY

The field of tumor immunology is over 100 years old. During the past century, environmental, physical, genetic, hormonal, and viral factors have been associated with cellular transformation leading to tumor formation. Although antigens had been identified on some tumors, it has only been during the past decade that advances in molecular biology have allowed identification of TAA in individual patient tumors. The humoral and cell-mediated responses to tumors have also been described, and the concept of immunosurveillance was developed. Since it is obvious that the immune response does not eradicate all tumors that arise and that tumors have evolved strategies allowing escape from the host immune response, this concept is currently the subject of active debate. Research on TAA and the immune response has led to the development of experimental immunotherapeutic protocols and vaccines. Although these strategies are not yet considered front-line therapy for cancer, they hold considerable promise for the future.

POINTS TO REMEMBER

▶ Most tumor-associated antigens (TAA) represent modified or overexpressed self antigens and are inherently less immunogenic than viral or bacterial antigens.

▶ Common TAA can be expressed by human tumors of widely differing tissue types.

▶ A single tumor can express multiple TAA, each of which can be a target for immune recognition.

▶ Tumors have evolved a variety of mechanisms to escape immune recognition and destruction.

▶ Antibody or cellular-based immunotherapy of certain cancers is possible, if applied in an appropriate setting of "minimal residual disease."

▶ Immunotherapy against single TAA targets carries with it the risk of selecting "antigen loss variants" that may carry greater metastatic potential.

LEARNING ASSESSMENT QUESTIONS

1. The presence of a plantar wart on the sole of your foot is evidence of a
   a. metastatic cell.
   b. benign tumor.
   c. cancer.
   d. neoplasm.

2. The epithelial cells of the skin and the cells of the bone marrow are the most susceptible to ionizing radiation because they are
   a. part of the barrier function of the immune system.
   b. actively secreting cytokines.
   c. rapidly dividing cells.
   d. targeted by an immune response following exposure to radiation.

3. A young woman learns that she has a mutated form of the BRCA1 gene. What is the significance of this finding?
   a. She has breast cancer.
   b. She has an increased risk of breast cancer.

   c. She has a decreased risk of breast cancer.
   d. There is no particular significance to this finding.

4. Which of the following viruses have been shown to be associated with human cancers?
   a. certain strains of papilloma viruses
   b. Epstein-Barr virus
   c. hepatitis B and C viruses
   d. all of the above
   e. none of the above

5. Why weren't immunosuppressive therapies considered to be very effective during early clinical trials?
   a. Immunosuppressive therapies don't work.
   b. Immunosuppressive therapies have to be directed specifically against each patient's own tumor cells.
   c. The trials were performed as a last resort in patients with many clinical complications.
   d. Immunosuppressive therapies are primarily useful as debulking agents.

REFERENCES

Carter, P. 2001. Improving the efficacy of antibody-based therapies. *Nature Reviews Immunology* 1:118–29.

Parmiani, G., C. Castelli, P. Dalerba, and L. Rivoltini. 2001. T cell response to tumor antigens and its therapeutic use in cancer patients. *Advances in Experimental Medicine and Biology* 495:403–10.

Rammensee, H. G., T. Weinschenk, C. Gouttefangeas, and S. Stevanovic. 2002. Towards patient-specific tumor antigen selection for vaccination. *Immunology Reviews* 188:164–76.

Rosenberg, S. A. 2004. Shedding light on immunotherapy for cancer. *New England Journal of Medicine* 350:1461–63.

Stevanovic, S. 2002. Identification of tumour-associated T-cell epitopes for vaccine development. *Nature Reviews Cancer* 2:514–20.

Van Der Bruggen, P., Y. Zhang, P. Chaux et al. 2002. Tumor-specific shared antigenic peptides recognized by human T-cells. *Immunology Reviews* 188:51–64.

Waldmann, T. A. 2003. Immunotherapy: Past, present and future. *Nature Medicine* 9:269–77.

11

Clinical Applications of Flow Cytometry

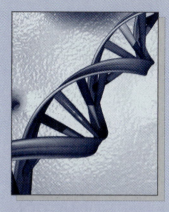

■ CHAPTER CHECKLIST

After reading and studying this chapter, the reader should be able to:

1. Explain the theory of standard flow cytometric instrumentation.
2. Describe the functions of the fluidics, optics, and electronic systems in a flow cytometer.
3. Describe the types of specimens that can be subjected to flow cytometric analysis, and discuss the standard approaches to specimen processing.
4. Describe common clinical applications of flow cytometric analysis.
5. Evaluate indications for the use of flow cytometric analysis and provide appropriate interpretation of results.
6. Determine the advantages and discuss the limitations of flow cytometric instrumentation.

● CASE IN POINT

The patient, an 18-year-old Caucasian male, was admitted to the hospital complaining of fatigue secondary to anemia. Analysis of a peripheral blood smear demonstrated a lymphocytosis with blasts. The blast cells constituted 70% of the white cells in the smear. A bone marrow biopsy was obtained and demonstrated a leukemic infiltrate.

Flow cytometric analysis of a bone marrow aspirate was performed to determine the phenotype of leukemic blasts. A flow cytometrichistogram is shown in Figure 11-1■. The patient's diagnosis was made, and he was started on chemotherapy.

ISSUES TO CONSIDER

After reading this patient's case history, consider

● The importance of flow cytometric analysis in the diagnosis of the patient presented in this case

● The basic principles of flow cytometric analysis

● Types of information that can be derived from the analysis

● How the information is utilized in clinical diagnosis and monitoring therapy

● Other clinical applications flow cytometric analysis can provide

IMPORTANT TERMS

Antigen
Clone
Dot plot
Flow cytometer
Fluorochrome
Forward scatter
Histogram

HLA
Hydrodynamically focused
  (hydrodynamic focusing)
Immunoglobulin
Laser
Light scattered (light scatter)

Lineage
Monoclonal antibody
Photodiode
Photomultiplier tube (PMT)
Side scatter
Stem cell

▶ INTRODUCTION

Flow cytometry is an important technology in the clinical laboratory with a broad range of applications employed in several areas of laboratory medicine. In the context of the clinical laboratory, the flow cytometer is, in the most basic sense, a particle counting instrument. However, the use of fluorescent-labeled monoclonal antibodies and other dyes allows the flow cytometer to identify and enumerate or characterize

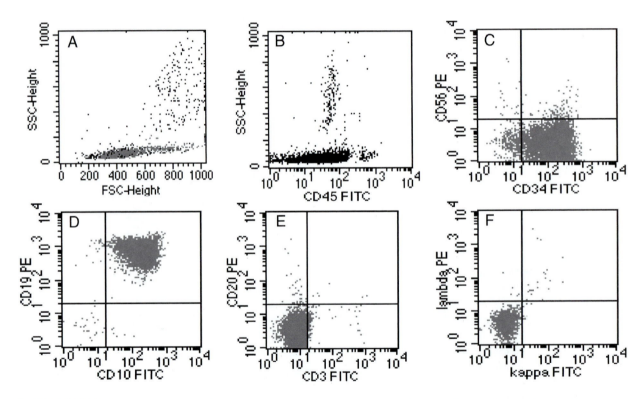

■ FIGURE 11-1 Flow cytometric dot plots from analysis of a bone marrow aspirate. (A) The forward vs. side scatter characteristics of the aspirate from this patient. Of note is the predominant population of small cells corresponding to lymphocytes (arrow). (B) The CD45 vs. side scatter plot demonstrates that the predominant population dimly expresses CD45. A small population of normal lymphocytes (bright CD45 expression) is indicated by the arrow. (C) A dot plot of CD34 vs. CD56 gated on the dim CD45 population demonstrates that the majority of the cells express the CD34 antigen that is characteristic of immature cells. (D) The same CD45 dim population also expresses both CD10 (present on immature B cells) and CD19 (a B cell antigen), which is characteristic of pre-B cells. One would not expect to see this large proportion of CD19 positive cells in the aspirate nor would they express CD10. (E) The dim CD45 positive cells do not express the CD3 (T cell antigen) or CD20 (a marker present on mature B cells). (F) The dim CD45 positive population does not express either class of immunoglobulin light chain, again, indicative of their immature stage of differentiation. The composite phenotype of the predominant population of lymphoid-sized cells in the aspirate is consistent with the morphologic appearance and supports a diagnosis of a pre-B acute lymphoblastic leukemia.

specific subsets of cells. The specificity imparted by the use of monoclonal antibodies allows one to enumerate specific cell subsets in complex (containing many different cell types) samples such as whole blood thus enhancing its usefulness. Not only can flow cytometry be used to enumerate the normal subsets of cells in fluids, it can also be used to identify "abnormal" cells. For example, cells lacking the expression of a key cell surface molecule or expressing a molecule not characteristic of a normal population of cells can be identified and enumerated by flow cytometry. This chapter provides an overview of the flow cytometry instrumentation, sampling requirements, types of reagents used, and data analysis. Clinical applications of flow cytometry in the clinical laboratory is also presented.

► BASIC PRINCIPLES OF FLOW CYTOMETRY

FLOW CYTOMETRY INSTRUMENTATION

The power of flow cytometric analysis lies in the ability to rapidly and precisely identify and enumerate large numbers of specific cell types in a complex suspension on a cell-by-cell basis. To accomplish this, a **flow cytometer** generates a stream of cells moving rapidly, one by one, through a focused beam of light from a **laser.** As the cells pass through the beam of light, photons are scattered in all directions. Several "photodetectors" capture the scattered light and generate digital signals that define characteristics of the cell such as size, internal complexity, and antigenic makeup. This information is stored and analyzed by a computer system. The coordinated functioning of three systems in the typical flow cytometer carry out these activities out: fluidics, optics and electronics/computer.

Fluidics System

The fluidics system of a flow cytometer is the sample handling system. When a suspension of cells is loaded on the cytometer, the cells are taken up through a probe and injected into a stream of pressurized sheath fluid (typically a buffered salt solution for mammalian cells) in the flow cell of the flow cytometer. The cells flow in the center of the stream of sheath fluid and are **hydrodynamically focused** into a rapidly moving, single file stream of cells. With cells at the right concentration and flow rate (number of cells passing through the laser beam per second), they will pass through the inter-

rogation point (the point at which the cells pass through the laser beam) of the flow cell one at a time in a highly reproducible fashion. The precise and reproducible delivery of cells to the laser beam is critical to the proper functioning of the instrument.

Optical System

As a cell passes through the focused beam of the laser, it causes light to scatter in all directions. The scattered light is detected and analyzed to characterize the cells in the sample (Figure 11-2■). Light that is refracted along the axis of the laser beam (**forward scatter**) is collected in the forward scatter **photodiode. Light scattered** at a 90° angle to the laser beam (side or orthogonal scatter) is collected by the side scatter **photomultiplier tube (PMT)**. The amount of forward scatter light is proportional to the cross-sectional area of the cell and is an indicator of cell size. Larger cells will refract more light in the forward direction and thus generate a stronger forward scatter signal. **Side scatter** is indicative of complexity of the cell surface and internal components. Cells such as polymorphonuclear neutrophils with many granules and a multilobed nucleus scatter more light at 90° and thus generate a stronger side scatter signal. These physical

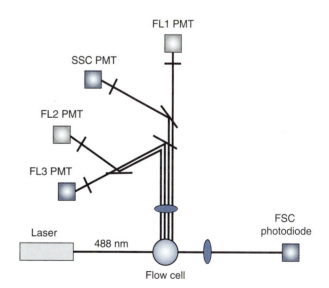

■ **FIGURE 11-2** Diagram of flow cytometer optical system. 488 nm laser light is shown interrogating a cell with resultant scattered laser and fluorescence emission. Scatter laser and fluorescent light are directed to specific detectors via a system of filters and mirrors such that light of defined wavelength is direct to each specific detector. FSC = forward scatter. SSC = side scatter. PMT = photomultiplier tube.

characteristics (forward and side scatter) are referred to as intrinsic parameters of the cells. One can also assess extrinsic parameters such as the presence of specific cell surface antigens that define a cell lineage, stage of maturation, or activation. Figure 11-2 is a schematic diagram of a flow cytometer.

To identify specific surface antigens of cells, one can "label" cells with reagents that bind specifically to the antigens. This is usually a **monoclonal antibody** that is labeled with a fluorescent molecule (**fluorochrome**). When a cell with a particular surface **antigen** labeled with a fluorescently tagged monoclonal antibody passes through the laser beam, the fluorochrome is excited and emits light of a wavelength specific to the particular fluorochrome. This light passes through optical mirrors and filters and is captured by additional PMTs, one for each type of fluorochrome (i.e., wavelength of light peculiar to a specific fluorochrome). In typical flow cytometers, 3 or 4 fluorescence detectors are used to capture light emitted from cells labeled with 3 or 4 different fluorochromes. Filters and mirrors dictate the range of wavelengths of light that reach any specific PMT. In this way, cells can be analyzed for 3 or 4 different cell surface molecules simultaneously. Thus, in total, one can assess 5 or 6 different characteristics of cells (size, complexity, and 3 to 4 specific antigens). Newer instruments can analyze even greater numbers of fluorescents parameters.

Fluorochromes emit light of a range (spectrum) of wavelengths. Many of the fluorochromes in common use have emission spectra that overlap. Because of this, PMTs and filter setups for one fluorochrome may detect some emission from a second fluorochrome due to spectral overlap. Fortunately, the electronics of the flow cytometer can be used to subtract a user defined amount of "contaminating" fluorescence from a second fluorochrome with an overlapping emission spectrum. This process is referred to as fluorescence compensation. It is necessary to optimize the flow cytometer setup for each group of fluorochromes employed in an assay to account for the spectral overlap.

Computer and Electronic System

The last step in the functioning of the electronics of a flow cytometer is to convert the signal generated by the collection of photons of light to a digital signal that is proportional to the amount of light scattered or emitted by the cell. This digital signal is then transmitted to the cytometer computer that stores and makes available the information for analysis. The digital sig-

nals are stored in "channels" that reflect the intensity of the signal. A strong digital signal is stored in a higher channel (usually on a scale of 1 to 256 or 1024 channels). The outcome of allocation of signals to channels is a frequency distribution of light scatter and/or fluorescence intensity. This data allows one to determine the number of cells that exhibit specific levels of scattered light or fluorescence.

Once a photodetector has generated an electrical signal proportional to the amount of light it receives and that signal has been classified into channels, what do we do with the information? This is the job of the computer analysis software of a flow cytometric system. The channel numbers that reflect the signal intensity of the parameter of interest are typically displayed in a one- or two-dimensional figure (single parameter **histograms** or dual parameter **dot plots**). Figure 11-3■ shows a single parameter dot plot while Figure 11-4■ is a dual parameter analysis of whole peripheral blood. A single parameter histogram provides a frequency distribution

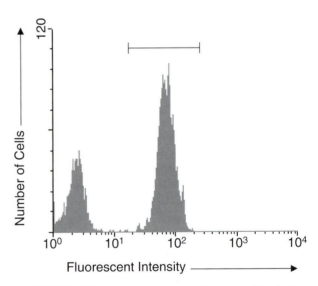

■ **FIGURE 11-3** A single parameter histogram. The light scatter or fluorescent signal from cells may be represented as a frequency distribution (a plot of signal intensity vs. cell number). This mixed population of cells (two or more) was stained with a monoclonal antibody to a single surface antigen. The predominant population of cells in the mixture expresses the antigen (defined by bracket). The remaining cells express only background levels of fluorescence (autofluorescence) and are located on the left end of the scale of fluorescent intensity. The Y axis indicates the number of cells at each level of fluorescent intensity.

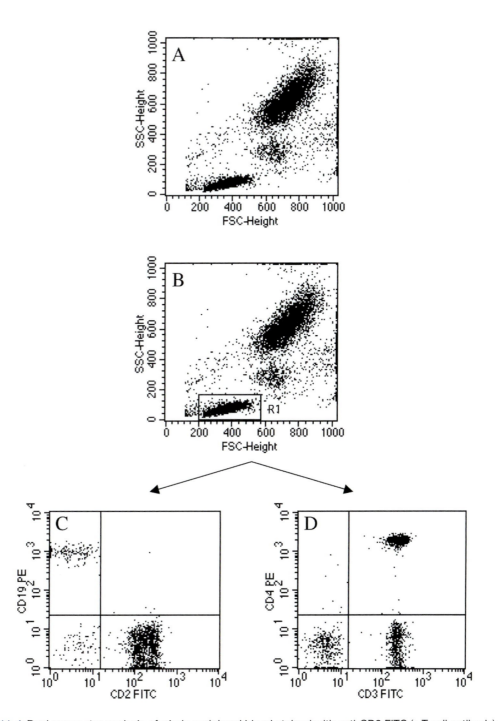

■ FIGURE 11-4 Dual parameter analysis of whole peripheral blood stained with anti-CD2 FITC (a T cell antibody) and anti-CD19 PE (a B cell antibody) in one tube. A second aliquot was stained with anti-CD3 FITC and anti-CD4 (a predominantly T helper cell antibody). The forward scatter (FSC; cell size) versus side scatter (SSC; cell complexity) dot plot A demonstrates the typical pattern of cell types in whole blood. One can distinguish lymphocytes, monocytes, and granulocytes based on these intrinsic parameters. Panel B shows the application of an analysis region (gate) (box labeled R1). Using computer software to identify cells of interest, in this case lymphocytes, the user restricts further analysis to lymphocytes. The porportion of T (82%; lower right quadrant) and B cells (12%; upper left quadrant) in the gated lymphocyte population is determined in the dot plot labeled C demonstrating the ability of flow cytometry to identify different cell types in a complex mixture with the use of monoclonal antibodies. The proportion of T helper cells (42%; upper right quadrant) in the gated lymphocyte population is determined in dot plot D, demonstrating the ability of flow cytometry to enumerate specific subtypes of cells based on detection of multiple antigens expressed by the cells of interest.

of the number of events in each channel. A dual parameter dot plots allows the user to assess two parameters simultaneously for each cell. Most flow cytometric software allows the user to restrict the analysis of various parameters to a specific population of cells via a process termed "gating." For example, in the analysis of the proportion of CD4 positive T lymphocytes in the peripheral blood, one can draw a "gate" around the lymphocyte population to restrict the analysis of the proportion of CD4 bearing cells to the lymphocyte population (see Figure 11-4). Additional information is needed if one wishes to determine the absolute number of CD4 positive T-lymphocytes. To determine this number, the concentration of total lymphocytes in the cell suspension must be known. In the case of CD4 T lymphocytes, multiply the proportion of CD4 and all of the total lymphocyte sums to determine the absolute number of CD4 and T-lymphocytes.

CELLULAR PROBES

As stated earlier, the intrinsic parameters of cells are assessed by their forward and side light scatter. However, most clinical applications of flow cytometry are aimed at identifying subsets of cells that may have similar light scatter characteristics. Thus, additional reagents to identify specific subtypes of cells are needed. For example, in an HIV-1 infected individual one needs to enumerate the T-helper subset of peripheral blood lymphocytes. While one can enumerate the lymphocyte population in a whole blood sample by assessing its light scatter properties, we cannot enumerate the number of CD4 T-lymphocytes in the lymphocyte population because it also contains CD8 T-lymphocytes, B-lymphocytes, natural-killer (NK) cells, and other, less frequent cell types. Monoclonal antibodies that specifically identify CD4 T-lymphocytes allow us to identify these or a multitude of other specific cell types by virtue of their line specificity for a target antigen.

MONOCLONAL ANTIBODIES

Antibodies, a product of B cells, are protein molecules that bind to a specific antigen. Antibodies in the blood of humans or animals represent a highly complex mixture of several different types of antibodies with a diverse range of antigen specificities. To effectively serve as a reagent to identify specific antigens, one must generate a **clone** of B cells that secrete a single antibody type with a defined target antigen specificity. Mono-

clonal antibodies fill this need. Through a complicated process of immunization to generate antigen specific B cells, fusion with a malignant cell line to generate an immortalized clone of cells, screening for production of the appropriate antibody, and expansion of the clone and purification, a preparation of antibody with a defined specificity is generated. Figure 11-5■ shows the preparation of monoclonal antibodies.

Thousands of monoclonal antibodies have been generated that recognize specific cell types and are useful for flow cytometric analyses. To be used for flow cytometric analysis, however, the monoclonal antibodies must be labeled so that we can determine if they bind to cells of interest. A variety of fluorochromes are available and useful for labeling monoclonal antibodies for flow cytometry. Cluster designations for commonly used monoclonal antibodies in flow cytometry and the cell types they bind to are shown on Table 11-1✪.

Fluorochromes are molecules that absorb light of one wavelength, for our purposes the wavelength of the laser in the flow cytometer, and emit light of higher wavelength. Emitted light is captured by the PMTs in the flow cytometer. One of the most commonly used fluorochromes is fluorescein isothiocyanate (FITC). The use of several fluorochromes with similar excitation but distinct emission wavelengths allows one to perform multicolor analyses (i.e., using two, three, or more different monoclonal antibodies each labeled with a different fluorochrome). In this way, very specific subsets of cells can be accurately defined in complex mixtures by the concomitant detection of multiple cell surface or intracellular antigens. Table 11-2✪ shows fluorochromes commonly used for flow cytometry and the absorption and emission spectra.

It should be noted that fluorescently labeled monoclonal antibodies are not the only reagents useful in flow cytometry. A variety of fluorescent dyes can be used to study various properties of cells. For example, dyes that bind to nucleic acids can be used to estimate the DNA content of a population of cells. Other dyes that are taken up by cells and react to changes in the activation state of cells can be used to assess aspects of cell function.

SAMPLE PROCESSING

Staining cells with monoclonal antibodies or other dyes is a relatively straightforward process. Two types of staining protocols are typically employed for flow cytometric analysis (direct and indirect antibody staining). Direct fluorescent staining employs a mon-

1. INOCULATION

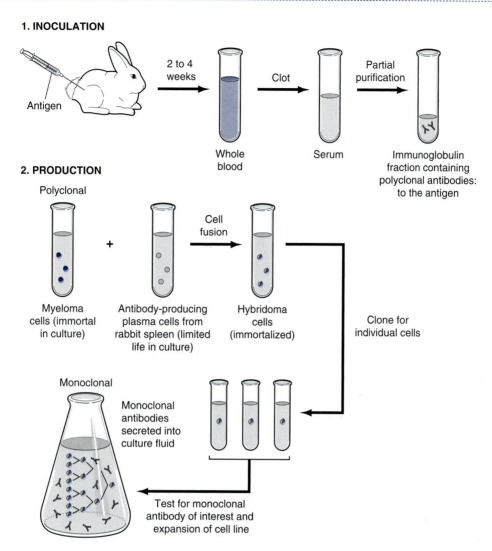

2. PRODUCTION

■ **FIGURE 11-5** A laboratory animal, such as a rabbit or mouse, is immunized with a specific antigen (the desired target of the monoclonal antibody to be made). After 2 to 4 weeks, the success of immunization is verified by the detection of polyclonal antibodies in the animal's serum. To produce the monoclonal antibody, spleen cells from the animal are fused to myeloma cells that are then subjected to cloning and screening for the antibody of interest.

oclonal antibody that is covalently linked to a fluorochrome. Indirect staining employs an unlabeled monoclonal antibody which, binding to target antigen, requires a second step using an anti-immunoglobulin antibody (an antibody that binds to another antibody, usually of a different species) that is conjugated to a fluorochrome. Figure 11-6■ shows the difference between direct and indirect antibody staining. In indirect staining, the cell mixture is first incubated with the unlabeled monoclonal antibody,

unbound antibody is washed away, and then the cells are incubated with fluorochrome labeled secondary antibody.

The drawbacks to this approach are the increased background staining sometimes seen, as well as more complicated assay setup. The advantages include the ability to assess markers for which no directly labeled primary antibody are available and typically a brighter staining intensity which may be useful for assessment of dimly expressed antigens. Directly labeled mono-

⊘ TABLE 11-1

Cluster Designations for Commonly Used Monoclonal Antibodies in Flow Cytometry and the Cell Types Recognized

Monoclonal Antibody Designation	Target Cell Type
CD2	T cells; NK cells
CD3	T cells
CD4	T helper cells, monocytes (dimly expressed)
CD5	T cells; some B cells
CD8	T cytotoxic cells, macrophages
CD10	Immature T, B cells; PMN s
CD13	Monocytes, PMN s
CD14	Monocytes, PMN s (dimly expressed)
CD16	NK cells, PMN s, monocytes
CD19	B cells
CD20	B cells
CD25	Activated T cells
CD33	Monocytes
CD34	Stem/Progenitor cells
CD45	Leukocytes
CD56	NK cells, monocytes (dimly expressed)
Anti-Kappa	B cells
Anti-Lambda	B cells
Tdt	Immature Lymphocytes

Each monoclonal antibody binds to a specific target molecule. However, the target molecule may be expressed on several different cell types as indicated. NK = natural killer cell; PMN = polymorphonuclear neutrophil.

clonal antibodies have the advantage of a shorter assay setup time and typically a reduced amount of background (nonspecific) staining of cells in the suspension.

SPECIMEN TYPES FOR FLOW CYTOMETRY ANALYSIS

The types of specimens that can be analyzed by flow cytometry are limited only be the availability of single cell suspensions and the availability of reagents with defined specificity for the cells of interest. Because flow cytometry is based on analysis of single cells, any sample in which the cells are in suspension is likely suitable for the flow analysis. Clinical samples such as peripheral flood or bone marrow are common samples. Other samples, such as bronchoalveolar lavage fluids,

are also appropriate. In certain circumstances, samples may be subjected to purification (to remove unwanted cells) or enrichment (to increase the frequency of cells interest) procedures.

Solid tissue (lymph nodes, tumor) may also be subjected to flow cytometric analysis; however, they must be processed to generate single cell suspensions. This is most commonly achieved by physical disaggregation of the tissue to generate a suspension of cells.

Two parameters of sample adequacy are critically important to assess. First, one must have a sufficient number of cells to stain and acquire. For typical clinical applications, 2×10^5 cells/ml or more are required for processing. Second, for samples that are greater than 24 hours old or have been processed from tissues it is important to assess cell viability. Dead cells are prone to nonspecific uptake of fluorochrome-labeled

✪ TABLE 11-2

Fluorochromes Commonly Used for Flow Cytometry and the Absorption and Emission Spectra

Fluorochrome	Absorption Maximum	Emission Maximum
FITC	492	520–530
PE	480–565	575–585
PerCP	490	677
APC	650	660
PE-Cy5	480–565	620

As can be seen, all except APC can be excited with the 488nm lasers of typical clinical flow cytometers. If APC is used, a second laser must be employed to provide the correct light source for excitation. Also, it can be seen that some of the fluorochromes have emission maxima that are relatively close. As such, it is important that compensation be optimized for assays in which 2 or more of these fluorochromes are used for analysis. FITC = fluorescein isothiocyanate; PE = phycoery-thrin; PerCP = peridinin chlorophyll; APC = allophycocyanin; PE-Cy5 = phycoerythrin-CY5 tandem conjugate.

Direct staining   Indirect staining

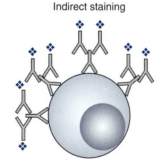

■ FIGURE 11-6 The direct fluorescent antibody staining technique employs a monoclonal antibody that is covalently linked to a fluorochrome. In the case where the monoclonal antibody of interest is not available in a directly conjugated fashion, an indirect staining method can be used. In this approach, the antibody to the target antigen (primary antibody) is incubated with the cell suspension. The cells are then washed to remove unbound primary antibody and the fluorescently labeled secondary antibody is added. This antibody binds specifically to antibodies of a particular isotype and species (e.g., goat anti-mouse IgG). After incubation, unbound secondary antibody is washed away, and the cells are fixed. Indirect staining, in addition to providing a method for use of unlabeled primary antibodies, is also useful for staining antigens that are dimly expressed (antigens that are present in low amounts on or in a cell). As depicted, several secondary antibodies may bind to a single primary antibody thus amplifying the fluorescent signal from the dimly expressed antigen.

antibodies and may interfere with the accurate enumerates of cells of interest.

When staining cell preparations, the use of purified cells, such as peripheral blood mononuclear cells, requires no additional manipulations except for fixation. However, whole anticoagulated peripheral blood is commonly used for immunophenotyping. The number of red blood cells (RBCs) is very high in whole blood and can complicate analysis of flow cytometric data. As such, it is typical to lyse the RBCs before fixation and analysis of whole blood. Commercially available lysing agents may be used for this purpose. Alternatively, one can prepare and use an ammonium chloride lysing solution. After lysing RBCs, a wash step to remove the lysing agent is often performed. More recently, methods that do not require a wash step have been developed.

The final step in sample preparation is to "fix" cells in a solution of paraformaldehyde to inactivate infectious agents and to stabilize the labeled cell surface antigens. Typically, stained cells are resuspended in a 1% paraformaldehyde solution. After fixation, stained cell preparations can be held at 4°C for some period of time before acquisition on the flow cytometer. This provides some flexibility in workload management for the laboratory. Figure 11-7■ shows the schematic flow diagram for the procedure for preparing blood sample for flow cytometric analysis.

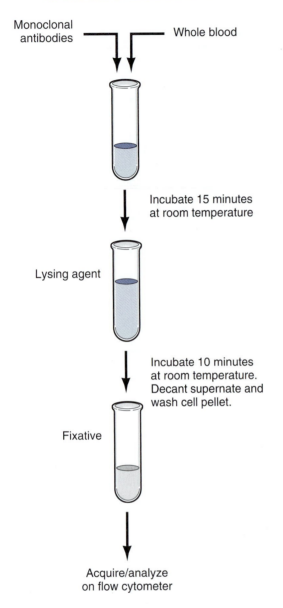

Monoclonal antibodies

Whole blood

Incubate 15 minutes at room temperature

Lysing agent

Incubate 10 minutes at room temperature. Decant supernate and wash cell pellet.

Fixative

Acquire/analyze on flow cytometer

■ **FIGURE 11-7** The standard procedure for staining whole blood with monoclonal antibodies for flow cytometric analysis involves mixing monoclonal antibodies with the an aliquot of anticoagulated blood and incubating for a short period followed by a short incubation with an agent that will lyse RBCs. After centrifugation the resultant cell pellet is washed to remove cell debris and residual lysing agent. Finally a fixative, typically a 1% paraformaldehyde solution, is added to the cells to stabilize the antibodies bound to the cell surface and inactivate infectious agents that may be present in the sample.

▶ CLINICAL APPLICATIONS OF FLOW CYTOMETRY

ENUMERATION OF CD4 T-LYMPHOCYTES IN PERIPHERAL BLOOD

AIDS (acquired immunodeficiency syndrome) is the outcome of infection with human immunodeficiency virus type 1 (HIV-1). The hallmark of this infection is the loss of CD4 T lymphocytes, a key cell type involved in the development of immune responses to foreign antigens. Typically, patients infected with HIV undergo a gradual decline in the number of CD4 T cells. As disease progresses, patients lose the ability to fight off common infections (opportunistic infections) and malignancies.

Serial monitoring of CD4 T-cells provides several important pieces of information for management of HIV-infected individuals. The CD4 level is reflective of the degree of immunosuppression. A level of 200 CD4 T cells per microliter of blood is indicative of substantial immunosuppression and is a criterion for the diagnosis of AIDs. Additionally, this is the level at which administration of prophylactic antibiotics for various opportunistic infections is often begun. Serial monitoring also allows the physician to gauge the kinetics of CD4 decline and thus infer the rate of disease progression. It is also useful to monitor CD4 counts after initiation of antiretroviral therapy. Successful therapy usually results in increases in CD4 levels. When patients experience an increase in CD4 T cells with effective therapy, they may be able to stop taking prophylactic medicines for opportunistic infections.

There are a number of approaches to the enumeration of CD4 T cells. Most commonly, a three- or four-color method is used to determine the proportion (percentage) of CD4 T cells in the blood. Determination of the absolute number of CD4 T lymphocytes (number of cells/ul of blood) can be accomplished by combining flow cytometric determination of the proportion of CD4 T lymphocytes with the absolute lymphocyte count from a hematology analyzer. The absolute number of CD4 T cells is the product of the CD3 and CD4 dual positive cell percentage and the absolute lymphocyte count. More recently, other methods have been developed for absolute counting that obviate the need of hematologic analyses. A known number of beads can be added to tubes and used to calculate the absolute CD4 count. Alternatively, there are flow cytometric instruments that count the number of cells in a defined volume and thus generate an absolute CD4 count. An example of a CD4 analysis is shown in Figure 11-8■.

ENUMERATION OF FETAL HEMOGLOBIN CONTAINING CELLS

A newer application of flow cytometry is for the enumeration of fetal hemoglobin containing RBCs. The standard method for enumeration of fetal hemoglobin containing cells, the Kleinhauer-Betke test, is a microscopic-based assay that is notoriously subjective and imprecise. The ability of flow cytometry to rapidly and objectively assess large numbers of cells for the presence of fetal hemoglobin makes it an attractive alternative. Enumeration of fetal hemoglobin containing cells is employed primarily for quantitating the level of fetal bleed in mothers at risk for sensitization to fetal Rhesus D (RhD) positive RBCs and to assist in the management of patients undergoing intrauterine transfusions.

Sensitization of an RhD-negative mother to an RhD-positive fetus can result in hemolytic disease of the newborn (HDN). This serious disease can be prevented by identification of RhD-negative mothers bearing RhD-positive fetuses and administration of anti-RhD immune globulin. To prevent sensitization, the number of fetal hemoglobin containing cells in the peripheral blood is determined and used to determine the amount of anti-Rh immune globulin that she receives.

The detection of fetal hemoglobin is accomplished with a hemoglobin F specific monoclonal antibody in much the same fashion as determination of other antigens. However, hemoglobin is intracellular; thus, an additional step of cell permeabilization is required prior to addition of antibody. Permeabilization allows the antibody to diffuse inside the cell and bind to fetal hemoglobin if present. The RBCs are fixed, permeabilized, then incubated with the anti-HbF monoclonal antibody.

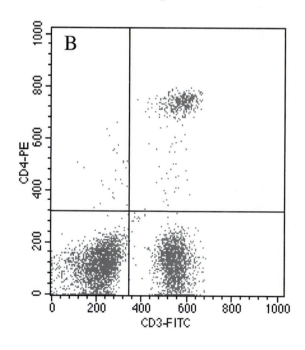

FIGURE 11-8 Dual parameter dot plots from a representative HIV seronegative (A) and HIV seropositive (B) donor. The reduced frequency of dual positive CD3/CD4 cells is apparent when one compares the density of dots in the upper right quadrants of A versus B. The actual percent CD3/4 dual positive cells in the lymphocytes population is below the plots. The absolute CD4 T-lymphocyte count is the product of the CD4 percent and the absolute lymphocyte count.

FLOW CYTOMETRY IN TRANSPLANTATION

Flow cytometry has become an important tool in **stem cell** and solid organ transplantation. Enumeration of CD34 expressing stem/progenitor cells has emerged as a common assay in stem cell transplantation. For solid organ transplantation, the detection of preformed antibodies in the recipients' blood to HLA molecules of the potential donor is an important application. Flow cytometry is well suited for these analyses.

As hematopoietic stem cells mature in the bone marrow, they express a variety of cell surface proteins in a coordinated fashion. One of the earliest appearing markers on the cell surface is the CD34 antigen, which is subsequently lost with maturation of the cell. Thus, the presence of CD34 is a marker of stem/progenitor cells. Enumerating the number of CD34 bearing cells provides an estimate of the repopulating capacity of a stem progenitor cell product. The ability to enumerate CD34 bearing cells has proven advantageous over the previously employed approach of determining the total mononuclear cell dose as the guide for the quantity of stem cell preparation to infuse.

A straightforward immunophenotyping panel can be used to determine the proportion and absolute number of CD34 bearing cells in the total white cell population (CD45 positive) of bone marrow or peripheral blood stem cell preparations. These numbers are then used to determine the amount of stem cell product required for infusion.

In solid organ transplantation, flow cytometry has three major applications. In renal transplant candidates, the presence of preformed antibodies to **HLA** (human leukocyte antigen) molecules of the donor are markers of immunologic sensitization and associated with an increased risk for graft rejection. Because of the significance of preformed HLA antibodies (also termed alloantibodies), patients awaiting a renal transplant submit serum samples on a monthly basis to be screened for the presence of HLA antibodies and to determine their specificity (i.e., which HLA antigens they recognize). In this way donors with unacceptable HLA antigens (those to which the patient has specific antibodies) can be deferred from donation. Antibody screening can be accomplished by a number of distinct techniques. Flow cytometry–based antibody screening has the advantage of being the most sensitive method for detection and characterization of alloantibodies.

Flow cytometric–antibody screening involves the incubation of the potential recipient serum with a panel of lymphocytes (which express HLA molecules) or latex beads (with HLA molecules coupled to the beads). The panel of cells or beads is large so that many different HLA types are represented. If the patient serum has HLA antibodies, they will bind to the target cells/beads. After removal of unbound antibodies by a wash step, bound antibodies are detected by addition of an antihuman IgG antibody that is labeled with a fluorochrome such as FITC. Using this assay the frequency of specific HLA types that the recipients serum recognizes as well as the specific HLA types can be determined.

When a potential donor is identified for a kidney recipient, it is necessary to perform a pretransplant crossmatch. This involves mixing recipient serum with donor lymphocytes to detect the presence of donor specific HLA antibodies which, if present, bind to the donor cells. Figure 11-9■ shows a single parameter dot plot demonstrating the results from a flow cytometry cross-match. Binding is detected by addition of a fluorochrome-labeled antihuman IgG antibody. When pre-

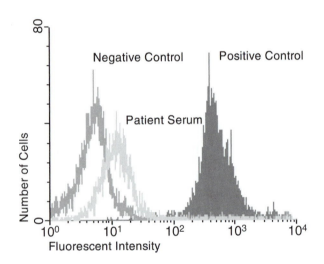

■ FIGURE 11-9 A single parameter dot plot demonstrating the results from a flow cytometry cross-match. The distribution of fluorescent intensities for the positive control, negative control, and recipient sera have been overlayed on the same plot for comparison. In this assay (an indirect staining method) donor lymphocytes are incubated with patient serum or controls, washed, then incubated with an FITC-labeled goat antihuman IgG antibody preparation. Unbound secondary antibody was washed away, and the cells were fixed. The strong FITC fluorescence of the positive control serum indicates binding of the control antibody. The negative control serum shows only background levels of fluorescence. The patient serum shows an intermediate, but significant, level of fluorescence. Thus, this patient was determined to have antibodies that specifically recognize donor lymphocytes (a positive cross-match).

sent, donor specific antibodies impart an increased risk of rejection episodes or immunologic graft failure. When this risk is high, transplant centers may elect not to proceed with the transplant. As with antibody screening, there are a number of methods in use to perform donor cross-matching. Flow cytometry has become an important member of this list because of its high sensitivity. The flow cytometric cross-match is performed in a similar manner to the antibody screen except that the target cells are the potential donors lymphocytes (T and/or B cells) and not a large panel of cells or beads.

A final application of flow cytometry in the transplant field is as an aid to physicians prescribing antirejection therapy. Patients that are experiencing severe rejection episodes, not responsive to first-line therapies such as steroids, may be treated with antibodies that deplete T cells from the patient. Depleting T cells is a highly potent way to suppress antigraft immune responses. Examples of these types of therapies include OKT3 (an antibody to the epsilon chain of the CD3 antigen on T cells) or thymoglobulin (a rabbit polyclonal antiserum to thymocytes). In order to appropriately manage patients receiving these therapies, it is necessary to determine that they are working appropriately. As such, patients receiving one of these agents typically have peripheral blood samples analyzed by flow cytometry to determine the absolute number of CD3 positive T cells. This assay is usually conducted as a standard whole blood immunophenotyping assay with directly labeled anti-CD3 monoclonal antibodies. In successfully treated patients, the CD3T cell numbers are very low (less than 10 per microliter), even undetectable.

APPLICATIONS OF FLOW CYTOMETRY IN HEMATOLOGY

Flow cytometry can be utilized to enumerate cells other than lymphocytes, sometimes without the use of monoclonal antibodies. Reticulocyte enumeration is an application that uses a nucleic acid binding dye instead of a monoclonal antibody to identify the cells of interest. The basis of this assay is that reticulocytes contain residual ribosomes (which contain RNA). Thiazole orange is an RNA-binding dye that fluoresces when excited by standard flow cytometry lasers. When incubated with blood, it diffuses into cells and binds RNA. Flow cytometric analysis can then be used to determine the frequency of fluorescent RBCs (reticulocytes). The reticulocyte percentage is used as a measure

of erythropoesis and release of RBCs from the bone marrow in patients with anemia.

Another application is for the diagnosis of paroxysmal nocturnal hemoglobinuria (PNH). In this disorder RBCs are unusually susceptible to complement-mediated lysis. It has been determined that this susceptibility is due to the lack of cell surface complement regulatory proteins (CD55 and CD59). These proteins are linked to the cell surface by specific proteins that anchor them to the cell surface. There is a lack of these anchors in patients with PNH and thus a lack of cell surface expression of the complement regulatory proteins. When this occurs, patients exhibit uncontrolled complement mediate lysis of RBCs. The lack of these anchor proteins can be assessed by staining for the presence of cell surface CD55 and CD59 on RBCs or neutrophils. This assay is more accurate and precise than the manual sugar water test, the alternative method employed to test for PNH.

FLOW CYTOMETRY IN HEMATOPATHOLOGY

Another major application of flow cytometry in the clinical laboratory is for the phenotypic characterization of hematologic malignancies (leukemias and lymphomas). These malignancies are clonal proliferations of lymphoid or myeloid cells at varying degrees of maturation. Flow cytometry using monoclonal antibodies to cell surface and intracellular antigens that define the lineage (e.g., T cell, B cell, or myeloid cell) and stage of maturation (e.g., pre-B cell, mature B cell) is useful as an aid in the diagnosis, classification, and monitoring of these diseases. As presented in the case study at the beginning of this chapter, flow cytometric analysis of the bone marrow taken from the patient showed light scatter gating (Figure 11-1) that demonstrated a marrow aspirate with a predominant population of low side scatter cells with a broad size (forward scatter) distribution. The low side scatter cells were predominantly dimly CD45 positive (Figure 11-1 arrow), characteristic of immature cells, in contrast to the few brightly CD45 staining cells (encircled) that likely represent mature lymphocytes in the marrow sample. The dim CD45 positive cells had the phenotype of immature B cells. They expressed CD34 and CD19 but were negative for the mature B and T cell markers, CD20 and CD3, respectively. They were also negative for surface **immunoglobulin,** further supporting the immature classification. Finally, the leukemic population had dual expression of CD19 and

CD10, a typical characteristic of B cell acute lymphoblastic leukemia.

The patient was given the diagnosis of pre-B cell acute lymphoblastic leukemia. He was started on chemotherapy and subsequently demonstrated a decline in the proportion of blast cells to 3%.

Hematopoeitic cells arise from bone marrow precursors that undergo a tightly regulated developmental pathway, resulting in mature cells that populate the blood and secondary lymphoid organs. During the process of maturation, cells express a variety of antigens. Some antigens are present early in development and lost with maturation, some are absent in early precursors and are expressed as the cells mature, and some are present throughout the developmental process. The pattern of expression of these various antigens define the **lineage** and state of maturation of hematologic cells. Table 11-1 provides a listing of cell surface and intracellular antigens that are commonly assessed to define the lineage and maturation state of hematologic cells.

During the process of malignant transformation, this tightly regulated pattern of expression of antigens may be disrupted. Detection and enumeration of cells with an altered phenotype or cells accounting for inappropriate proportion of the total population is the basis by which flow cytometry can aid in the diagnosis of these diseases. There are several types of changes that can occur in malignant cells: (1) lack or decreased expression of an expected antigen; (2) expression of an antigen at the wrong stage of development; (3) expression of an inappropriate lineage specific antigen; and (4) uniform expression of a clonal specific antigen (light chain restriction).

Panels of monoclonal antibodies are typically used in the clinical laboratory to define these abnormal patterns of antigen expression. A short list of hematologic malignancies and characteristic antigen profiles is given in Table 11-3✪. Antibodies to these antigens are utilized in flow cytometric assays in a fashion similar to that of Figure 11-1. Figure 11-10■ shows the analysis of peripheral blood from a patient with chronic lymphocytic leukemia. Common specimen types for analysis include blood, bone marrow, and lymph node cells. No processing requirements specific for these cells sources are necessary other than those required to maintain cell viability if staining and analysis are delayed. The increased background staining in samples with low viability may interfere with the ability to detect the low-frequency malignant cells. As such, viability determinations are important if aged samples are used.

✪ TABLE 11-3

Hematologic Malignancies with Associated Immunophenotypes

Malignancy	Immunophenotype
B-ALL	CD10, CD13 some, CD19, CD22, CD33 some, CD34, CD45 dim or negative, HLA-DR, Tdt
T-ALL	CD1a, CD2, CD3, CD4, CD5, CD7, CD8, CD10 some, CD13 some, CD33 some, CD34, CD45 dim
AML	CD4 some, CD5 some, CD7 some, CD11b some, CD13, CD14 some, CD15 some, CD19 some, CD33, CD34, CD45 dim, CD56 some, CD117, HLA-DR
B-CLL	CD5, CD20 dim, CD23, CD45, Ig light clonality
HCL	CD10, CD20, CD22, CD25, CD103, Ig light chain clonality
SLL	CD5, CD20 dim, CD23, CD45, Ig light chain clonality
FCC	CD10 some, CD19 dim, CD20 bright, Ig light chain clonality

It should be noted that the immunophenotypes can vary as indicated (some). B-ALL = B cell acute lymphoblastic leukemia; T-ALL = T cell acute lymphoblastic leukemia; AML = acute myeloid leukemia; B-CLL = B cell chronic lymphocytic leukemia; HCL = hairy cell leukemia; SLL = small lymphocytic lymphoma; FCC = follicular center cell lymphoma; Tdt = terminal nucleotidyl transferase; Ig = immunoglobulin

▶ FUTURE TRENDS IN FLOW CYTOMETRY

Flowcytometry is a common technique in the clinical laboratory used for enumeration of normal and abnormal cells in blood and other tissues of the body. The ability to rapidly and precisely assess large numbers of cell on a single-cell basis coupled with the specificity imparted by the use of monoclonal antibodies has proven useful in many specialties within the clinical laboratory. Although not addressed in this chapter, study of cell function is a growing area of flow cytometry, and while predominantly of research interest, will likely make its way into clinical application. The development of additional applications and new monoclonal antibodies with specificities relevant to particular cells types will serve to continue expanding the clinical utility of flow cytometric analysis.

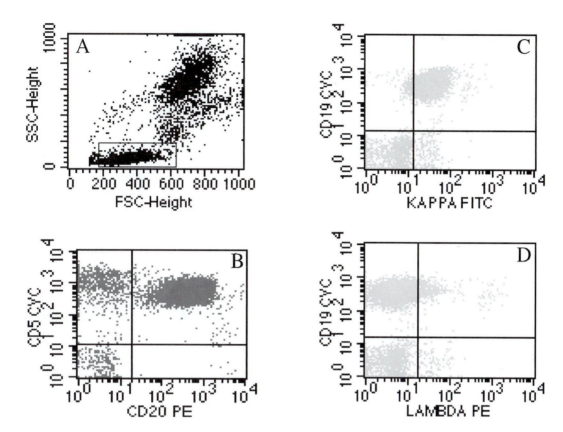

■ FIGURE 11-10 Analysis of peripheral blood from a patient with chronic lymphocytic leukemia. Peripheral blood was stained with directly labeled antibodies to T and B lymphocyte antigens to define the predominant population of cells and also to determine if they were clonal (i.e., derived from the malignant transformation of a single cell). The forward versus side scatter plot (A) demonstrates a pattern typical of peripheral blood. A gated lymphocyte analysis (B) demonstrates a predominant population of CD20 and CD5 dual positive cells (encircled). This is not typical of normal peripheral blood in which the frequency of CD20 positive B lymphocytes would be expected to be less than 15%. Also, these B cells all co-express CD5 (a T cell marker that is normally expressed on only a small subset of normal B lymphocytes). This example demonstrates the ability of flow cytometry to detect antigens not expressed by the normal counterparts of peripheral blood B lymphocytes. Additionally, panels C and D demonstrate the ability of flow cytometry to define a clonal population of cells. In panel C the malignant cells are shown to uniformly express kappa light chains on the cell surface (encircled). Staining for lambda light chains (D) was negative (encircled) except for a few residual normal B lymphocytes (arrow). In a normal population of B lymphocytes, one would detect both kappa and lambda light chain positive cells at a ratio of approximately 1.5:1.

SUMMARY

Flow cytometry is a technology that allows the clinical laboratory to identify and enumerate specific cell types in complex biologic samples. The flow cytometer accomplishes this effective analysis by the generation of a stream of cells that pass single file through a laser beam. When cells pass through the laser beam, they scatter light in amounts that reflect the size and complexity of the cell. In addition, cells can be stained with dyes or fluorescently labeled monoclonal antibodies to cell surface or intracellular antigens to identify specific cell types. Scattered light and fluorescence signals collected by the optical system of the flow cytometer and converted to digital signals are stored for later computer analysis. The ability of flow cytometry to enumerate specific cells types has made it a widely applicable technology to many areas of the clinical laboratory, including immunology, hematology, and transplantation.

POINTS TO REMEMBER

▶ Flow cytometry has the advantage of providing a rapid analysis of large numbers of cells in an objective and precise fashion. The types of cells that can be identified and enumerated is limited only by the availability of reagents, monoclonal antibodies, or fluorescent dyes that identify the cell type of interest.

▶ Many different types of samples can be subjected to flow cytometric analysis as long as they are in a single cell suspension. As cells pass through the flow cytometer, they intersect the beam of a laser and scatter the laser light. This scattered light is captured by several "detectors" that convert the energy from the light to electrical signals that are proportional to the size and complexity of the cells. Cells stained with fluorescent monoclonal anti-bodies fluoresce when they pass through the laser. The fluorescent light is also captured by the optical system of the cytometer. The patterns of signals from the scattered light and fluorescence provide a "picture" of the cell's size, complexity, and antigenic makeup that is used to classify and enumeration the cell type.

▶ Flow cytometry provides a rapid, precise analysis of cells in complex mixtures on a single cell basis. This information is used to enumerate normal and/or abnormal components of a cell suspension. In the patient case, flow cytometry identified an abnormal population of immature B lymphocytes based on reactivity with a panel of monoclonal antibodies that define the lineage and maturation state of the cells.

LEARNING ASSESSMENT QUESTIONS

1. What are the advantages of flow cytometric enumeration of cell subsets compared with a microscopic based enumeration?

2. What is a monoclonal antibody and why is it useful for flow cytometry?

3. What is the difference between a histogram and dual parameter dot plot?

4. How would one calculate the absolute CD4 T cell count in a blood sample that had 20% CD4 T cells and an absolute lymphocyte count of 950 cells/ul? What are the most frequent cell types, other than CD4 T-cells that account for the remainder of the lymphocytes in the blood?

5. If you were asked to analyze a five-day-old peripheral blood sample for the presence of leukemic blasts, what would be a major consideration in interpreting the results?

REFERENCES

Bray, R. A. 2001. Flow cytometry in human leukocyte antigen testing. *Semin Hematol* 38:194–200.

Givan, A. L. 2001. *Flow Cytometry First Principles,* 2nd ed. Wiley-Liss, New York.

Gratama, J. W., D. R. Sutherland, and M. Keeney. 2001 Flow cytometric enumeration and immunophenotyping of hematopoietic stem and progenitor cells. *Semin Hematol* 38:139–47.

Mandy, F. F., J. K. Nicholson, and J. S. McDougal. 2003. Guidelines for performing single-platform absolute CD4+ T-cell determinations with CD45 gating for persons infected with human immunodeficiency virus. Centers for Disease Control and Prevention. *MMWR Recomm Rep* 52(RR-2):1–13.

Mundee, Y., N. C. Bigelow, B. H. Davis, and J. B. Porter. 2000. Simplified flow cytometric method for fetal hemoglobin containing red blood cells. *Cytometry* 42:389–93.

Nguyen, D., L. W. Diamond, and R. C. Braylan. 2003. *Flow Cytometry in Hematopathology. A Visual Approach to Data Analysis and Interpretation.* Humana Press, Totowa, NJ.

1997 revised guidelines for performing CD4+ T-cell determinations in persons infected with human immunodeficiency virus (HIV). 1997, Centers for Disease Control and Prevention. *MMWR Recomm Rep* 46(RR-2):1–29.

Richards, S. J., A. C. Rawstron, and P. Hillmen. 2000. Application of flow cytometry to the diagnosis of paroxysmal nocturnal hemoglobinuria. *Cytometry* (Communications in Clinical Cytometry) 42:223–33.

Riley, R. S., J. M. Ben-Ezra, A. Tidwell, and G. Romagnoli. 2002. Reticulocyte analysis by flow cytometry and other techniques. *Hematol Oncol Clin North Am* 16:373–420.

Schellekens, P. T., M. Koot, M. T. Roos et al. 1995. Immunologic and virologic markers determining progression to AIDS. *J Acquir Immune Defic Syndr Hum Retrovirol* 10 suppl 2:S62–6.

Sharpiro, H. M. 2003. *Practical Flow Cytometry,* 4th ed. Wiley-Liss, Hoboken, NJ.

12

Hybridization Techniques

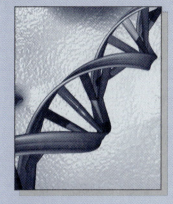

■ CHAPTER CHECKLIST

After reading and studying this chapter, the reader should be able to:

1. Describe the structures of both DNA and RNA, and explain how each is used in clinical diagnosis.
2. Describe and differentiate the processes of transcription, translation, and replication.
3. Explain how differences between prokaryotic and eukaryotic DNA may be exploited for diagnostic purposes by hybridization technology.
4. Explain the rationale behind the use of restriction enzymes for DNA isolation and sequencing.
5. Discuss the general concept of nucleic acid blotting.
6. List the shared characteristic(s) of Southern blotting, Northern blotting, and in situ hybridization.
7. Describe the application of hybridization techniques to the diagnosis of infectious disease, genetic disorders, and histocompatibility testing.
8. Describe proper specimen collection and preparation for hybridization testing.
9. Diagram the steps required for in vitro hybridization methods.
10. Describe Southern blot and the clinical applications of this technique.
11. Describe Northern blot and the clinical applications of this technique.
12. Describe in situ hybridization and the clinical applications of this technique.
13. List the general factors that affect in vitro hybridization assays.
14. Compare the basic concepts of hybridization assays with other techniques.
15. Diagram the basic procedures for DNA purification, RNA purification, preparation of DNA probes, Southern blotting, Northern blotting, and in situ hybridization.

ⓔ CASE IN POINT

The trail was cold—really cold. The "ladies of the evening" who had been murdered had drawn their last breath a century and a half ago. But, a few fragments of what they had been remained. With twenty-first-century molecular techniques, the DNA in a few long-dead cells could be amplified into a great enough quantity to be compared with DNA from other cells. The murderer was about to be revealed.

CASE IN POINT *(continued)*

ISSUES TO CONSIDER:

After reading the case history, consider

- The techniques would be used to extract the DNA from the samples
- Problems that might be encountered in dealing with small samples of very old tissues
- The usefulness and rationale of whether or not to use in situ hybridization techniques in this case
- Hybridization techniques that would be used
- The results you would expect to see if the DNA recovered from the victims matched that of the proposed murderer

IMPORTANT TERMS

Anticodon

Base triplet

Codon

Digest

DNA (deoxyribonucleic acid)

DNA polymerase

DNase

Endonuclease

Enhancer

Hybridization

Intron

mRNA (messenger RNA)

Nick translation

Nitrogenous base

Nucleic acid probe

Nucleotide

Oligonucleotide

Operon

Primer

Probe

Purine

Pyrimidine

Random primer extension

Restriction enzyme

RFLP (restriction fragment-length polymorphism)

Ribosome

RNA polymerase

RNA (ribonucleic acid)

RNase

rRNA (ribosomal RNA)

Semiconservative replication

Transcription

Translation

tRNA (transfer RNA)

▶ INTRODUCTION

Advances in molecular biology techniques have led to a better understanding of the genetic mechanisms underlying the immune response. Although precipitation reactions are useful for quantitation of antibody production, and T and B cells might be identified by their surface antigens, analysis of the specific genes active during a response to an antigen requires sorting out of those genes undergoing transcription and those that remain silent. Molecular biology has also helped elucidate mechanisms underlying inherited deficits in the immune system and those portions of the immune response responsible for allograft rejection. New approaches to correcting immunodeficiencies and to development of novel approaches to immunosuppression have had a direct effect on advances in the understanding of the immune response at the molecular level. This chapter begins with the basic concepts and principles of molecular biology, providing an overview of the structures and functions of DNA and RNA and how they are used in clinical diagnosis. Then the chapter describes the processes of transcription, translation,

and replication. Purification and analysis of nucleic acids and their uses are also discussed. In addition, this chapter provides an overview of the different hybridization techniques and their applications in clinical immunology and in research.

▶ BASIC MOLECULAR BIOLOGY

HISTORY

The foundations of molecular biology date back to the first half of the twentieth century when it was first determined that the "beads on a string" appearance of eukaryotic chromosomes was the product of **DNA (deoxyribonucleic acid)** and protein. An experiment in 1952 by Alfred Hershey and Martha Chase demonstrated that DNA was genetic material, rather than protein. These investigators grew the bacteriophage T2 along with the target organism *Escherichia coli* in radioactive sulfur. They found that the sulfur was incorporated into the protein components of the phage but not into the DNA. Conversely, when the experiment was conducted using radioactive phosphorus, uptake was seen in DNA but not in protein. Furthermore, if the bacteria were lysed, only radioactive phosphorus could be detected. The conclusion drawn from these results was that phage DNA was the genetic material infecting the bacteria. The function of DNA was further elucidated when George W. Beadle, E. L. Tatum, and Joshua Lederberg were awarded a Nobel Prize in 1958 for their discovery of genetic recombination in *E. coli,* proving the relationship of genes to enzymes.

While these experiments suggested the function of DNA, they did not address the structure of the molecule. In a seminal article in *Nature* in 1953, James Watson and Francis Crick proposed the double helix as a model for the structure of DNA. They drew extensively upon the X-ray crystallography structures of DNA done by Rosalind Franklin in Maurice Wilkins's laboratory at King's College in London. Watson and Crick hypothesized that, given the physical constraints superimposed on the molecule, the helix must be 2 nm in diameter, and that there should be two strands (the double helix). Nitrogenous bases would be stacked 1/3 nm apart, and the uniform diameter of the structure meant that **purines** (guanine or adenine) in one strand would have to pair with **pyrimidines** (cytosine or thymine) in the other strand. Since the specific pairing was thus determined by the structure of the base, complementary base pairing was indicated. This hypothesis was corroborated by experimental data from Erwin Chargoff, who had found the amount of adenine in a given quantity of DNA was matched by the amount of thymine.

In the *Nature* paper, Watson and Crick mentioned, "It has not escaped our notice that the specific pairing we have postulated immediately suggests a possible copying mechanism for the genetic material." Severo Ochoa and Arthur Kornberg were awarded a Nobel Prize in 1959 for their fundamental discoveries on synthesis of DNA and RNA. Watson, Crick, and Wilkins were rewarded with a Nobel Prize for their research in 1962.

Later Nobel Prizes awarded for work in molecular biology demonstrate the continuing importance and interaction of the field with others, including immunology. David Baltimore, Howard Temin, and Renato Dulbecco were honored in 1975 for their discovery of the viral enzyme reverse transcriptase, a substance that would lay the foundation for the 1993 prize to Kary Mullis for the development of the polymerase chain reaction technique. In 1978 prizes to Daniel Nathans, H. O. Smith, and Werner Aber for the use of restriction enzymes in the mapping of viral genomes, in 1980 to Paul Berg for fundamental contri-

butions to the biochemistry of recombinant DNA, and in 1980 to Walter Gilbert and Frederick Sanger for fundamental contributions to the sequencing of DNA further underscore the importance of the basic theories and techniques of molecular biology.

STRUCTURE AND FUNCTION OF DNA

From the description of DNA structure by Watson and Crick and the work of many other investigators, the precise structure and function of DNA has been elucidated. DNA is a polynucleotide with a deoxyribose sugar-phosphate backbone linked by covalent bonds (Figure 12-1■). By convention, the sugar's carbon

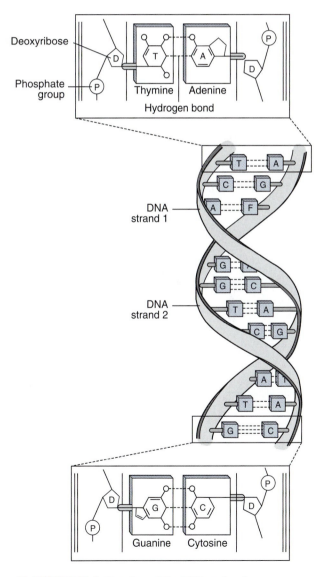

■ FIGURE 12-1 Structure of the DNA molecule.

atom attached to a hydroxyl group (−OH) is termed the 3′ end of the molecule, while the phosphate group is termed the 5′ end. Each **nucleotide** in this molecule is in turn comprised of a phosphate group, a deoxyribose sugar, and a **nitrogenous base** (Figure 12-2■). Although there are only four nitrogenous bases and, therefore, four nucleotides from which to chose—adenine, thymine, cytosine, and guanine—the combination of these in polynucleotides of varied lengths is virtually endless. The required interaction of adenine with thymine and guanine with cytosine in the complementary strands of DNA allows a series of hydrogen bonds to form "stair steps" to hold those strands together.

It is this sequence of nucleotides within each DNA molecule that makes each gene, or functional portion, of the molecule unique. Through a series of intermediate steps, a gene may be transcribed into RNA and then translated into a protein. Because of the double helix structure of DNA, each chain may also be replicated into another DNA molecule. It is this **semiconservative replication,** where each newly formed DNA strand reanneals with a parent strand, that allows DNA to serve as the heritable genetic material of a cell. Replication begins at the origin of replication.

It is just as important to consider what DNA cannot do, as well as the functions of DNA. The unique series of nucleotides in each gene in a DNA molecule encodes the sequence of amino acids required to make a particular protein. Because of the mechanisms of transcription and translation, DNA does not contain any heritable information for carbohydrates or lipids. Some genes in DNA do, however, code for enzymes necessary for the synthesis of some carbohydrates or lipids within an organism, thus allowing the genes within DNA to control metabolic function in the organism.

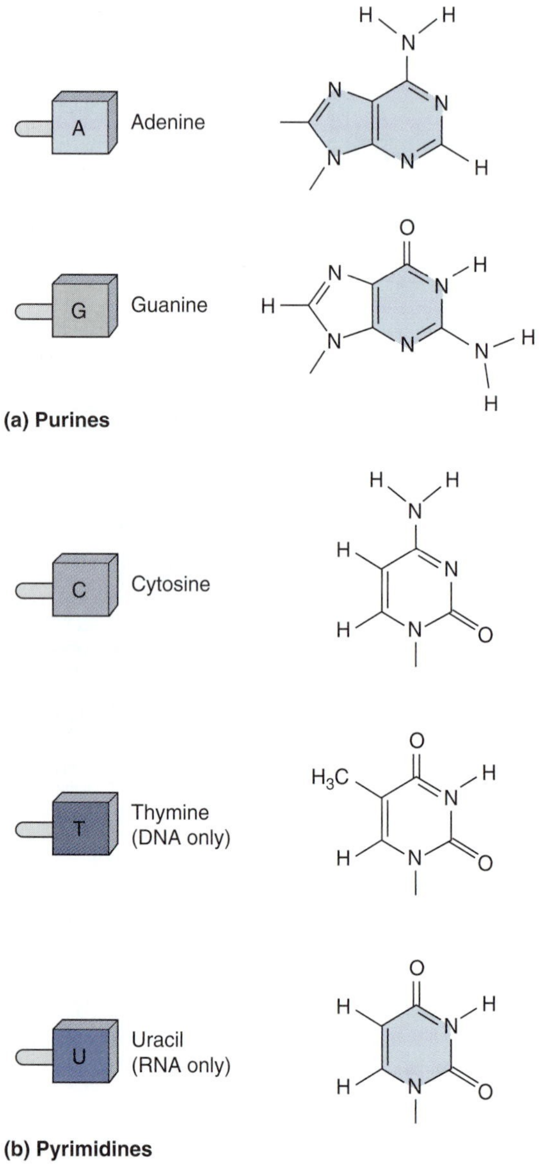

STRUCTURE AND FUNCTION OF RNA

RNA (ribonucleic acid) occurs in three forms— **messenger RNA (mRNA), ribosomal RNA (rRNA),** and **transfer RNA (tRNA)** (Figure 12-3■). Although none of the three forms have two complementary strands forming the characteristic double

(a) Purines

Adenine
A

Guanine
G

(b) Pyrimidines

Cytosine
C

Thymine
(DNA only)
T

Uracil
(RNA only)
U

■ FIGURE 12-2 Structure of purines and pyrimidines.

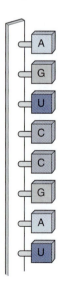

■ FIGURE 12-3 Structure of mRNA, rRNA, and tRNA.

helix of DNA, RNA does have a similar primary structure. In RNA, ribose replaces the deoxyribose sugar found in DNA, and uracil replaces thymine as a nitrogenous base. mRNA occurs as a long strand that can leave the nucleus prior to protein translation and carries the genetic information of the DNA to be used for protein synthesis in the cytoplasm of the cell. rRNA is found combined with protein within the ribosomes active in protein production. tRNAs, at least one for each amino acid, are found free in the cytoplasm. These molecules have a characteristic shape and are used to carry amino acids to the ribosome during protein synthesis. The tRNA cannot pick up the amino acids unaided, but rather require specific enzymes to link the specific amino acid to its attachment site.

THE UNIVERSAL GENETIC CODE

The genetic message contained within the DNA and carried to the cytoplasm by mRNA is critical for protein production. Proteins are comprised of amino acids, and the unique sequence of amino acids gives a particular protein its individual function and identity. This amino acid sequence is specified within the DNA by a three **base triplet** sequence, which in turn is transcribed into a complementary **codon** in mRNA. For example, the sequence "thymine-adenine-cytosine" or TAC in the DNA would be "adenine-uracil-guanine" or AUG in mRNA. During protein synthesis, or **translation,** the tRNA would carry the amino acid methionine and would pair with AUG on the mRNA via its **anticodon** UAC. Calculation of all combinations of four nucleotides gives 64 possible base triplets. Three of these triplets code for RNA (UAA, UAG, UGA), and act as stop codons during translation. The remaining 61 base triplets code for amino acids. Therefore, there is considerable redundancy in this genetic code, with two or even three base triplets coding for one amino acid.

TRANSCRIPTION, TRANSLATION, AND REPLICATION

DNA acts as a template for production of RNA during a process called **transcription.** (Figure 12-4■). The process begins when a portion of DNA is uncoiled and the hydrogen bonds between the two strands in a limited area are broken. Purines and pyrimidines within the nucleus form hydrogen bonds with their complement

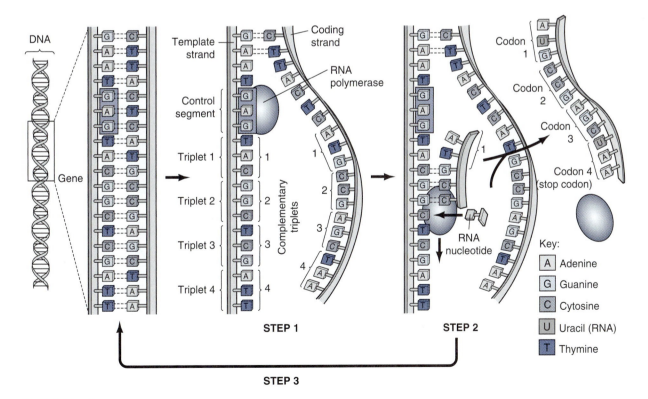

■ FIGURE 12-4 Transcription of mRNA from a DNA template.

on one strand of the exposed DNA. An enzyme called **RNA polymerase** binds to a specific site called the promoter within the gene to be transcribed then catalyzes formation of the covalent bonds necessary for connection of one nucleotide to the next. The mechanism of transcription is such that multiple pre-mRNA molecules may be synthesized at one time from one gene, thus allowing amplification of a limited amount of genetic information contained in the DNA molecule. Following transcription, splicing out of **introns** (sequences of DNA scattered throughout a gene that do not code for protein) and other modifications of the RNA are required before it leaves the nucleus to be used as the "message" for protein production. The DNA used as a template during transcription reforms its hydrogen bonds when transcription is complete, and the RNA polymerase is recycled as well.

The finished mRNA template is then used during protein translation (Figure 12-5■). The **ribosomes,** containing protein and rRNA, coordinate this event. During initiation, the small subunit of the ribosome binds the mRNA, while the large subunit binds tRNA, and the large subunit binds to the small subunit. The initiator tRNA binds to the start codon UAG on the mRNA via its anticodon UAC. This start sequence is universal in mammalian cells and is critical to establish the correct reading frame for transcription and translation. During elongation of the growing peptide chain, codon recognition occurs at the A site of the ribosome, while peptide bond formation and translocation occurs at the P site. As each peptide bond is

formed, the tRNA responsible for delivering that particular amino acid leaves the ribosome while the ribosome moves the tRNA in the A site into the P site for formation of the next peptide bond and translocation event. Three different sequences can serve as stop codons. In the final state of translation, chain termination, the stop codon is reached, the newly formed polypeptide chain released, and the ribosome split into subunits for future use.

DNA replication is both bidirectional and semiconservative (Figure 12-6■). The process is very accurate in mammals, with an estimated error rate of only one per one billion nucleotides. This accuracy is due in part to the proofreading function of **DNA polymerase.** This enzyme, along with other DNA polymerases, enzymes, and proteins, is found in the replisome, which bonds proteins to the origin of replication, specific regions of DNA about 250 nucleotides long. The DNA in the area of replication undergoes localized denaturation. DNA helicases are responsible for this "unzipping" of the two replication forks, while DNA gyrase relieves the tension generated by the supercoiling found in nonreplicating DNA. DNA polymerase adds nucleotides to the 3′ end of the DNA, so the daughter DNA strand grows from 5′ to 3′. Since replication is bidirectional, there is continuous synthesis of the daughter DNA strand in this direction. Synthesis of new DNA 3′ to 5′ using the other strand as a template is discontinuous. A variety of enzymes, both polymerases and ligases, are needed to add nucleotides to the growing DNA daughter strands, to link pieces of the discontinuous DNA, to

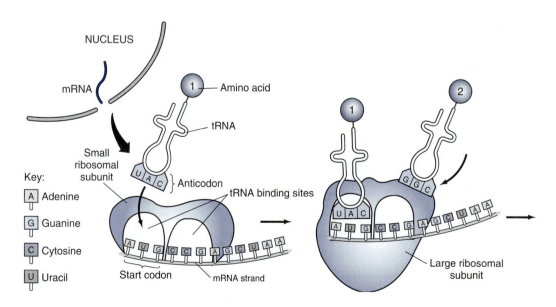

■ FIGURE 12-5 Translation of protein from an mRNA template.

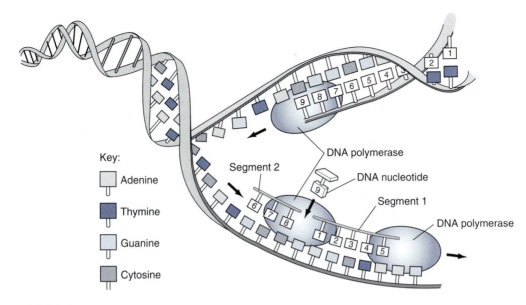

Key:

☐ Adenine

☐ Thymine

☐ Guanine

☐ Cytosine

DNA polymerase

Segment 2

DNA nucleotide

Segment 1

DNA polymerase

■ **FIGURE 12-6** Replication of DNA.

proofread the nascent DNA, and to repair any damaged DNA. When replication is complete, each new DNA molecule will have one parent strand and one daughter strand aligned through hydrogen bonds by complementary base pairing—semiconservative replication.

DIFFERENCES BETWEEN PROKARYOTIC AND EUKARYOTIC DNA

DNA in mammals occurs in long strands called chromatin. Human beings have about three meters of DNA packed into 46 chromosomes. This DNA is wound around nucleosomes comprised of a core of eight histone proteins, giving the DNA a "beaded string" appearance. This beaded string of histones and DNA is further organized into a helical fiber, then supercoiled. In contrast, while prokaryotic DNA does have proteins analogous to histones, the packing is not as extensive as that seen in eukaryotic cells.

Eukaryotes, whose metabolism requires a greater number of regulatory proteins, also have more control sequences in their DNA than do prokaryotes. Each eukaryotic gene generally has its own promoter (section of the gene where transcription of that particular gene begins) and control sequences. Activation of a eukaryotic gene generally requires RNA polymerase plus a number of transcription factors that must bind to control sequences called **enhancers,** which are located far from the gene to be transcribed. Activator proteins are thus much more important in control of eukaryotic

transcription than are repressor proteins. Eukaryotic genes also contain noncoding sections. These introns are removed from the newly formed mRNA in the nucleus during posttranscriptional modification. A cap (guanine) is added to one end of the molecule, and a tail (multiple adenine residues) is added to the other end prior to translocation to the nucleus.

In contrast, there are no introns in prokaryotic DNA and no need for extensive posttranscriptional modification. Genes and their control elements are located into **operons,** where a cluster of genes with related functions are in the same location as a promoter and an operator. Regulator genes coding for repressor proteins are generally more important for turning off transcription than are activator proteins. Also, translation begins as soon as transcription starts since prokaryotic mRNA does not need to be translocated out of a nucleus to the cytoplasm.

▶ PURIFICATION AND ANALYSIS OF NUCLEIC ACIDS

DNA PURIFICATION AND QUANTITATION

Since DNA is contained in the nucleus of a eukaryotic cell, and within the cytoplasm of a prokaryotic cell, DNA purification must begin with lysis of the cells. Bacterial specimens may be obtained from broth cultures, while mammalian cells may be procured from tissue culture, or the actual tissue itself may be homogenized. Although the approach to DNA purification differs depending on the starting specimen and species, all techniques require gentle lysis of the cell, separation of nucleic acids from contaminating protein, and purification of DNA from contaminating RNA. The precise techniques used depend on the starting specimen and the final purpose of the isolation, but in all cases, sample collection and preparation must be meticulous and must avoid activation of **DNase** or any other treatment which would result in sheared DNA.

Purification of DNA from bacterial plasmids begins with a pellet of bacterial cells containing the desired plasmid. Cell lysis and release of the plasmids is commonly achieved by addition of Tris hydrochloride, sodium EDTA, lithium chloride, and Triton-X 100. Extraction with a mixture of phenol and chloroform gives an upper aqueous layer containing the DNA along with protein and RNA. Repeated ethanol precipitation and phenol:chloroform extraction removes the residual protein. After drying, the remaining pellet contains DNA and some RNA. Contaminating RNA may then be removed by incubation with **RNase** A.

An alternate technique for preparation of plasmid DNA degrades the bacterial cell wall with lysozyme. RNase A is included early in the procedure to degrade RNA. This first incubation step is carried out at a low temperature to minimize shearing of DNA by endogenous DNase activity. Addition of sodium hydroxide results in a high pH which denatures double-stranded DNA to single-stranded DNA, while concomitant addition of sodium dodecyl sulfate (SDS) denatures proteins. Incubation and gentle rocking avoids shearing of high-molecular weight DNA. DNA is precipitated and renatured to double-stranded DNA by the addition of potassium acetate. Final purification of the DNA from any remaining RNA is accomplished by precipitation in isopropanol followed by ethanol precipitation. Further protein denaturation and removal requires an additional phenol:chloroform extraction step, with one final ethanol precipitation to clean up the resulting DNA.

The goal of protocols for preparation of prokaryotic DNA (such as that from bacteria) is to isolate high-molecular weight with a minimum of breakage. Cells are mixed with EDTA, which will chelate the cofactors needed by DNase. This treatment stops the action of that enzyme, and protects the DNA from shearing. Addition of an ionic detergent such as sarkosyl will dissolve the cell membrane and denature proteins. Early addition of RNase and protease degrades high-molecular weight RNA and digests proteins. The DNA and remaining RNA are then precipitated by use of either a high salt buffer plus isopropanol or by ethanol precipitation. Overlay of the precipitate with isopropanol results in a viscous mass containing DNA which can then be spooled (wound) onto a glass rod.

Isolation of DNA from eukaryotic cells proceeds in a similar fashion. Once again, addition of EDTA chelates the magnesium and calcium ions needed as cofactors by DNase, and also weakens the plasma and nuclear membranes of the cell. Because DNA is contained within the nucleus of a eukaryotic cell, a centrifugation step to isolate the nuclei is then required. This portion of the procedure was not required for isolation of DNA from prokaryotic cells, where the DNA is not contained within a discrete nucleus. Addition of SDS disrupts the nuclear membranes and denatures the nucleoproteins contained within. Addition of sodium chloride and sodium citrate helps to remove denatured proteins by disrupting the ionic bonds between DNA and protein, and decreases the solubility of DNA in ethanol for effective precipitation of relatively pure DNA. The DNA is then removed from the ethanol precipitate by spooling onto a glass rod. If DNA of higher purity is required, additional extraction with phenol:chloroform and further ethanol precipitation may be used.

The purity of the DNA extracted can be assessed with agarose gel electrophoresis. Different forms of DNA (circular, single-stranded, double-stranded) migrate differently. The resulting bands may be visualized with ethidium bromide, which intercalates between the stacked bases of double-stranded DNA. Although nucleic acids themselves absorb ultraviolet light at 260 nm and 280 nm, ethidium bromide will have optimal fluorescence at 300 nm when it is intercalated, allowing the DNA to be seen within the agarose gel. This technique is useful for small quantities of DNA. Larger quantities spooled off may be quantitated directly by spectrophotometry.

mRNA PURIFICATION AND QUANTITATION

The ultimate goal is RNA purification is isolation of pure, full-length mRNA. This goal is not easy to achieve, since structural RNA contaminates the preparation. In addition, endogenous RNases are a major problem. These enzymes, which will degrade RNA, must be inactivated during the procedure. Since RNases are ubiquitous, glassware and solutions must be treated with a solution of diethlypyrocarbonate. If Tris, which inactivates the diethlypyrocarbonate, is to be used, glassware must be baked and plasticware treated with chloroform. RNases are present on human skin, so gloves must be worn during all parts of the procedure.

DNA may be procured from eukaryotic cells in culture, but preparation from tissue is often desired. The tissue must first be homogenized. Cells in the resulting suspension are then lysed with a detergent such as sarkosyl. If there are high levels of endogenous RNases, or if very clean RNA is desired, cells can be lysed with guanidium isothiocyante and the RNA separated on a cesium chloride gradient. In an alternate procedure, digestion with protease and nuclease will denature proteins and digest DNA. Extraction with phenol and chloroform can then remove the denatured proteins. The remaining nucleic acids are precipitated with ethanol, and the product of that reaction treated with lithium chloride to remove polysaccharides, tRNAs, and some DNA. Large RNA is insoluble in lithium chloride and will remain in the precipitate.

Most protocols for purification of eukaryotic RNA result in a product containing total RNA, which is primarily ribosomal and transfer RNA. mRNA may be purified from this mix by a further ethanol precipitation followed by passage through an oligo(dT)-cellulose column. Most mRNA, but not structural RNA, contains a tail of adenine residues—a poly-A tail. This poly-A tail will form hydrogen bonds with the oligo(dT) on the cellulose beads, and will remain behind on the column while the structural RNAs lacking the poly-A tail will be eluted from the column. A low-salt wash will elute the mRNA, which can then be precipitated in ethanol.

After purification, spectrophotometry may be used to quantitate the purified RNA.

RESTRICTION ENZYMES AND THEIR USES

Restriction enzymes, also known as Type II **endonucleases,** occur naturally in bacteria as a defense mechanism, and the name of each enzyme reflects the genus and species of the bacteria from which it was isolated. If more than one enzyme has been isolated from a particular bacterial strain, Roman numerals are used. These enzymes are analogous to molecular scissors and have the ability to hydrolyze phosphodiester bonds at internal locations within a polynucleotide chain. As implied by the synonymous name "sequence-specific endonuclease," these enzymes cleave DNA only at a particular sequence or recognition site (Table 12-1✪). These recognition sites are generally at least four base pairs long, and have twofold symmetry,

✪ TABLE 12-1

Recognition Sequences of Some Common Restriction Endonucleases

Enzyme	Recognition Site
Taq I	T/CGA
Hae III	GG/CC
Hind III	A/AGCTT
Eco RI	G/AATTC
Bam HI	G/GATCC
Bcl I	T/GATCA

meaning that nucleotides at one end are complementary to the other end. Some may cut within a palindrome (a sequence reading the same as their inverse complement) to generate cohesive or "sticky" ends. These ends may be staggered with a protruding 5' phosphate group or staggered with a recessed 5' phosphate end and a 3' OH protruding end. Other enzymes cut symmetrically in the exact center of the sequence to generate blunt ends. Reaction of a restriction enzyme or multiple enzymes with double-stranded DNA results in a mixture of various length fragments of DNA called a **digest.**

These enzymes have become essential tools in molecular biology because of their ability to precisely and predictably cut double-stranded DNA. They may be used to determine the length of a DNA molecule. They may also be used to cleave DNA from disparate sources to be ligated with other DNA to make a chimeric DNA molecule—an application used when insertion of a foreign gene into a vector for transfection is desired. Restriction digests are also used in DNA typing (also known as DNA profile analysis or DNA fingerprinting) for forensic use or paternity testing. The utility of this DNA fingerprinting was illustrated in the Case in Point presented in this chapter.

The probability of any particular enzyme acting upon a DNA molecule is influenced by the reaction time, since reaction times may be altered to produce partial cleavage. The length of the recognition sequence and the size of the DNA to be studied also affect the chance of recognition since short recognition sequences and long DNA strands increase the probability of having cleavage sites. The number of possible cuts within a given length of DNA can be estimated by the formula $N/4^n$, where N equals the number of base pairs in the DNA strand and n is the number of bases in the recognition sequence of the enzyme. Although enzyme activity is affected by salt concentration, many are active over a wide range of salt concentrations, so multiple compatible enzymes may be used to produce a digest. If cleavage of DNA by a particular restriction endonuclease is not desired, that DNA may be methylated for protection.

The technique for digesting DNA with either a single enzyme or with multiple enzymes is far less complicated than is the choice of enzymes. Either crude or purified DNA may be used although more enzyme must be used if the specimen is crude DNA. The specimen and enzyme(s) (1 U enzyme per 1 μg DNA is a common mixture) are incubated in buffer for one hour, usually at 37°C. The reaction is then stopped with a gel loading buffer, EDTA, or heat inactivation, dependent on which enzyme was used and the ultimate purpose of the digest.

The fragments produced in the digest can then be analyzed by gel electrophoresis. The agarose concentration can be adjusted to accommodate the expected range in size of the fragments. Depending on the origin of the DNA, there may not only be fragments of varying lengths, but also a variety of DNA structures including supercoiled DNA, nicked DNA, dimers, and higher catenanes. Visualization may be achieved with ethidium bromide and UV illumination. Alternate approaches to gel electrophoresis include pulsed field gel electrophoresis useful for large fragments generated by infrequent cutter enzymes or the high-speed, high-resolution technique of capillary electrophoresis. Alternative to ethidium bromide staining include silver stains for polyacrylamide gels and brilliant cresyl blue or methylene blue for agarose gels.

DNA SEQUENCING

There are two primary techniques used to sequence DNA. The general strategy is generation of a set of single-stranded **oligonucleotides** in four separate reactions (A, T, G, and C). Each olignucleotide generated will have one fixed end and one terminating at each A, T, G, or C. These may then be resolved on high-resolution denaturing polyacrylamide (sequencing) gels. Although these gels can resolve up to 500 bases differing only by one nucleotide, most protocols are reliable only to about 300 nucleotides. Therefore, if larger DNA strands are to be sequenced, they must first be broken into smaller units.

The dideoxy chain termination method, or Sanger method after its developer, is based on the principle that DNA polymerization (replication) of a complementary copy of a template strand of single-stranded DNA by DNA polymerase can be interrupted by dideoxyribonucleoside triphosphates (ddNTP). These will terminate polymerization of that particular fragment. A **primer** (a short piece of DNA that forms hydrogen bonds with the complementary bases of the template) is required to allow addition of nucleotides by DNA polymerase. A typical reaction mixture will have a relatively high concentration of dNTP mixed with small quantities of one of the four ddNTPs: dATP, dGTP, dCTP, and dTTP. In appropriate concentrations the ddNTPs will compete with the dNTPs during polymerization. The result will be pieces of DNA of identical sequence terminated at different points. The four different reaction mixtures containing all possible fragment lengths can then be separated by electrophoresis on a polyacrylamide gel. The separation results in a "ladder," the steps of which can be read after autoradiography or some other visualization technique. Although the sequence of the other strand can be inferred by complementarity, both strands are generally sequenced to ensure that technical difficulties did not introduce an error in the sequence.

The Sanger procedure used *E. coli* DNA polymerase I large fragment (also known as a Klenow fragment). With the enzyme, the average length of the sequencing products is controlled by the dideoxynucleotide:deoxynucleotide ratio, with a higher ratio yielding shorter products. An alternate labeling/termination method uses modified T7 DNA polymerase. In this procedure, the primer is labeled and then terminated by incorporating dideoxynucleotides. In this case, the length of the fragments generated is controlled by the concentration of deoxynucleotides in the labeling reaction, with a high concentration yielding longer fragments or by the dideoxynucleotide:deoxynucleotide ratio in the termination reaction.

The dideoxy chain termination method has both advantages and disadvantages. It is rapid, and gives good resolution of the bands formed by the DNA fragments on the polyacrylamide gel. However, there may be premature chain termination by the DNA polymerase.

Because of the disadvantages, an automated chemical degradation method (Maxam-Gilbert sequencing) was devised. In this method, premature termination is not a problem. The preparation time required for DNA purification in this procedure is time consuming, but specialized cloning vectors have decreased the time required. This method is the sequencing method of choice for small oligonucleotides.

In the chemical degradation method, labeled DNA is cleaved with rare-cutter restriction enzymes. Alternatively, base-specific modification of four aliquots of radioactively labeled DNA can be set up, with piperidine used to catalyze cutting of the DNA strands at the modified bases. With either technique, the resulting fragments can then be separated on by polyacrylamide gel electrophoresis. Visualization of the separated fragments can then be achieved by autoradiography.

Autoradiography requires the use of P^{32} or S^{35} labeled DNA. This procedure may use autoradiographic film or emulsion. In either case, the film/emulsion is exposed to the gel. Any area containing the radioactive probe will expose the film. The film or emulsion is then developed in the same manner as film from a camera.

If the use of radioactive materials is to be avoided, fragments can be identified with Southern blotting and pulse-field electrophoresis. In this scenario, fluorescent dye is attached to the ddNTP, with a different color for each of the four nucleotides. A laser can then detect the colors of the bands as they occur on the gel. The intensity of a particular color is recorded as a peak, and the order of the peaks indicates the nucleotide sequence of the DNA strand.

Commercial kits are now readily available for sequencing. Sequencing machines are capable of automating gel electrophoresis, detection of bands, and, with the appropriate computer hardware and software, can analyze the bands and deduce the DNA sequence. A fluorescent label or P^{32} is commonly used.

▶ HYBRIDIZATION TECHNIQUES

OVERVIEW OF HYBRIDIZATION AND BASIC BLOTTING TECHNIQUES

The two complementary strands of DNA making up the double helix are held together by hydrogen bonds. Because of this, the structure is not stable under temperatures greater than 90°C or at a pH of greater than 10.5, or in the presence of formaldehyde, and will denature in these conditions. If denatured DNA is returned to favorable conditions (lower temperature and pH), complementary strands will reform hydrogen bonds by complementary base pairing. If the reannealing DNA strands are from different sources, the process is termed **hybridization.** If the sequence of one strand is known, the degree of similarity of an unknown strand can be deduced. Areas of the unknown strand that reanneal to the sequenced strand are complementary, indicating the presence of similar or identical genes.

Hybridization reactions can be carried out in solution, or may be performed as mixed-phase hybridization with nucleic acids immobilized in a procedure known as blotting onto some sort of solid support such as a nitrocellulose membrane. **Probes** (DNA of known sequence) can also be hybridized to nucleic acids in a dry gel without blotting to a membrane. This technique is restricted to oligonucleotide probes but has numerous advantages, including less expense, more sensitivity, and a more efficient transfer of large amounts of DNA.

There are many variations in blotting techniques, but all immobilize the nucleic acids onto some type of solid support. Blotting simply means the transfer of the resolved DNA to the support, and Southern blotting refers specifically to the transfer of single-stranded DNA separated on an agarose gel to a nitrocellulose membrane. Blotting of this type is commonly achieved through capillary blotting with the gel to be blotted covered with the transfer membrane and layered with filter paper. As the transfer buffer is absorbed upward into the filter paper, the DNA is carried from the gel onto the membrane. The exact mechanism of binding of nucleic acids to nitrocellulose membranes has not been completely defined, but they appear to bind through a combination of hydrophobic interactions, hydrogen bonding, and salt bridge formation.

The capillary blotting method used with agarose gels and its variations are not effective for transferring DNA from polyacrylamide gels to nylon filters. An alternative technique called electroblotting has been found to be highly effective if used with ultraviolet crosslinking, and can transfer and retain small DNA fragments on the filter. This technique has been found to be very useful for genome sequencing and for polymerase chain reactions (PCR) used to quantitate rare DNA.

Preparation of Nucleic Acid Probes

The use of specific sequences of DNA as probes for a DNA or RNA sequence of interest began in 1961 when Spiegelman and Hall observed that single-stranded DNA could anneal through hydrogen bonding to complementary RNA to make a chimeric double-stranded DNA-RNA molecule. This seminal work was expanded upon, and short, single-strand **nucleic acid probes** linked to a radioisotope for detection are now isolated or synthesized to detect genes of interest for many applications. These probes have been used for identification of infectious diseases (often combined with PCR) such as human immunodeficiency virus (HIV), tuberculosis, and Lyme disease. Identification of genetic diseases such as cystic fibrosis, Duchenne's muscular dystrophy, Huntington's disease, and a variety of immunodeficiencies has also employed nucleic acid probes. Probes are also used in combination with PCR for **restriction-fragment length polymorphism (RFLP)** analysis.

If the sequence of the gene of interest is known, a probe can be synthesized. However, the specific sequence of the gene is often unknown. Therefore, probe generation generally begins with a restriction enzyme digestion of DNA. After agarose gel electrophoresis separation of the DNA fragments on the basis of size and visualization of the bands with ethidium bromide and UV light, the DNA in question can be eluted by some technique from the gel to be used for hybridization. There are several different ways to retrieve the DNA from the gel. Electroelution is effective, and results in a pure preparation of the probe. For this technique, a trough is cut into the gel on the positive side of the DNA and lined with dialysis tubing. Further electrophoresis causes the DNA to run into the trough, from which it can be extracted along with the electrophoresis buffer. Addition of salt and ethanol will concentrate the sample by precipitation. For some applications, an alternative technique is to cut the band from the gel and freeze the agarose slice. The liquid can then be squeezed out, and the DNA harvested in relatively pure form from the supernatant. DNA can also be retrieved if low melting-point agarose is used for the gel, since the temperature needed to melt the gel will not denature the double-stranded DNA. DNA retrieved by this technique is generally then extracted by phenol. Other possibilities include electrophoresis onto DEAE cellulose paper. This procedure is followed by elution, phenol extraction, and ethanol precipitation. A rapid method of isolating DNA fragments from linkers or synthetic oligonucleotides is to remove the oligonucleotide fragments by passage over a Sephacryl S-300 column.

Although probes may be labeled with radioisotopes for detection by autoradiography, other techniques have been devised to synthesize and label probe DNA with nonradioactive substances. One such technique is **nick translation** labeling. This procedure incorporates biotinylated (biotin-labeled) nucleotides into an oligonucleotide probe. Double-stranded oligonucleotides are labeled using DNase I, DNA polymerase I, and dTNPs, one of which is labeled with biotin. The DNase I makes random nicks along backbone of double-stranded DNA to be labeled. This exposes the 3'OH within the nicked strand. Nicked strands have one strand intact with a break of the phosphodiester bond in the other strand. DNA polymerase then adds nucleotides from the pool of dNTPs with template strand used for complementary base pairing. The 5'>3' exonuclease activity of DNA polymerase I removes the existing strand as synthesis continues. This particular procedure works best at temperatures no greater than 15°C since higher temperatures may make the nicked strand separate from the complementary strand, generating nonspecific probes in the process. Incorporated nucleotides can be separated from unincorporated nucleotides by ethanol precipitation or by gel exclusion chromatography. If ethanol precipitation is used, oligonucleotides greater than 15–20 nucleotides in length will be precipitated, while shorter sequences will remain in solution. The probes can be separated on a gel and visualized by a reaction with strepavidin, which forms a covalently linked complex with the biotin-labeled DNA when incubated in the presence of alkaline phosphatase. Reaction with a chromogenic substrate such as 5-bromo-4-chloro-3-indoyl phosphate produces a blue color which can be intensified with the addition of nitroblue tetrazolium chloride.

Oligonucleotide labeling, or **random primer extension** labeling, is very useful in only a small amount of template is available. The technique allows amplification and labeling of the template to generate high specific-activity probes. Double-stranded DNA is denatured, and short random oligonucleotides are added to the mixture to act as primers. DNA synthesis is initiated by a DNA polymerase with both 5'>3' polymerase activity and 3'>5' exonuclease activity (Klenow fragment). DNA synthesis initiated in this fashion will occur only by primer extension. Because the hybridized primers are not degraded, the labeling is random. The technique generally copies all parts of template DNA with equal frequency, and separation of unlabeled precursors may not be necessary since as much as 90% of the labeled precursors may be incorporated. Problems with the technique may arise if too much unincorporated label or template DNA remains.

Southern Blot

The ability to detect hybridization of unknown DNA with known probes was greatly enhanced when, in 1975, E. M. Southern described a technique for transferring DNA separated by electrophoresis on agarose gels onto nitrocellulose membranes. This technique was particularly useful for samples with a large number of fragments, such as those generated by a restriction digest, which make a continuous smear on electrophoresis.

Many variations on this technique have been developed to accommodate the type of detection system to be used, the amount of DNA to be transferred, and the speed of transfer desired. The traditional technique begins with isolation and restriction enzyme digestion of DNA. The restriction digest is then separated by gel electrophoresis, with incorporation of a known size standard. The DNA bands are visualized with ethidium bromide and UV light. The gel is then soaked in an alkaline solution to denature the DNA (only single-stranded DNA will bind to the membrane) and then blotted by capillary action. This traditional transfer method is time consuming, and new variations have speeded up the transfer process by use of a vacuum apparatus (vacuum blot) or by electrophoresis (electroblot). After transfer of the DNA to the membrane, the labeled probe is added to hybridize to the immobilized DNA. The results are read by autoradiography. The techniques and its variations are efficient and sensitive, but variations in gel preparation and DNA concentration can result in different migration patterns for the same size fragments. Inclusion of known standards as controls is therefore critical.

If the use of radioactivity is to be avoided, there are alternatives to isotope-labeled probes. Probe DNA incubated with photoactivatible biotin under a heat lamp followed by extraction of the unreacted biotin with 2-butanol and ethanol precipitation of DNA will result in a labeled probe. After hybridization, addition of avidin-alkaline phosphatase will bind the avidin to the biotin. The resulting "sandwich" may then be visualized colorimetrically by addition of 5-bromo-4-chloro-3-indoly phosphate (BCIP) and nitroblue tetrazolium. The alkaline phosphatase bound to the avidin catalyzes the hydrolysis of phosphate from the BCIP, which then undergoes a redox reaction with the nitroblue tetrazolium to form a visible blue precipitate.

Other nonradioactive labeling and detection systems include horseradish peroxidase or digoxigenin–anti-digoxigenin. Detection systems may be colorimetric for substrates which produce a colored product, or by chemiluminescence for products that give off light.

Northern Blot

Contrary to popular wisdom, the Northern blot was not developed by anyone named Northern. Rather, this method is analogous to the Southern blot in procedure, but instead of detecting hybridization of DNA molecules, it allows detection of small RNA molecules. The method is extremely sensitive, and can determine both the size and amount of a specific RNA if a labeled specific probe is available. However, the structure of the RNA cannot be determined by a Northern blot. Northern blots are used in particular when the transcription of a particular gene or the quantity of mRNA resulting from that transcription is in question.

The overall procedure for Southern blots and Northern blots is similar. The RNA specimen is separated on the basis of size by electrophoresis on a denaturing gel (generally formaldehyde agarose, glyoxal, or methyl mercury gel). After hybridization with a labeled probe for the gene, the RNA is blotted onto nitrocellulose with the appropriate buffers (different from those used for Southern blot since RNA does not bind to nitrocellulose with the standard buffers) or onto a diazoenzylmethol filter membrane. The detection systems used are the same as those used for Southern blot, depending on whether the probe is labeled with a radioisotope or biotin.

IN SITU HYBRIDIZATION

Development of the Technique

Southern blots are useful for determining the extent of hybridization of the DNA in question to a specific sequence of interest, and Northern blots are useful for determining the amount of mRNA transcribed for a particular gene. However, many genes of interest are expressed in cells not easily isolated from a tissue, or present in too few cells to produce adequate amounts of DNA. Other genes may be expressed only briefly during differentiation of a cell. In situ hybridization provides a method of hybridizing DNA or mRNA in a tissue without requiring isolation of the cells containing that nucleic acid. The relationship of those cells to the surrounding tissue can be seen following counterstaining. Either paraffin sections or frozen sections may be used, and the procedure may be combined with immunohistochemistry to localize both mRNA and the protein products of the particular gene of interest. As long as a specific labeled nucleic acid probe is available, the technique is sensitive enough to detect gene deletions and rearrangements since these will give altered hybridization patterns. If appropriate detection systems are chosen, both DNA and mRNA can be detected in the same tissue section.

Basic In Situ Procedures

The basic protocol for in situ hybridization begins either with fixation of tissues or pelleted cells in paraformaldehyde or infusion with sucrose. Paraformaldehyde fixed cells are then dehydrated with ethanol and xylene and embedded in paraffin. These tissue blocks may then be sectioned with a microtome. The sucrose-infused tissues should be immediately embedded in OCT gel and snap-frozen. These may then be sectioned with a cryostat. The resulting tissue sections will then require fixation with paraformaldehyde and dehydration with ethanol and xylene.

Paraffin sections to be hybridized are first deparaffinized in xylene. The sections are then rehydrated in ethanol and denatured in hydrochloric acid. Postfixation is performed with paraformaldehyde and blocked with iodoacetamide and N-ethylmaleimide. The sections are then again dehydrated in ethanol and are ready for hybridization.

Hybridization is performed on the tissue sections on the slides in a moist chamber. Specific labeled probes suitable for Southern blot or Northern blot are also suitable for in situ hybridization. After hybridization, the slides are treated with RNase, dehydrated with ethanol and ammonium acetate, dried, and visualized with emulsion autoradiography.

Hybridization with cryosections is similar, but does not require deparaffinization of the slides prior to hybridization. The thawed, fixed sections are acetylated, after which the procedure identical to that of the paraffin sections.

After hybridization, the hybridized probes may be visualized either by film autoradiography or by emulsion autoradiography. If film is to be used, the slides are exposed at 4°C to the film with the emulsion side facing. As an alternative, slides may be dipped into emulsion, exposed at 4°C, developed, and fixed. After fixation, the emulsion is scraped off and the slides counterstained and mounted. When the tissue is observed under dark-field microscopy, the developed silver grains appear as white dots on a black background.

The slides may also be counterstained to define the tissue and to help localize those cells or areas of tissue where hybridization occurred. Common counterstains include Giemsa, which will stain nuclei, hematoxylin/eosin or toluidine blue to stain both nuclei and cytoplasm, or Hoechst staining of the nuclei.

Nonradioactive detection systems may also be used for in situ hybridization. Fluorescent in situ hybridization (FISH) uses fluorescence to detect the signal rather than isotope labeled probes and autoradiography.

▶ APPLICATIONS OF HYBRIDIZATION TECHNIQUES IN IMMUNOLOGY

CLINICAL IMMUNOLOGY AND MICROBIAL IMMUNOLOGY

Hybridization techniques are currently used in clinical practice. These techniques allow direct detection of a variety of microorganisms, and are particularly used for specimens that may contain multiple organisms, organisms for which culture techniques are not available, or those that are difficult to culture, or when subspecies characterization is needed. DNA hybridization can be used to detect the present of DNA coding for enterotoxin in E. coli. Probes for RNA have been used successfully to detect both bacteria (L. pneumophilia and M. pneumoniae) and viruses (papillomavirus subtypes). Northern and Western blots are commonly used for detection of human immunodeficiency virus RNA and protein in order to determine the viral load in a patient.

RFLP may be used to detect a variety of mutations, including deletions, rearrangements, point mutations, or an increase or decrease in gene repeat copy number. Since the mutated gene will not be cut in the same places by restriction enzymes as a wild type gene, Southern blots or RFLP analysis can be useful for diagnosis of immunodeficiencies caused by genetic error.

RFLP analysis may also be used to detect polymorphisms in histocompatibility locus antigens. Although these polymorphisms are not mutations, the altered DNA sequences will result in different length fragments generated during restriction enzyme digest. This analysis is widely used in paternity testing and in forensic science.

RESEARCH APPLICATIONS

The application of hybridization techniques and DNA sequencing in research is limited only by the imagination of the investigator. Gene polymorphisms may be defined, as in analysis of HLA polymorphisms. Northern blot or in situ hybridization are frequently used to determine which genes are active during an immune response. Immunocytochemistry is often combined with in situ hybridization to localize both mRNA and protein production from a gene of interest in tissue. Gene expression may also be studied through preparation of DNA and transfection.

DNA and RNA preparation and hybridization techniques may be used whenever a gene sequence or expression is in question. The combination of techniques or variations may be tailored to suit both the specimen and the research question.

SUMMARY

Advances in molecular biology technique have led to a better understanding of the genetic mechanisms underlying the immune response. Molecular biology has also helped elucidate mechanisms underlying inherited deficits in the immune system and those portions of the immune response responsible for allograft rejection. New approaches to correcting immunodeficiencies and to development of novel approaches to immunosuppression have had direct results on advances in the understanding of the immune response at the molecular level. The unique structures and properties of DNA and RNA have been exploited to determine the DNA sequence of genes, detect similarities in sequence between cells from different individuals, analyze genetic abnormalities, and dozens of other clinical and research applications.

POINTS TO REMEMBER

▶ Only protein sequences are encoded within the DNA.

▶ mRNA for a particular gene is transcribed from a limited section of the DNA molecule.

▶ Proteins are produced by translation of the mRNA molecule.

▶ Differences between prokaryotic and eukaryotic DNA may be exploited for diagnostic and research purposes by molecular biology techniques.

▶ DNA purification procedures require lysis of the cell and nuclear membrane, organic solvent extraction of nucleic acids, and ethanol precipitation of the DNA.

▶ RNA purification procedures are similar to those used for DNA purification, but great care to avoid degradation of the RNA by ubiquitous RNases must be taken during specimen handling and preparation.

▶ Restriction enzymes act as molecular scissors and are able to cut double-stranded DNA at precise locations.

▶ Southern blot, Northern blot, and in situ hybridization all require labeled probes for the gene or gene product in question.

▶ Only in situ hybridization allows simultaneous analysis of DNA hybridization and mRNA expression, or mRNA expression and protein production.

▶ The techniques of molecular biology may be modified or combined in novel ways in order to utilize different types of specimens or to answer new questions.

LEARNING ASSESSMENT QUESTIONS

1. Using in situ hybridization and immunohistochemistry, you have detected both mRNA and protein related to the new gene you are investigating. Beginning with transcription of RNA, explain how the protein was produced in the cells in which it was located.

2. You have isolated and have obtained the sequence of a protein found only in the serum of patients with a currently undefined immunodeficiency syndrome. What steps would you take to resolve the question of whether this syndrome is of genetic or microbial origin?

REFERENCES

Barch, M., T. Knutsen, and J. Spurbeck, eds. 1997. *The AGT Cytogenetics Laboratory Manual,* 3rd ed. Lippincott-Raven Publishers, New York.

Block, A. W. 1999. Cancer cytogenetics. In: *The Principles of Clinical Cytogenetics,* ed. S. L. Gersen and M. B. Keagle. Humana Press, Totowa, NJ.

Fan, Y. S., ed. 2002. *Molecular Cytogenetics: Protocols and Applications.* Humana Press, Totowa, NJ.

Gall, J. G. and M. L. Pardue. 1969. Formation and detection of RNA-DNA hybrid molecules in cytological preparations. *Proc Natl Acad Sci USA* 63:378–83.

Kocher, T. D. and A.C. Wilson. 1991. DNA amplification by the polymerase chain reaction. In: *Essential Molecular Biology: A Practical Approach,* Vol. II, ed. T. A. Brown. IRL Press, Oxford.

Lowery, M. C. 2000. *Application of FISH Technology on Paraffin-Embedded Tissue, Procedural Tips and Trouble-Shooting Guide,* Vysis, Ed., Downers Grove, IL.

NCCLS. 2002. *Fluorescence in Situ Hybridization (FISH) Methods for Medical Genetics,* Approved Guideline, MM7-P, Vol. 21, No. 6.

Pardue, M. L. and J. G. Gall. 1969. Molecular hybridization of radioactive DNA to the DNA of cytological preparations. *Proc Natl Acad Sci USA* 64:600–604.

Trask, B. and D. Pinkel. 1990. Fluorescence in situ hybridization with DNA probes. *Methods Cell Biol* 33:383–400.

13

Amplification Techniques

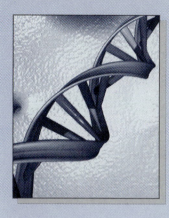

■ CHAPTER CHECKLIST

After reading and studying this chapter, the reader will be able to:

1. Provide an overview of amplification technology and how it is used in clinical diagnosis.
2. List and discuss the advantages and disadvantages of using amplification technology in clinical diagnosis.
3. Explain PCR technology and profile the advantages and disadvantages.
4. Discuss the general concepts, components, and conditions of amplification testing.
5. Describe the steps required in contamination prevention in PCR techniques.
6. Describe RT-PCR and its clinical applications.
7. Describe other means of amplification testing and thir clinical applications.
8. List the general factors that affect amplification assays.
9. Compare the basic concepts of amplification assays with other molecular-based techniques.
10. Apply quality control concepts as they are used in hybridization testing.

℮ CASE IN POINT

A 30-year-old female presented to the emergency room with a history of two days of fever, nausea, vomiting, and a very intense headache. She had a slightly stiff neck. On physical exam, her neck was sore but not rigid. Her temperature was 99.8° F. A CT scan was normal. A lumbar puncture was then performed, and the following results were obtained from her cerebrospinal fluid (CSF): glucose, 60 mg/dl (normal range, 40–70 mg/dl); protein, 75 mg/dl (normal range, 12–60 mg/dl); white blood cell (WBC) count 40/mm^3 (normal range, 0–5/mm^3) with 80% lymphocytes. A Gram stain was negative for bacteria, and a latex antigen meningitis panel was negative for *Haemophilus influenzae* type B, *Streptococcus pneumoniae*, *Streptococcus agalactiae*, *Neisseria meningitidis*, and *Escherichia coli*. Bacterial cultures were submitted. Cerebrospinal fluid was submitted for herpes virus (HSV) polymerase chain reaction (PCR) and for enterovirus reverse transcriptase PCR (RT-PCR). She was admitted for observation; antibiotic therapy was previously initiated in the emergency room and maintained. The HSV PCR was

CASE IN POINT (continued)

negative, but the enterovirus RT-PCR was positive, using generic enterovirus primers. Antibiotic therapy was discontinued, and the patient started recovering a day later and was discharged; she made a full recovery in about a week. Bacterial cultures never became positive.

ISSUES TO CONSIDER

After reading the patient's case history, consider

- The laboratory findings that may indicate the etiology of the patient's clinical condition
- The clinical applications of molecular methods for detecting pathogens to provide rapid diagnosis
- The advantages and disadvantages of amplification techniques in clinical diagnosis of diseases
- The benefits of molecular-based technology in patient care

IMPORTANT TERMS

Anneal
bDNA (branched DNA) detection
cDNA (complementary DNA)
Denaturation (denature)
dNTP (deoxynucleotide triphosphate)
DNA (deoxynucleic acid)
DNA polymerase
Downstream (primer)
Electrophoresis
Ethidium bromide
Gene
Image analysis

ISA (In situ amplification)
LCR (ligase chain reaction)
NASBA (nucleic acid sequence based amplification)
Oligonucleotide
PCR (polymerase chain reaction)
PCR amplicon product
PCR product
Primer
Primer annealing
Primer extension
Probe

RACE
Real-time PCR
RNase (ribonuclease)
RNA (ribonucleic acid)
RNA template
RT (reverse transcriptase)
RT-PCR (reverse transcriptase PCR)
Template
Template DNA
Thermal cycler
Tm
Transcription
Upstream (primer)

▶ INTRODUCTION

Clinical microbiology and immunology laboratories have adapted to several new techniques and detection/identification methodologies over the years. Advances in automation and rapid detection techniques have revolutionized the clinical microbiology and immunology laboratory—physicians are able to receive patient results from specimens faster now than, say, 30 years ago. These advances have enabled the clinical microbiology and the clinical immunology laboratory to keep pace with the advances that have occurred in

other clinical diagnostic laboratory sections, such as clinical chemistry.

In the past decade or so, a new revolution has occurred, or has been occurring in, the clinical diagnostic laboratory. This new revolution is the rapid progress in the field of molecular biology, and the extremely rapid, specific, and sensitive detection and identification techniques that are possible by exploiting the nature of biomolecules such as **DNA, RNA,** and protein. Now, early in the twenty-first century, many hospitals have molecular diagnostic laboratories, and these laboratories employ such methods as the **polymerase chain** reaction **(PCR)**, reverse transcriptase **PCR (RT-PCR)**, the **ligase chain reaction (LCR)**, and many other techniques. This chapter covers basic principles of some of these molecular-based tests, applications of these tests, and what the future may hold in molecular diagnostics for the clinical immunology laboratory.

▶ AMPLIFICATION TECHNOLOGY: AN OVERVIEW

In general, there are two basic areas of molecular diagnostic testing—detecting a specific target directly with the use of labeled **probes** and amplifying a specific nucleic acid target for detection or characterization. The use of labeled probes was an important step in molecular diagnostics; however, the advent of the PCR has not only revolutionized molecular diagnostics, but it also has completely revolutionized science. Both research and clinical laboratories can now amplify and detect a vast array of **genes** and transcripts of genes by using the PCR or a variant of the PCR. Clinical laboratories can now detect many different genetic diseases and infectious disease agents with the PCR and other amplification tests.

There are various advantages and disadvantages to employing molecular diagnostic techniques in the clinical laboratory. Most molecular diagnostic methods—especially when amplified methods are used—are far more sensitive than standard tests used in the laboratory. Amplification methods are more sensitive than direct hybridization-based tests because target nucleic acid may not be present in high enough amounts for detection. Molecular techniques are also more specific than standard laboratory tests. A typical molecular assay will not only detect that an organism is present in the disease process, but also it will give the identity of that organism as well, which can save time in a clinical setting. As shown in the opening case study, where the etiology of the disease may have been recovered by a viral culture, molecular methods of detecting viral pathogens, in particular, provides a more rapid diagnosis. Amplification techniques can rapidly detect nearly any microorganism. Unlike most molecular-based tests that yield qualitative results—that is, a yes or no answer—many amplification techniques give quantitative data, or numbers that are relative to a standard or control and can give meaningful information on the progression of a disease state, for example, the number of virus particles present in a given test sample. However, the use of a molecular technique to detect only one organism may not rule out other microorganisms

in a disease process. Amplification techniques can also be used to detect and identify human genetic diseases and cancers.

Many molecular tests are also difficult to perform, and interpretation can be difficult. For example, a given microorganism may be detected in a specimen, but it may not necessarily be involved in actual disease. Many molecular-based tests require special equipment that many clinical laboratories do not ordinarily use, and the costs associated with setting up a molecular diagnostic laboratory can be prohibitive.

POLYMERASE CHAIN REACTION

History and Evolution

PCR is the most widely used amplification technique in molecular biology and molecular diagnostics, and is the basis for many tests. A typical PCR test can amplify a single copy of target DNA into an exponential amount of product over the course of several (25–40) cycles of PCR, using a pair of **primers,** the correct buffer, the four **deoxynucleotide phosphates (dNTPs;** dA, dC, dG, and dT), a source of **template DNA,** and an enzyme called **DNA polymerase** in three separate steps: (1) **denaturation,** (2) **primer annealing,** and (3) **primer extension.** This powerful tool is now a staple of the molecular diagnostics lab.

The concept of the PCR as a molecular biology technique was first thought of by Kary B. Mullis, a chemist at the Cetus Corporation in Emeryville, California, in 1983; this new technique was first published in 1985. The original description of replicating DNA using a pair of primers was described in 1971 by Gobind Khorana. Mullis, though, developed the theory and application of the PCR. Mullis's early method was labor intensive. It involved using two different heat blocks set at different temperatures for separate reactions—95°C to denature double-stranded DNA and 30°C to anneal primers and also to extend the reaction—so the reaction tubes were manually transferred from heat block to heat block over several cycles. The DNA polymerase employed (the Klenow fragment of *Escherichia coli* DNA polymerase I) to synthesize new strands of DNA was not thermostable at 95°C, and had to be added after each step. In addition, the low 30°C reaction temperature resulted in the formation of nonspecific PCR products.

One important breakthrough in PCR methodology occurred in 1986, when the **thermal cycler** was first developed by Perkin Elmer-Cetus Instruments. A thermal cycler is essentially a programmable heat block that can rapidly cycle between different temperatures.

The introduction of the thermal cycler was a step toward standardizing PCR; it also saved time for the researcher or laboratorian.

The next important advance in PCR technology occurred in 1988, when a special DNA polymerase was described from *Thermus aquaticus,* a bacterium that lives in hot springs in Yellowstone National Park. This enzyme is called *Taq* DNA polymerase. This DNA polymerase has key features that are discussed in a later section.

Since the advent of the PCR in the mid-1980s, many different applications of the technique have been developed, including reverse transcriptase PCR (RT-PCR), **real-time PCR,** and other variations. Many of these variations are discussed further, and several are used in molecular immunology in lieu of standard PCR.

Basic Technique

The PCR is an amplification tool to detect and/or characterize a target of interest. There are three basic steps of the PCR: denaturation, primer annealing, and primer extension (Figure 13-1■). These steps are cycled many times (25–40) to synthesize a detectable amount of amplified target.

Denaturation Denaturation is performed to separate target double-stranded DNA into single strands, so that primers may anneal to their target sequences in the second step. Denaturation must be performed at a high temperature—94°C or 95°C—to break the bonds of double-stranded DNA. During cycles of the PCR, denaturation is usually accomplished for 15 to 30 seconds. Typically laboratories employ an initial denaturation step (usually 2–5 minutes at 94–95°C) before PCR cycles begin to ensure proper separation of the template (target) DNA.

Primer Annealing The second step of the PCR is primer annealing. The primers—single-stranded pieces of DNA, about 15–30 bases in length (**oligonucleotides**)—will **anneal** to their complement sequence at a range of temperatures, depending on the DNA base composition and length of the primers. Typically, primers will anneal best to the template DNA between 50–60°C. Once the primers are annealed to the template DNA, the DNA polymerase in the reaction will proceed with the third general step of the PCR, primer extension. Primer annealing is usually performed for 30-60 seconds, depending on the protocol employed.

Primer Extension Primer extension refers to the addition of individual DNA bases (dNTPs) to the primers by DNA polymerase to synthesize a new strand of DNA. This new strand of DNA is complemen-

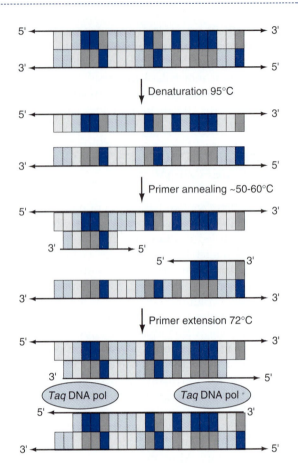

■ **FIGURE 13-1** The polymerase chain reaction (PCR). Double-stranded DNA is heat denatured, then primers anneal to each strand of DNA at specific sequences at a lower temperature. *Taq* DNA polymerase then adds dNTPs to each primer to synthesize new strands of DNA during primer extension. The reaction undergoes several cycles (25–40) of denaturation, primer annealing, and primer extension to amplify the DNA target.

tary to the template strand of DNA. Primer extension is normally performed at 72°C when *Taq* DNA polymerase is utilized in the reaction—this is the optimal temperature for *Taq* DNA polymerase activity. The amount of time necessary for each primer extension reaction during the PCR depends on the size of the expected **PCR amplicon product** and the rate of activity of the DNA polymerase used in the reaction; a given DNA polymerase will add a given number of dNTPs to a growing DNA chain per second. In general, primer extension is performed for 1–2 minutes per cycle during the PCR.

Finally, most researchers and laboratories include a final primer extension step at 72°C for 2 to 10 minutes to fully extend any remaining annealed primers in solution—this ensures that all DNA in the final reaction mixture is double stranded.

Thus, a "typical" PCR protocol is shown in Box 13-1✱.

Components and Reaction Conditions of the PCR

As described earlier, several components are necessary to perform the PCR. These components, and a brief description of their use, are listed in Table 13-1✪.

Taq **DNA Polymerase** There are many commercially available DNA polymerases. The most commonly used is *Taq* DNA polymerase. This enzyme, isolated from the thermophilic bacterium *T. aquaticus,* does not lose function at the high temperature (94–95°C) necessary to denature double-stranded DNA, unlike DNA polymerases from many other organisms. As already described, this enzyme functions best at a temperature of 72°C. It functions in a broad pH range, and works best at pH 7.0–7.5; under proper conditions, it will add about 100 dNTPs per second during primer extension. However, the exact rate of primer extension may vary according to the manufacturer of the enzyme. There are also several versions of *Taq* DNA polymerase available on the market, many of which have specialized uses in either research or diagnostic laboratories.

Buffer For proper function of *Taq* DNA polymerase, each PCR assay requires the appropriate buffer conditions. Nearly always, the buffer is supplied by a manufacturer for their particular DNA polymerase. The buffer is typically supplied in a concentrated form (often "10×," meaning the buffer must be diluted by a factor of 10 in the final PCR mixture). Most of the time the buffer is Tris buffer, and the concentrated form of the buffer usually has a pH of 8.0–9.0. The pH of Tris buffers decreases when the temperature of a reaction is increased—the pH decreases by 0.3 for every 10°C increase in temperature. Thus, a supplied Tris buffer with a pH of 8.4 at 25°C will have a pH of 7.0 at 72°C.

✪ TABLE 13-1

Components of the PCR

Component	Use
DNA polymerase	Enzyme that catalyzes the PCR
Oligonucleotide primers	DNA polymerase extends new DNA from primers
Mg^{2+}	DNA polymerase requires Mg^{2+} to function
Buffer, with or without Mg^{2+}	DNA polymerase requires correct buffer to function
Deoxynucleotides (dNTPs)	Used by DNA polymerase to synthesize new DNA
Template DNA	The target DNA of the reaction

Magnesium Buffer may be purchased or supplied with or without magnesium (Mg^{2+} in the form of $MgCl_2$). Magnesium is essential for the function of *Taq* DNA polymerase; the enzyme is inactive in the absence of free magnesium in the reaction buffer. Magnesium concentration also affects primer annealing efficiency during the PCR. Since some of the other components of the reaction mixture will bind free magnesium ions, such as dNTPs, template DNA, and chelating agents such as EDTA, magnesium must be present in excess in the reaction mixture. If there is too low an amount of magnesium in solution, no PCR products may form. However, too much magnesium reduces *Taq* DNA polymerase fidelity (error rate—the incorporation of incorrect dNTPs) and nonspecific amplification products may result. Thus, the concentration of magnesium may have to be adjusted for a particular PCR protocol. Typically, a final concentration of 1.0–3.0 mM is used; 1.5 mM is about average for most reactions.

Deoxynucleotide Triphosphates (dNTPs) Like the other components discussed earlier, the concentration of dNTPs is also important to the PCR. High concentrations—above 800 μM of a mixture of all four dNTPs—will increase the error rate of *Taq* DNA polymerase. Normal PCR assays utilize concentrations of between 800 μM and 800 μM of each dNTP (between 800 μM and 800 μM total dNTP mix); 800 μM of each dNTP is often used.

Primers Primers are the starting points of a PCR assay—DNA polymerase uses primers annealed to a template DNA sequence to add individual dNTPs to during a reaction. Final concentrations of 0.1–0.5M are usually used for primers in the PCR. High concentrations

✱ Box 13-1 PCR Protocol

Initial denaturation step: 94°C for 5 minutes

30 cycles of:

    Denaturation: 94°C for 15 seconds

    Primer annealing: 55°C for 30 seconds

    Primer extension: 72°C for 1 minute

Final extension step: 72°C for 5 minutes

of primer may lead to mispriming and the formation of nonspecific PCR products, and/or may promote the formation of primer-dimers (primers pairing with each other in solution). Success of a PCR assay depends on the proper design of the primers. Two primers are used in a standard PCR assay. Each is complimentary to one of the strands of double-stranded DNA. When designing primers form a known sequence (i.e., a published sequence), only one strand of DNA is usually depicted. The individual designing the primers must realize that there is an antiparallel strand of DNA to the published sequence. One primer, sometimes referred to as the "forward" primer, or the **"upstream"** primer, is designed from the published sequence. The other primer has been referred to as the "reverse" or **"downstream"** primer, and is the inverted complement of the published sequence. See Figure 13-2■ for an example of upstream and downstream primers based on target sequence. Once the primers have been designed, the size of the expected PCR product can be determined by counting the DNA bases from primer to primer (be sure to include the primers themselves). Primers are

designed from a known target sequence—usually a unique region of the target. Published known sequences can be attained from a variety of sources, including literature and from Internet databases. One public domain internet database used often is Gen-Bank, on the National Center for Biotechnology Information (NCBI) Web site, at http://www.ncbi.nlm.nih .gov/. Nearly all published sequences can be found through searches on this Web site. There are some general rules that should be followed when designing primers. These include

■ Design primers so that they are about 15–30 bases in length (20–25 bases is typical). Nonspecific primer annealing may result if primers of shorter length are used—the primer sequences may match more than the desired target(s).

■ Design both primers with about the same guanine-cytosine (GC) base composition—about 40% to 60% GC. Guanine (G) and cytosine (C) base pair with three hydrogen bonds, while adenine (A) and thymine (T) base pair with two hydrogen bonds. De-

```
541    caccgtttcg caggtgtggt tcggccaccg ctactcccag tttatgggga tctttgagga
       gtggcaaagc gtccacacca agccggtggc gatgagggtc aaatacccct agaaactcct
601  ccgcgccccc gtcccttcg aggaggtgat cgacaagatc aacgccaagg gggtctgtcg
       ggcgcggggg caggggaagc tcctccacta gctgttctag ttgcggttcc cccagacagc
661  gtccacggcc aagtacgtgc gcaacaacct ggagaccacc gcgtttcacc gggacgacca
       caggtgccgg ttcatgcacg cgttgttgga cctctggtgg cgcaaagtgg ccctgctggt
721 cgagaccgac atggagctga aaccggccaa cgccgcgacc cgcacgagcc ggggctggca
       gctctggctg tacctcgact ttggccggtt gcggcgctgg gcgtgctcgg ccccgaccgt
781  caccaccgac ctcaagtaca acccctcgcg ggtggaggcg ttccaccggt acgggacgac
       gtggtggctg gagttcatgt tggggagcgc ccacctccgc aaggtggcca tgccctgctg
841    ggtaaactgc atcgtcgagg aggtggacgc gcgctcggtg tacccgtaca acgagtttgt
       ccatttgacg tagcagctcc tccacctgcg cgcgagccac atgggcatgt tgctcaaaca
901    gctggcgact ggcgactttg tgtacatgtc ccccgttttac ggctaccggg aggggtcgca
       cgaccgctga ccgctgaaac acatgtacag gggcaaaatg ccgatggccc tccccagcgt
961 caccgaacaac accagctacg ccgccgaccg cttcaagcag gtcgacggct tctacgcgcg
       gtggcttgtg tggtcgatgc ggcggctggc gaagttcgtc cagctgccga agatgcgcgc
1021 cgacctcacc accaaggccc gggccacggc gccgaccacc cggaacctgc tcacgacccc
       gctggagtgg tggttccggg cccggtgccg cggctggtgg gccttggacg agtgctgggg
```

■ FIGURE 13-2 Portion of the human herpesvirus I glycoprotein B (UL27) gene, GenBank assession number AF259899, submitted by Ling, J.-Y., Chen, T.-M. and Stroop, W. G., April 24, 2000. The published sequence is the top strand (black text). The complimentary strand (not published) is the bottom strand (blue text). Two potential primers are illustrated in the sequence. The gray shaded upstream primer, from bases 781–800, is the same as the published sequence. The downstream primer, shaded in blue, is the inverted complement of the published sequence, and would be correctly written as "gtaaaacggggacatgtaca"; it would be referred to as spanning bases 940–921. The two primers would theoretically form a PCR product of 160 base pairs after successful amplification.

signing both primers with approximately the same %GC will mean that both will anneal with about the same efficiency to target DNA. The base composition, and the length of the primers, will dictate the annealing temperature (specifically, the melting temperature, **Tm**) of the primers. The Tm is the temperature at which 50% of primer has annealed to its target. There are various ways to calculate Tm based on the length and base composition of a primer. One easy calculation method is $Tm = 2(A+T) + 4(G+C)$. Using this formula, a 50% GC primer that is 20 bases in length would have a Tm of 60°C ($Tm = 2(10) + 4(10) = 20 + 40 = 60$). Since most laboratories would prefer that more than 50% of primer anneal to its target, many individuals use an annealing temperature lower than the Tm; one such annealing temperature (Ta) that is often used is $Ta = Tm - 5°C$. For the aforementioned 50% GC, 20-base long primer with a Tm of 60°C, the annealing temperature would thus be 55°C. If PCR product does not form at this temperature, experimenting with other annealing temperatures may be performed.

■ Design primers to avoid the formation of secondary structures within the primer. Secondary structures (such as hairpin loops) may form if complementarity (regions within the primer sequence that base pair together) occurs within the primer. Primers that form secondary structures will not anneal efficiently to template DNA, so the amount of "free" primer in solution is markedly reduced.

■ Design primers so that they do not complement each other near their 3' ends. If they do, they may form a primer-dimer in solution; this also reduces the amount of primer for reaction. Primers that are rich in GC bases at their 3' ends have a better chance of forming primer-dimers.

Template Nucleic Acid   **Template** is sometimes referred to as the target of a PCR or other amplification procedure. The template serves as a blueprint for the reaction. Primers are designed to recognize specific template sequences, and will anneal to the template during the PCR and other amplification reactions. Complementary DNA formed during standard PCR is based on the template sequence.

Template DNA for standard PCR can be isolated by a variety of laboratory methods; there are many procedures in the literature for all specimen types. In addition, there are many kits available on the market designed for nucleic acid isolation. Commercially available kits have several advantages, although they can be expensive. They are simple to use; provide con-

sistent, quality isolation results; and usually do not use hazardous chemicals or reagents. Some commercially available kits are adaptable to nearly any type of specimen, whereas others are developed for specific specimen types.

Specimens that nucleic acids are isolated from include (but are not limited to) tissue, blood, other body fluids, stool, bacterial colony matter, broth-cultured bacteria, and cells from tissue culture. There are procedures for the isolation of nucleic acids from paraffin-embedded, fixed tissues. There are also methods available to isolate viral nucleic acid from a variety of sources.

Quantitation of Nucleic Acids

Quantitation of isolated nucleic acids is important for some procedures including during amplification methods where the amount of formed PCR products is important (such as in some applications of reverse transcriptase PCR). Quantitation of nucleic acids can be achieved by ultraviolet (UV) light spectrophotometry. Nucleic acids absorb UV light readily at 260 nm (depicted as A_{260}); the concentration of DNA or RNA can be determined by measuring the absorbancy of the isolated sample at this wavelength. The calculations are based also on the extinction coefficient of either DNA or RNA (the theoretical concentration of either DNA or RNA at an absorbancy of 1.0 at 260 nm; this number is 50.0 μg/ml for DNA and 40.0 μg/ml for RNA) and the dilution factor of the sample. The concentration, then, of DNA can be determined with the formula shown in Box 13-2✳.

For example, an unknown sample is measured by UV spectrophotometry for concentration. The A_{260} for a 1:100 dilution of the sample is 0.34; the concentration of DNA would be (0.34) (100) (50 μg/ml), or 1,700 μg/ml. However, since template nucleic acid is usually used in microliter (μl) amounts in amplification procedures, the concentration must be divided by 1000 to yield, for the above example, a working concentration of 1.7 μg/μl.

The relative purity of a sample is also important for some amplification procedures. Cellular proteins and/or cellular debris and excess salts/solvents used in

---

✳ Box 13-2   Concentration of DNA

$$[DNA] + A_{260} \times dilution \times 50.0 \ \mu g/ml$$

Similarly, the concentration of RNA in a sample is determined with the formula:

$$[RNA] = A_{260} \times dilution \times 40.0 \ \mu g/ml$$

the isolation procedure may contaminate nucleic acid preparations. Purity can be determined by measuring the absorbancy at 280 nm (A_{280})—proteins absorb well at A_{280}. The ratio of A_{260}/A_{280} gives the relative purity of a sample. A pure sample of DNA has an A_{260}/A_{280} ratio of 1.8 ± 0.15, while a pure sample of RNA has an A_{260}/A_{280} ratio of 2.0 ± 0.15. Contaminants, however, will skew the A_{260}/A_{280} ratio.

Contamination Prevention in PCR Techniques

The PCR is an extremely sensitive detection technique; even a small amount of contaminating nucleic acid may be amplified, resulting in a false positive result. Extracted DNA from a specimen must be maintained intact and separate from other specimens, and must also not be allowed to contaminate PCR components. In addition, operator (i.e., human) DNA must not be allowed to contaminate specimen DNA or reaction components. There are methods and equipment that may be used to minimize the risk of contamination in a molecular diagnostics laboratory. These are summarized in Box 13-3✳ and include the following:

- Extract DNA at a different bench from where PCR assay components are assembled. It is preferable to perform these two functions in different rooms in the laboratory, if possible. Some labs will also add DNA template to reaction tubes on a third bench (or in a third room). The analysis of PCR products should also be done on a separate bench from all other functions, or in a different room.

- Utilize separate equipment and supplies for each bench—that is, maintain separate pipettes, microcentrifuge tubes, pipette tips, and so on.

- Use only aerosol-resistant pipette tips. These pipette tips have filters in them that greatly reduce the spread of aerosols during pipetting. These tips can be purchased prepackaged and presterilized.

- Wear a lab coat, and always use gloves during all phases of the PCR procedures. Change gloves when handling different specimens, and change gloves between samples or if the gloves may have become contaminated.

- Clean all laboratory areas and equipment with a decontaminating solution such as freshly prepared 10% bleach before and after all procedures. There are solutions available for purchase that are designed to eliminate contaminating nucleic acids and enzymes that destroy nucleic acids from bench tops and equipment.

- Keep all sample tubes and reagent tubes capped at all times when they are not being handled.

- Use UV light to destroy contaminating nucleic acids if it is feasible to use on a particular bench. If some (or all) of the procedures are performed in biosafety cabinets, UV light is a good choice for decontamination. UV light will cross-link and nick nucleic acids, rendering them unamplifiable. Do not expose PCR components and primer solutions to UV light since this may damage them. Always use care when using UV light.

Detection Methods for PCR Products

The DNA products that result from the PCR can be detected by agarose gel **electrophoresis** and real-time PCR.

Agarose Gel Electrophoresis This method is simple to perform, and is essentially an extra step after a PCR assay has been run. DNA and other biomolecules can be easily separated on the basis of charge, size, and shape. DNA has a net negative charge, so it will migrate toward a positive pole (the anode) in an electrical field. Agarose, which is somewhat like a molecular sieve, is often used to separate DNA fragments of 100–2000 bp size. The agarose gel is usually prepared by mixing solid agarose powder with a buffer, such as Tris-boric acid-EDTA buffer (TBE buffer) or Tris-acetate-EDTA buffer (TAE buffer). The agarose is heated until it is molten, then poured into a casting tray to solidify. A comb is placed into the molten agarose, and

---

✳ Box 13-3   Preventing Contamination in PCR Techniques

Extract DNA at a different bench from where PCR assay components are assembled.	Clean all laboratory areas and equipment with a decontaminating solution.
Use only aerosol-resistant pipette tips.	Keep all sample tubes and reagent tubes capped at all times when they are not being handled.
Utilize separate equipment and supplies for each bench.	Use UV light to destroy contaminating nucleic acids if it is feasible to use on a particular bench.
Wear a lab coat and always use gloves during all phases of the PCR procedures.	

the agarose will form around it while it solidifies. The comb is pulled out before electrophoresis is started, and this leaves wells that **PCR product** can be loaded into to run through the gel matrix. The same buffer (TBE or TAE) that is used to prepare the agarose gel is used as a tank buffer during electrophoresis; the gel is completely covered by buffer. PCR product samples are then mixed with a loading dye, which contains a marking dye such as bromophenol blue, and a heavy ingredient, such as sucrose or glycerol. The marking dye will correspond to a certain size of DNA as it runs through the gel, and thus will give one a rough idea of where the PCR products have migrated. The heavy ingredient keeps the PCR products weighted down in the wells in the agarose, until the electrical field is turned on and the samples enter the agarose matrix. When the samples have separated, they can be stained with a dye. Nearly always the dye used is **ethidium bromide.** Ethidium bromide intercalates into nucleic acids and will fluoresce orange under UV irridiation. An **image analysis** instrument that uses UV light to capture computer images of the PCR products is often used now. See Figure 13-3■ for an image of PCR products separated in an agarose gel.

Real-Time PCR   Real-time PCR is a variant of standard PCR that incorporates a detection method in the procedure—PCR product formation is measured throughout the procedure. An extra detection step is not necessary when amplification is completed. This is a procedure that saves time compared with standard PCR analyzed by agarose gel electrophoresis. Real-time PCR is also very sensitive and just as specific as standard PCR.

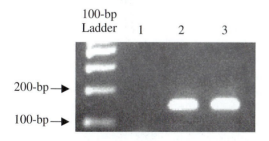

100-bp
Ladder   1   2   3

200-bp →

100-bp →

■ **FIGURE 13-3** Separation of human herpesvirus 1 and 2 glycoprotein B PCR products in a 2% agarose gel. Generic HSV primers were used. The 100-bp ladder is a molecular sizing marker; 100-bp and 200-bp sizes of double-stranded DNA are shown with arrows. (1) Negative control (no DNA template used); (2) HSV-1; (3) HSV-2. PCR products were stained with ethidium bromide. The image was captured with a Biorad Fluor-S MultiImager in the author's laboratory.

Detection of formed PCR products can be accomplished with dyes or with fluorescent-labeled probes. One dye that is often used for detection of PCR products during real-time PCR is SYBR Green. This dye fluoresces when it is bound to the sample. It can also be used to stain nucleic acids separated by agarose gel electrophoresis. There are two commonly used types of SYBR Green: SYBR Green I, which binds to double-stranded DNA, and SYBR Green II, which binds to single-stranded DNA and RNA. SYBR Green I is used in real-time PCR applications, since formed PCR product is double-stranded. While SYBR Green is very sensitive, it is generally not as specific as fluorescent-labeled probes for detection of PCR product. The dye will bind to formed primer-dimers if any are formed and give false fluorescent results.

There are different methods of real-time PCR that use a fluorescent-labeled probe for detection of target nucleic acid. The probes, regardless of method, are usually designed with a reporter dye (the fluorescent dye) and a quencher. The quencher keeps the reporter dye from fluorescing until the probe has bound to target DNA. The real-time system that is used (e.g., the LightCycler from Roche Instruments, the SmartCycler from Cepheid Instruments, etc.) will detect fluorescence from the labeled probe when this happens. When the level of fluorescence rises exponentially above background fluorescence, a positive result is obtained—that is, PCR product has formed. Two real-time PCR methods are briefly discussed here, TaqMan and the use of molecular beacons.

TaqMan   TaqMan uses a probe with a fluorescent dye on the 5′ end and a quencher dye on the 3′ end. Fluorescent energy transfer (FRET) is the principle behind the method, and TaqMan relies on the 5′ → 3′ exonuclease activity of *Taq* DNA polymerase. The probe is used in conjunction with a pair of primers; the probe is specific for an internal region to both primers on the target DNA. The probe will anneal one of the PCR products formed during PCR, and *Taq* DNA polymerase will cleave the fluorescent dye from the quencher dye during extension. Once the fluorescent dye is free of the quencher, a fluorescent signal is detectable. The *Taq* DNA polymerase exonuclease activity only acts when the probe is bound to the target. Thus, an increase in fluorescence represents a concomitant increase of PCR product in the sample.

Molecular Beacons   A molecular beacon is a single-stranded probe in the shape of a hairpin. The fluorescent and quencher dyes—one on the end of each strand of the probe—are held in close proximity to each other because the hairpin is folded back onto itself. Fluorescence is quenched by energy transfer. During denaturation, the hairpin structure of the molecular beacon denatures (along with target DNA). The probe will then anneal to one of the strands of the PCR product; in the process, the fluorescent dye is physically removed from the quenching dye, and fluorescence is released. The probe will release when the temperature is raised for primer extension; it does not interfere with PCR cycling. As PCR product accumulates, an increase in the level of fluorescence is also observed.

Applications of the PCR in Immunology

There are many applications of the PCR in a clinical immunology laboratory. Several different organisms, such as *Chlamydia trachomatis, Neisseria gonorrhoeae,* hepatitis A virus, hepatitis B virus, hepatitis C virus, HIV-1, and many others, may be identified by the use of standard PCR or a derivative. The case represented in this chapter is an example of aseptic (viral) meningitis. Most cases of aseptic meningitis are caused by enteroviruses; most people recover after about a week. Other causes of aseptic meningitis include HSV, cytomegalovirus (CMV), and other viruses. The standard of testing for enteroviruses is viral culture. However, viral culture takes time and has limited clinical use. With the advent of molecular methods of detecting enteroviruses and most other viruses, diagnosis can be made more rapidly than culture. Because antibiotics are ineffective against viruses, and cannot be used to treat enterovirus infections, treatment is symptomatic. While this may not provide a treatment benefit for the patient in this case, early diagnosis of this virus would avoid unnecessary antibiotic treatment for the patient. In addition, additional and expensive laboratory testing can be avoided.

Many of the other amplification methods discussed in this chapter have been adapted for the detection of many bacteria and viruses; some are FDA approved and should receive consideration for use in a molecular immunology laboratory.

REVERSE TRANSCRIPTASE PCR (RT-PCR)

The enzyme **reverse transcriptase (RT)** is used by retroviruses to convert viral RNA into a complimentary DNA copy (cDNA) that can integrate into the host cells genome. Reverse transcriptase PCR (RT-PCR) is an extremely sensitive method of detecting and quantifying messenger RNA (mRNA; also called transcript). The technique has many uses. It is used to analyze gene expression, and can also be used to detect RNA viruses, so this technique has applicability in the molecular immunology laboratory.

History and Basic Technique

Retroviruses, such as avian myeloblastosis virus (AMV), have been known since the early 1900s. The special nature of these viruses was not known, however until the 1960s when Howard Temin observed that replication of viruses with RNA genomes was inhibited by actinomycin D which inhibits DNA synthesis. This unusual phenomenon led to the concept of reverse **transcription**—a process where RNA is converted into DNA. Many retroviruses capable of infecting nearly all organisms have been discovered. All of these retroviruses use RT, properly known as RNA-dependent DNA polymerase, to convert genomic RNA into cDNA. There are various commercially available RT enzymes. Two of the most used RTs include enzymes isolated from AMV and Moloney murine leukemia virus (MMLV). However, many of the commercially available RT enzymes are proprietary constructs, many of which have not only RT capability but also DNA polymerase activity; that is, once the initial reverse transcription step is completed, the cDNA is used for standard PCR. Detection of PCR products from RT-PCR is the same as for standard PCR.

Isolation and Purification of RNA

A source of high-quality RNA is essential for successful RT-PCR. Usually RT-PCR is so sensitive and specific that only total RNA must be extracted from specimens rather than isolation of mRNA. This is useful since mRNA is present in relatively small amounts in total RNA preparations—the majority (80%–85%) of total RNA is represented by ribosomal RNA (rRNA); the remainder is transfer RNA (tRNA) and mRNA. Only small amounts of total RNA (less than 1 ng) are required for successful RT-PCR.

The isolation of intact quality RNA can be problematic since RNA is chemically and biologically less stable than DNA. In addition, **ribonucleases (RNases)** that digest RNA are nearly ubiquitous and are very resilient to destruction. Also, mRNA by its nature has a short half-life—it will degrade rapidly. All these factors demand special attention to recover and properly store quality RNA.

Attention should be made to creating a working environment that is as free from RNases as possible. Since RNases are nearly ubiquitous, nothing should be automatically assumed to be free of RNases, unless reagents and/or RNA isolation kits are purchased by a company that ensures its products are RNase free. Human hands are excellent sources of RNase, therefore, gloves should always be worn when isolating and handling RNA. It is possible now to purchase RNase-free supplies (such as microcentrifuge tubes, pipette tips, etc.) and solutions, so the elimination of RNases introduced from the working environment and laboratory personnel should be the highest concern. Solutions designed to eliminate RNase from bench top surfaces, equipment, and even glassware and plasticware are now available for purchase.

There are many methods of RNA isolation depending on the specimen source and type. It is probably more convenient and practical to use RNA isolation kits that can be purchased from several different manufacturers. These kits allow standardization of the RNA isolation technique for laboratory personnel and usually yield high-quality RNA free from RNases. Kits also reduce the need for storage and use of hazardous chemicals used in nucleic acid isolation. Laboratories that utilize their own RNA isolation protocols typically treat all prepared solutions with diethylpyrocarbonate that will effectively remove RNases. There are many RNA isolation protocols available in the literature.

Once intact quality RNA is prepared, it must be stored properly so that mRNA degradation does not occur rapidly. Generally, RNA should be stored at −70°C in aliquots to avoid damaging multiple freeze-thaw cycles. RNA that is stored in an RNase-free buffer can usually be held at −20°C and 4°C for several weeks before degradation will occur.

Synthesis of cDNA

Once total RNA has been isolated, the initial step of synthesizing **cDNA** from transcript is performed. In standard PCR a pair of primers is used to synthesize new copies of DNA from the template material. In RT-PCR the same pair of primers may be used. Initially, however, only one primer is used in the reaction to produce a cDNA copy of the mRNA template. With most available RT enzymes, the synthesis of cDNA proceeds at 42°C for 30 minutes. Incubation at 42°C alleviates secondary structure, which occurs commonly in RNA and impedes production of cDNA. This first-strand synthesis produces a single DNA strand that is complementary to the mRNA template. Once this first strand of DNA is produced, standard PCR is used to amplify the cDNA for detection. Many commercially available RTs are inactivated at 95°C, so the samples are heated from 42°C to 95°C. This also activates the DNA polymerase activity of many commercially available RTs. Then, standard PCR cycles are run.

Quantitation

One of the useful applications of RT-PCR is the possibility of quantifying transcript from different samples to depict differences in gene expression or to quantify levels of virus from clinical specimens. Because of sample-to-sample variation, quantitation can be difficult. Samples must be normalized to each other, and usually an internal control is utilized to compare the amount of unknown samples. For example, the amount of total RNA used in each RT-PCR assay for each specimen must be the same. In addition, an internal control of transcript that is expressed equally under most conditions and in high amount is also amplified. One example of an internal control (a "housekeeping" gene transcript) is the β-actin transcript of eukaryotic organisms; for prokaryotic organisms, 16S rRNA may be used. During analysis, unknown sample amounts are compared and normalized to the internal control amount for each sample. To complicate quantitation, the efficiency of both the RT and the DNA polymerase used in the reaction may have to be accounted for. The determination of viral load of some RNA viruses (such as hepatitis C virus) is performed by quantitative RT-PCR.

5′ and 3′ RACE

One of the problems of RT-PCR is that cDNA that complements the 5′ end and the 3′ end of mRNA is not often produced. A modification of RT-PCR, called rapid amplification of cDNA ends (**RACE**) was developed in 1988 to characterize transcripts at the 5′ and 3′ ends. There are several different available protocols for both 5′ and 3′ RACE. 5′ RACE, sometimes called "anchored" PCR, enables the characterization of the 5 end of transcripts. Generally, a gene-specific antisense oligonucleotide (primer 1) that base pairs as close to the 5′ end of the transcript as possible primes first-strand synthesis of cDNA. After first-strand synthesis, a homopolymeric tail (all of one type of dNTP such as dC) is placed onto the 3′ end of the cDNA, often using the enzyme called terminal deoxynucleotidyl transferase (TdT); this tail is the "anchor." Then, a primer (primer 2) specific for the anchor is used in conjunction with a primer located 3′ to primer 1 in a PCR assay. This amplifies cDNA of the 5′ end of the original transcript. There are variations to this theme as well, and several 5′ RACE kits are available commercially. In 3′ RACE, the 3′ poly (A) tail of eukaryotic transcripts is exploited. An oligo (dT) primer (primer 1) with a unique 5′ sequence is used for initial cDNA first-strand synthesis. Then, the produced cDNA is used in a PCR using a primer complimentary to the unique sequence in primer 1 and a gene-specific primer.

Contamination Problems and Concerns

In addition to the omnipresent potential for RNase contamination during RNA isolation, handling, and storage, RNA preparations must also be free of contaminating DNA. Even extremely small amounts of contaminating DNA from total RNA preparations can be amplified during RT-PCR and yield false results. DNA is typically removed from RNA preparations with deoxyribonucleases (DNases) that can be purchased commercially. Most kits available on the market include a DNase in the kit for just this purpose. Other sources of DNA contamination include genomic DNA and other PCR products. Maintaining a clean laboratory will reduce the potential for DNA contamination, as will the use of separate rooms for the different PCR procedures.

Applications of RT-PCR in Immunology

There are several applications of RT-PCR in the clinical immunology laboratory. Most involve the detection of different viruses from specimen samples, as with standard PCR. For example, RT-PCR can be used to detect and to monitor viral load in patients infected with hepatitis C virus or to detect rabies virus from tissue from both human and animal material.

LIGASE CHAIN REACTION

LCR was first described in 1989 when it was originally called the ligation amplification reaction (LAR). This method varies from the PCR in that it uses pairs of probes and DNA ligase for amplification.

Basic Theory and Reaction

The LCR is a technique where gene sequences are amplified by a thermostable DNA ligase; a thermostable DNA polymerase is also used in the procedure. Typically, two pairs of probes are annealed to target DNA with short gaps between them—the probes are designed to anneal to the template DNA in a head to tail manner. Each pair of probes is specific for one of the strands of target DNA. Once annealed, DNA polymerase will add the missing nucleotides between the probes, and then DNA ligase joins the probes to form an amplified product. The formed ligation products are then used as template for still more ligase reactions—the process continues exponentially during several cycles of LCR. The LCR is performed in a thermal cycler, like the PCR.

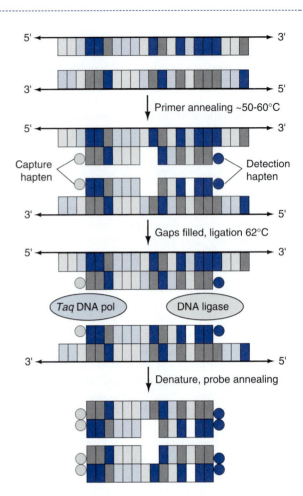

■ **FIGURE 13-4** Ligase chain reaction. Target DNA is initially heat denatured. Then, pairs of labeled probes anneal to each strand of target DNA, with a small gap in between each pair. *Taq* DNA polymerase adds missing nucleotides to fill the gaps in between the probes, then DNA ligase seals the probes together. The DNA is again heat denatured, and probe will anneal to both template DNA and to ligated probe fragments. The haptens are used for capture and detection (see text description).

Figure 13-4■ depicts a typical LCR. First, template DNA is briefly denatured (this requires only about one second) by heating to about 94–95°C. Then as in standard PCR, the reaction mixture is cooled so that the two sets of probes anneal to their target sequences. The annealing temperature is dependent on the sequence and length of the probes, like in standard PCR. The annealing step is usually only performed for about 1 second. Then DNA polymerase fills the short gaps (typically designed to be only a few nucleotides in length) between the probes at a temperature of 62°C for about one minute; at this same temperature, the

DNA ligase will join the probes. Depending on the protocol, there will be about 40 cycles of LCR. Detection of amplified products is often fluorescence based. For example, Abbot Laboratories utilizes hapten groups attached to each probe. Some of the probes have an attached capture hapten, and some of the probes have an attached detection hapten. The probes are designed in a manner that when they are joined together, there will be a capture hapten on one end and a detection hapten on the other end. Antibodies on microbeads will capture the amplified products, and noncaptured probes are washed away. An alkaline-phosphatase conjugate is added that is specific for the detection hapten on the amplified product. The substrate 4-methylumbelliferyl phosphate is added to the mixture and produces a fluorescent signal when cleaved. An automated detection instrument (the LCx analyzer) detects the fluorescent signal.

Applications of the LCR in Immunology

The LCR has been used very successfully for detection of pathogens such as *C. trachomatis* and *N. gonorrhoeae* in clinical immunology laboratories. The LCx system from Abbott Laboratories is FDA approved for detection of these two organisms from clinical samples. The LCR has also been used to detect point mutations in human genes.

NUCLEIC ACID SEQUENCE BASED AMPLIFICATION

NASBA is a method that can be used to detect both DNA and RNA targets. It is also known as self-sustained sequence replication (3SR). NASBA is a method that proceeds under isothermal conditions, that is, a thermal cycler is not necessary.

History and Basic Technique

In 1989, Kwoh et al. described a non-PCR based nucleic acid amplification technique which they referred to as a transcription-based amplification system (TAS). TAS was used to amplify mRNA by repeated two-cycle reactions of cDNA synthesis. The cDNA was then transcribed back into multiple copies of RNA. Heat was required to denature the RNA:DNA hybrids formed during the process, and this inactivated the enzymes used in TAS. *Escherichia coli* RNase H was later added to TAS to degrade the RNA template of the RNA:DNA hybrid, leaving the DNA copy free as template for cycling reactions. The addition of *E. coli* RNase H meant that

heat was not required, and the reaction could thus proceed isothermally (i.e., at 41°C). NASBA is a result of this early work and can be used as a detection system.

The reaction uses the combined activities of a ribonuclease (RNase H), an RNA-dependent DNA polymerase (AMV-RT), and a DNA-dependent RNA polymerase (from bacteriophage T7); a temperature of 41°C is used. First, a primer is annealed to the template nucleic acid. The 3′ end of the primer is specific for the target; the 5′ end of the primer incorporates the promoter region of the T7 RNA polymerase. Then cDNA of the target is produced by AMV-RT. The RNA from the resulting RNA:DNA hybrid is then denatured by RNase H. A second primer, complimentary to the synthesized cDNA strand, then anneals. Extension takes place from this primer by DNA-dependent DNA polymerse activity from AMV-RT. This double-stranded cDNA has a functional T7 RNA polymerase promoter on one end. The RNA polymerase then uses the cDNA as a transcriptional template to produce mRNA. A large amount of mRNA is produced from a single double-stranded cDNA template—approximately 10–1000 copies of transcript per cDNA. This newly synthesized transcript corresponds to the original target RNA in the sample. The new transcripts then are used as template for additional reactions. The observed amplified increase is about 10^9-fold.

DNA can also be used as template; the process is essentially the same, except that the target DNA is first denatured at 95–100°C before the enzyme mixture is added and the reaction is allowed to proceed.

Applications of NASBA in Immunology

This technique may be used to detect several different pathogens in the clinical immunology laboratory. Bio-Merieux offers testing for several viruses, bacteria, fungi, and parasites with its NucliSens NASBA system, including but not limited to HIV-1, cytomegalovirus, enteroviruses, human papillomavirus, dengue virus, measles virus, *C. trachomatis,* and *N. gonorrheae.*

BRANCHED DNA DETECTION

While most genetic amplification techniques detect an exponential increase of target nucleic acid, **branched DNA (bDNA) detection** relies on amplification of signal. Since signal is detected, quantitation is possible and accurate, and the technique has been utilized for several years in clinical diagnostic laboratories. Branched DNA detection is sensitive and reliable.

History and Basic Technique

Urdea et al. published branched DNA detection methodology in 1991, using alkaline phosphatase-labeled oligonucleotides specific for hepatitis B virus and hepatitis C virus. The target nucleic acid is not amplified. There are several bDNA detection techniques in use now, along with commercially available detection systems.

The target nucleic acid is initially denatured, like in other amplification procedures, to single strands. Then several gene-specific probes are hybridized to the target nucleic acid. There are different types of probes and oligonucleotides used, somewhat like in the LCR. One set of oligonucleotides are called capture extenders (CE) that capture the target nucleic acid to a solid support matrix, like a microtiter plate well. Another set of oligonucleotides are the label extenders (LE). Many of these are hybridized to the target nucleic acid. In early bDNA assays, a bDNA amplifier probe would then anneal to the LE oligonucleotides; the amplifier then binds several labeled probes (labeled with an enzyme such as alkaline phosphatase). In more recent adaptations of the bDNA assay, a preamplifier is first annealed to the LE oligonucleotides. Then many amplifiers bind to the preamplifier, followed by annealing of many labeled probes to the amplifiers. The preamplifier/amplifier structure is a branched molecule and can be labeled potentially thousands of times. The newer bDNA assays have stronger signal amplification and are more sensitive. Figure 13-5■ shows a schematic of the bDNA assay technique.

Use of bDNA-Based Detection in Immunology

Because bDNA-based detection systems produce sensitive and specific quantifiable data, these assays are useful for following loads of viruses such as HIV and hepatitis C virus. Branched DNA assays have been used successfully for several years in this capacity in the clinical immunology laboratory.

IN SITU AMPLIFICATION

In situ amplification (ISA) is a technique used to associate genetic abnormalities or alterations associated with human disease by nucleic acid amplification. With ISA, a laboratory is able to detect low-copy nucleic acid sequences of genetic abnormalities and amplify them to detectable levels directly from tissue or related specimens. It is also used to detect low copies of viral nucleic acid in tissues and cells. The method is based on combining the techniques of in situ hybridization (ISH) and the PCR.

History and Theory of ISA

In 1969, Pardue and Gall introduced the method of hybridization of labeled RNA and DNA fragments to cytologic specimens on slides. This technique became known as ISH, and the method has been greatly refined since its introduction. It is a valuable research and diagnostic method—it allows for diagnosis of viral and neoplastic diseases and also is capable of quantification. The method of ISH essentially uses labeled nucleic acid probes to detect specific nucleic acid targets in tissue preparations, intact cells, or chromosomal material. One of the drawbacks of ISH, though, is that the threshold of sensitivity is about 10 copies of transcript or viral DNA per cell. Thus, low-level gene expressions, or low levels of viral load (or latent viral infections), are difficult to detect by ISH.

An alternative to the sensitivity issues of ISH was apparent when the PCR was introduced in the mid-1980s. Haase et al. first reported the amplification of lentiviral nucleic acid from inside cells in 1990, and ISA was born. Essentially a target sequence is amplified during ISA to detectable levels from the same specimen types as ISH (tissue, intact cells, and chromosomes). The technique, like the PCR, is sensitive and specific. In fact, Zehbe et al. reported in 1992 of amplification of single copies of human papillomavirus DNA in tissue cells by ISA. Any amplification technique, such as the PCR, RT-PCR, NASBA, and so on, may be used for ISA. There are many available ISA protocols. There are two general ISA methods. In one method, cells are fixed and permeabilized, then suspended in a PCR assay mixture in tubes and target is amplified in a standard thermal cycler. The resulting PCR products are cytocentrifuged onto glass slides. Finally, products are visualized on the glass slides by ISH or immunohistochemistry. ISA is also performed on glass slides. Tissues or cells on the glass slides are fixed and permeabilized, then covered with a PCR assay mixture. A coverslip is placed on top of the reaction mixture, and sealed to prevent evaporation. Alternatively, special chambers have been developed for reaction mixtures that clip onto the glass slides. Amplification is performed, and resulting products are analyzed either directly or indirectly. When using RT-PCR to amplify low amounts of transcript, the material should be treated with DNase prior to the procedure. Otherwise the reaction is similar to standard RT-PCR. It should be noted that ISA is

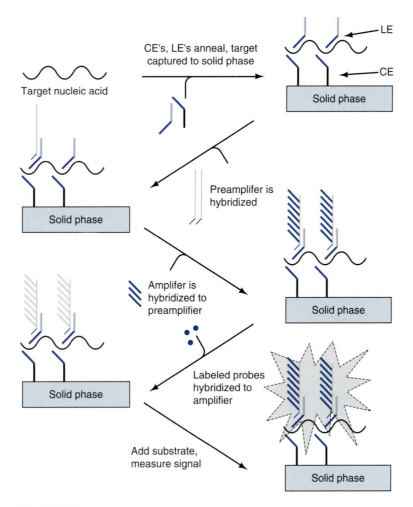

■ FIGURE 13-5 Branched DNA signal amplification. Capture extender (CE) oligonucleotides capture the target nucleic acid to a solid support platform, while many label extender (LE) oligonucleotides hybridize to the target. Preamplifier labels hybridize to the LE oligonucleotides; then several amplifier molecules bind to the preamplifiers. Many labeled probes then hybridize to the amplifiers. Substrate for the label is added, and generated signal is measured.

not as efficient as standard, solution-based PCR procedures. There are commercially available thermal cyclers for performing ISA on glass slides.

ISA Detection Methods
There are two basic methods of detecting ISA products: direct detection and indirect detection.

Direct Detection   Labeled nucleotides (with nonisotopic labels such as digoxigenin-11-dUTP or biotin-16-dUTP) are added to the ISA PCR assay at the start of the procedure during direct detection. The resulting amplified products are all directly labeled. There are some problems that occur with direct detection—false posi-

tive results can frequently occur. These problems include mispriming and labeled nucleotides incorporated nonspecifically due to DNA repair by DNA polymerase; the embedding process of paraffin-embedded tissues often results in damage to DNA. Thus, direct detection may not be a good detection option for ISA products.

Indirect Detection   Using ISH with labeled probes, detection of amplified product is usually performed by indirect detection. This procedure is also referred to as PCR ISH. Labeled probes (again, with a label such as digoxigenin-11-dUTP or biotin-16-dUTP) designed for the sequence of the amplification product are incubated with the ISA assay after PCR has been performed and visualized.

Use of Controls in ISA

Because both false-positive and false-negative results can readily occur with ISA, the use of proper controls is essential. As stated earlier, false positives can occur because of the DNA repair mechanism of damaged DNA in tissue sections or because of mispriming. False negatives also occur; these are typically the result of one of the several steps in the process not working correctly. The tissue fixation process cross-links protein and DNA, and this may interfere with primer access to its target. In addition, false negatives can occur due to poor heat conductance of the PCR mixture under the coverslip. Positive controls may include the following: the use of known cells or tissues that have a low copy number of the particular nucleic acid sequence that will be amplified to ensure proper function of the PCR; control for probe effectiveness by detecting the sequence of interest by ISH from cells or tissues that express the sequence in relatively high amounts; and/or run a conventional, non-ISA PCR assay with a low copy number of the target sequence—then separate the PCR products by electrophoresis, blot the products onto a membrane, and use the probes that will be used in ISA to detect the sequence on the membrane. This would ensure probe specificity. Negative controls may include the following: use tissue or cells known to not have the target sequence, purposely do not include one of the PCR reagents, and/or do not utilize the labeled probe in the detection step to ensure that endogenous enzymes (such as alkaline peroxidase) are not present in the cells or tissue.

▶ FUTURE TRENDS IN MOLECULAR IMMUNOLOGY

The incorporation of powerful molecular biological techniques has expanded the role of the clinical diagnostic laboratory; in the immunology laboratory, these methods are proving very useful for detection of a wide variety of microorganisms and disease states. One area that will become more advanced in the field of molecular immunology is an increase in the level—and reliance—of automation. For example, Roche Diagnostics has an automated nucleic acid extraction system on the market, the MagNA Pure LC System. The system will fill capillary tubes for real-time PCR analysis with the LightCycler instrument. Automated instruments will also become more compact to save

space in the laboratory. Gene chip technology is another area that will see future use in the clinical immunology laboratory.

GENE CHIP TECHNOLOGY

Generally most assays in molecular diagnostics target one gene, transcript, or protein. The concept runs along the lines of "one gene, one assay" and yields the conclusion that only a particular gene or gene product is involved in a particular disease state. However, organisms are complicated, and typically many genes and their products interact in a complex—and coordinated—fashion in cells and tissues. For a given disease state, thus, more than one gene or gene product may be involved. Standard molecular methods do not test for this "whole picture" phenonemen very well. Now, though, DNA microarrays and gene chip technology have made it possible to monitor entire genomes of organisms for genes or gene products that may be involved in disease processes.

Basic Theory and Schematic

There are several different names for gene chip technology that appear in the literature; these include DNA microarray, microarray, biochip, gene chip, DNA chip, and gene array, among others. In essence, an array is an ordered set of samples, attached to a solid support medium. A microarray can consist of hundreds, thousands, or even hundreds of thousands of DNA probes attached to a solid support (such as a glass background) using specialized, high-speed robotics and imaging equipment. Each DNA probe is spotted onto the support medium; on a microarray, the spots are usually less than 800 μM in diameter. The identity of the DNA probes attached to the solid support is known, and they are placed at a precise location. The DNA microarray can be used to identify sequences of genes (and/or gene mutations) and can be used to determine the level of expression of genes. With the potential of the microarray, a laboratory could test thousands of genes or sequences at one time. A microarray could be set up by spotting PCR products from targets of genes of interest onto a solid platform. Then test nucleic acid (perhaps transcript products from tumors, etc.) is labeled with fluorescent dyes and hybridized with the microarray DNA. Lasers that excite the fluorescent dyes are used on the microarray, and the signal is captured with a confocal laser microscope. Control samples are used. The excitation levels compared with the controls are viewed and may pro-

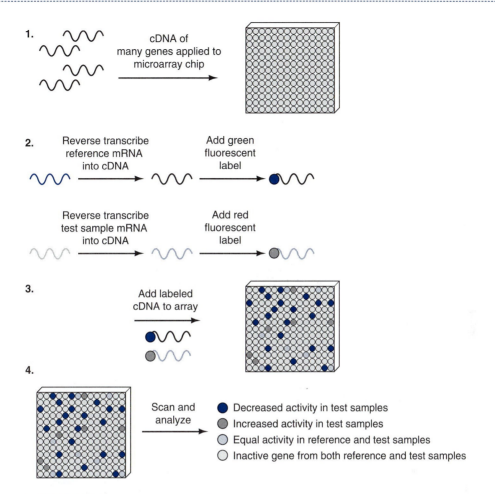

■ **FIGURE 13-6** Example of a DNA microarray. PCR products for specific genes are spotted onto a solid platform with the use of precise lasers and imaging equipment. Transcript from both a reference sample and from the test sample is reverse transcribed into cDNA and labeled with a fluorescent probe (in this case, green for reference sample cDNA is represented by blue and red for test sample cDNA is represented by gray). The labeled samples are hybridized to the DNA on the microarray, if applicable. A scanner analyzes fluorescent readings from the microarray and provides applicable data, such as the ratio of green and red fluorescence, to determine activity from each gene spot.

vide significant information as to what gene has increased or decreased amounts of transcript during the process being tested. Figure 13-6■ depicts a schematic of a microarray.

Applications of Gene Chip Technology in Immunology

While the possibilities of using microarray technology to identify gene sequences and gene expression are limitless, at this moment they are somewhat expensive to create and require expensive and special detection equipment. There are commercial gene chips available for HIV-1 genotyping and mutation analysis of some human genes, such as cytochrome p450 and the p53 tumor suppressor gene. Potentially probes for nearly all pathogenic microorganisms could be attached to a solid support medium and used to identify these organisms from samples. Probes could also be designed for nearly any disease process that occurs in humans, and the genes and/or their gene products that are involved in the process could be identified. Once identified, useful assays could be designed to readily detect these expressed genes or their products.

SUMMARY

Amplification reactions are very sensitive and specific techniques that are very useful for detecting, identifying, and quantifying nucleic acid from microorganisms and human diseases in the clinical laboratory. There are numerous advantages and disadvantages to employing molecular-based technology in the clinical laboratory. Most molecular diagnostic tests, although they can detect nearly any microbial agent and can identify human genetic disease, are difficult to perform and interpret results. Many molecular-based methods also require special equipment that most laboratories are not able to afford and the costs, for some, may still be prohibitive.

POINTS TO REMEMBER

▶ The polymerase chain reaction, the first amplification method used, is capable of amplifying very low amounts of nucleic acid to an exponential amount. PCR products can be detected by agarose gel electrophoresis or by real-time PCR.

▶ Reverse transcriptase (RT) is an enzyme that converts RNA into a complementary DNA (cDNA) strand. The enzyme is used in reverse transcriptase PCR (RT-PCR) to synthesize a strand of cDNA from RNA; the cDNA is then used in a standard PCR assay.

▶ The ligase chain reaction (LCR) is a technique that uses pairs of probes and amplifies them with DNA polymerase and DNA ligase. The probes are annealed to target DNA in pairs a few nucleotides apart. DNA polymerase will fill in the nucleotides between the probes and DNA ligase will join the probes together; this occurs on both strands of DNA. In this manner amplification of target occurs. The probes are labeled for detection.

▶ Nucleic acid sequence based amplification (NASBA) is an amplification technique that uses three enzymes in conjunction: a ribonuclease, a reverse transcriptase, and a DNA-dependent RNA polymerase. The reaction can proceed at one temperature, and does not need a thermal cycler.

▶ Branched DNA (bDNA) detection of nucleic acids is different from standard amplification tests in that the signal is amplified, not target nucleic acid. The generated signal from hybridized probes is quantifiable, and the test is very sensitive and accurate.

▶ In situ amplification (ISA) is a technique that is used to amplify nucleic acids from tissues, cells, and chromosomal material. Amplified products are detected with labeled probes.

▶ Gene chip technology (also called DNA microarrays) is a powerful technique that can be used to screen a population of transcripts against thousands of genes to determine gene activity. This technology can also be used in organism identification.

LEARNING ASSESSMENT QUESTIONS

1. Methods that may be used to reduce contamination problems in a PCR lab include
   a. the use of ribonucleases to decontaminate bench tops and equipment.
   b. the use of different rooms to perform the different steps of the procedure, if possible.
   c. performing all of the steps on the same bench, if possible.
   d. the use of UV light to decontaminate primers and other PCR components before and after use.

2. Which of the following is true about primers?
   a. should have GC-base compositions of less than 40%
   b. often form primer-dimers during the PCR by annealing to each other at their 5′ ends

   c. anneal to DNA in pairs next to each other during standard PCR
   d. anneal to their target sequence at a temperature based on sequence and length

3. Which of the following statements is incorrect regarding real-time PCR?
   a. SYBR Green I may be used to detect the formation of PCR products.
   b. Fluorescent-labeled probes usually have both a quencher and a reporter dye.
   c. PCR products are measured only when the entire reaction is complete.
   d. SYBR Green detection of PCR product formation tends to be less specific than fluorescent-labeled probe detection of PCR product formation.

4. True or false: The process of embedding tissue for histological analysis effectively destroys all nucleic acid present in the tissue.
   a. True
   b. False

5. Which of the following is true about *Taq* DNA polymerase?
   a. is an enzyme isolated from *Thermus aquaticus* that catalyzes the synthesis of new strands of DNA under appropriate reaction conditions.
   b. is an enzyme isolated from *Tetragenococcus aquaticus* that catalyzes the synthesis of new strands of DNA under appropriate reaction conditions.
   c. was originally isolated from a retrovirus.
   d. is used almost exclusively to reverse transcribe mRNA into cDNA.

6. The concentration of which of the following PCR reaction components is important to the success of a PCR assay?
   a. magnesium
   b. deoxynucleotide phosphates
   c. primers
   d. all of the above
   e. a and b only
   f. none of the above

7. Ribonucleases are:
   a. rarely problematic when working with RNA.
   b. nearly ubiquitous and must be managed when manipulating RNA.
   c. easily destroyed by gently heating RNA solutions.
   d. used as a reaction component in the ligase chain reaction (LCR).

8. Nucleic acid sequence based amplification (NASBA):
   a. has little application in a clinical molecular laboratory.
   b. uses a thermal cycler to rapidly change reaction temperatures.
   c. exploits signal amplification, not target amplification.
   d. uses three different enzymes in an isothermal reaction.

9. Which of the following statements is correct regarding in situ amplification (ISA)?
   a. ISA uses preamplifiers and amplifiers for detection.
   b. ISA can be performed from tissues, cells, and chromosomes.
   c. Most clinical laboratories use radiolabeled probes to detect ISA products.
   d. None of the above are correct.

10. A DNA microarray:
   a. could be used to test the level of expression of thousands of genes.
   b. can be used to test the level of expression from only one gene at a time.
   c. utilizes common laboratory equipment to design the microchip.
   d. cannot be used to test expression levels of genes.

REFERENCES

Eckert, K. A. and T. A. Kunkel. 1990. High fidelity DNA synthesis by the *Thermus aquaticus* DNA polymerase. *Nucleic Acids Res* 18:3739–44.

Gall, J. G. and M. L. Pardue. 1969. Formation and detection of RNA-DNA hybrid molecules in cytological preparations. *Proc Natl Acad Sci USA* 63:378–83.

Haase, A. T., E. F. Retzel, and K. A. Staskus. 1990. Amplification and detection of lentiviral DNA inside cells. *Proc Natl Acad Sci USA* 87:4971–75.

Kleppe, K., E. Ohstuka, R. Kleppe, I. Molineux, and H.G. Khorana. 1971. Studies on polynucleotides. XCVI. Repair replication of short synthetic DNAs as catalyzed by DNA polymerases. *J Mol Biol* 56:341–46.

Kocher, T. D. and A. C. Wilson. 1991. DNA amplification by the polymerase chain reaction. In: *Essential Molecular Biology: A Practical Approach*, Vol. II, ed. T. A. Brown. IRL Press, Oxford, pp. 185–207.

Kwoh, D. Y., G. R. Davis, K. M. Whitfield et al. 1989. Transcription-based amplification system and detection of amplified human immunodeficiency virus type I with a bead-based sandwich hybridization format. *Proc Natl Acad Sci USA* 86:1173–77.

Pardue, M. L. and J. G. Gall. 1969. Molecular hybridization of radioactive DNA to the DNA of cytological preparations. *Proc Natl Acad Sci USA* 64:600–604.

Saiki, R. K., D. H. Gelfand, S. Stoffel et al. 1988. Primer-directed enzymatic amplification of DNA with a thermostable DNA polymerase. *Science* 239:487–91.

Saiki, R. K., S. Scharf, F. Faloona et al. 1985. Enzymatic amplification of β-globin genomic sequences and restriction site analysis for diagnosis of sickle cell anemia. *Science* 230:1350–54.

Urdea, M. S., T. Horn, T. J. Fultz et al. 1991. Branched DNA amplification multimers for the sensitive, direct detection of human hepatitis viruses. *Nucleic Acids Symp Ser* 24:197–200.

Wu, D. Y. and R. B. Wallace. 1989. The ligation amplification reaction (LAR)—amplification of specific DNA sequences using sequential rounds of template dependent ligation. *Genomics* 4:560–69.

Zehbe, I. E., G. W. Hacker, J. Sallstrom, E. Rylander, and E. Wilander. 1992. Detection of single HPV copies in SiHa cells by *in situ* polymerase chain reaction combined with immunoperoxidase and immunogold-silver staining techniques. *Anticancer Res* 12: 2165–68.

14

Molecular Applications in Cytogenetics

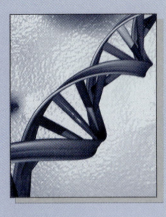

■ CHAPTER CHECKLIST

After reading and studying this chapter, the reader should be able to:

1. Describe cytogenetics as a discipline in laboratory medicine.
2. Describe the theory behind FISH and explain why FISH might be advantageous in cytogenetic analysis.
3. Summarize the classical cytogenetic techniques, along with clinical applications of these techniques.
4. Discuss the advantages and limitations of classical cytogenetics.
5. Develop a flow chart diagramming the protocol for FISH.
6. List at least five quality control considerations.
7. Describe the procedure used to report a cytogenetic study.
8. Discuss currently used clinical applications for both classical cytogenetics and for FISH.
9. Using the advantages and disadvantages of the procedure, discuss the utility of FISH.
10. List and describe advanced FISH techniques.

@ CASE IN POINT

A 32-year-old woman found a mass in her right breast during her routine monthly self-examination. After mammography and needle aspiration of the mass, an open biopsy was performed. Histologic examination of the specimen showed the presence of an adenocarcinoma. The mass was removed, along with draining lymph nodes. Examination of the mass showed it to be invasive, and evidence of tumor was found in three lymph nodes. There was no evidence of distant metastasis. The patient responded well to front-line chemotherapy. Three years later, there was a recurrence of the tumor, along with metastasis. Treatment with Herceptin was begun.

CASE IN POINT *(continued)*

ISSUES TO CONSIDER
After reading the patient's case history, consider

- Cytogenetic techniques that might be used to examine the initial tumor and lymph nodes
- Abnormalities that you might expect to find (Chapter 10 will also help you consider this point)
- The abnormality detected that suggests what form of therapy may be useful
- Techniques that could be used to monitor the success or failure of the therapy

IMPORTANT TERMS

Acquired genetic mutation
Alpha satellite
Amplification
Autosome
Background
Bacterial artificial
  chromosome (BAC)
Bands
Beta satellite
Birth defect
Break-apart probes
Cancer
Centromere
Chromosome
Chromosome band
Chromosome painting
Chromosome region p
Chromosome region q
Comparative genome
  hybridization
Congenital
Conserved sequence
Contiguous gene syndromes
Counterstain
Crossing over
Cytogenetics
Deletion

Denaturation
Deoxyribonucleic acid (DNA)
Direct labeling
Eukaryote
Fluorescent in situ
  hybridization (FISH)
Fluorochrome (fluor)
Fusion probes
Gene
Gene amplification
Genetic map
Genetic testing
Genomic DNA
Homolog
Hybridization
Imprinting
Indirect labeling
Inherit
Insertion
In situ hybridization
Interphase
Inversion
Isochromosome
Karyotype
Kilobase (kb)
Label
Meiosis

Metaphase
Microarray
Mitosis
Monosomy
Mosaic
Mutation
Noise
Oncogene
Paint
Polymorphism
Probe
Reporter molecule
Resolution
Satellite
Sex chromosome
Spectral karyotype (SKY)
Stringency conditions
Syndrome
Tandem repeat sequence
Target
Telomere
Telomeric repeats
Translocation
Trisomy
Uniparental disomy (UPD)
Vector
Whole chromosome paints

► INTRODUCTION

Cytogenetics is a specialized laboratory discipline that examines the structure and behavior of chromosomes at the cellular level. Classical cytogenetics requires viable, nucleated cells in cell cycle that are cultured anywhere from one day to two or more weeks, depending on the specimen type and preliminary diagnosis. It remains the gold standard in provid-

ing a whole genome scan. However, microscopic resolution limitations routinely prevent cytogenetic detection of certain genomic abnormalities. In addition, poor morphology associated with particular specimen types or complex rearrangements of genetic materials sometimes prevent identification of even larger abnormalities by standard techniques. Today, molecular-based techniques are being incorporated in cytogenetics laboratories. The principal molecular technique currently used in the clinical cytogenetic laboratory is **fluorescent in situ hybridization (FISH).** FISH has sometimes been called molecular cytogenetics, as it is a technique originally developed to enhance the resolution of chromosome observations. FISH may augment identification and diagnosis by increasing the sensitivity of detecting abnormalities several fold. This chapter presents the principles of chromosome analysis by classical cytogenetic studies and the advantages as well as limitations of traditional methods. This chapter covers the FISH procedure and its clinical applications in the cytogenetic laboratory. It also describes the difference between FISH and other molecular-based methods. The advantages and disadvantages of FISH methodology are presented.

▶ CLASSICAL CYTOGENETICS

CELL CULTURES AND HARVESTING

In classical cytogenetics, viable nucleated cycling cells in cultures are required. Individual cell types require different culture media, growth factors, and pH in order to obtain enough cells to perform chromosomal analysis. Cells are harvested from culture when an adequate number are in logarithmic growth phase.

There are three steps in harvesting cells from cultures. First, a mitotic inhibitor is added to the culture to arrest cells in metaphase and block progression of the cell cycle. Next, a hypotonic solution is added to lyse any red cells present and increase the volume of all other cells. Finally, the swollen cells are fixed using a modified Carnoy's fixative (3:1 absolute methanol:glacial acetic acid). The fixative alters the cell membranes and chromosomes by removing lipids and water molecules and denaturing proteins.

The fixed cell suspension is dispersed onto a glass slide under conditions of temperature and humidity that allows the swollen cells to flatten, pancakelike, onto the slide as the fixative evaporates. A properly prepared slide will have the majority of mitotic cells flattened or "spread" so the chromosomes are individually visible with few overlaps.

ENZYME TREATMENT AND STAINING

After aging the slide, naturally or artificially, to dehydrate the chromosomes, the preparation is treated with a proteolytic enzyme solution, then stained with a metachromatic dye. Enzyme treatment and staining elicit a repeatable pattern of horizontal light and dark

striations, called **bands,** along the chromosome length. A detailed, time-consuming comparison of the banding pattern between homologs allows detection of deleted, duplicated, or rearranged chromosomal segments (Figure 14-1■).

COUNTING CHROMOSOMES IN CELLS

The number of chromosomes present in intact cells is also determined. Individuals may present with **mosaicism** and contain multiple cell populations, each with a different chromosome complement. Mosaic phenotypes vary considerably depending on the involved chromosome or chromosome segment. To ensure detection of mosaicism of a specific parentage at a 95% confidence level, it is necessary to analyze from 15 to 100 mitotic cells per specimen, depending on the potential diagnosis. Once a mosaicism for a particular chromosome is suspected, hundreds of cells can be examined rapidly using FISH, greatly increasing the accuracy of the diagnosis.

COMPUTER IMAGING

Cytogenetics laboratories use computer-imaging systems with proprietary software to capture and **karyotype** two or more representative metaphase spreads per specimen. The software includes a laboratory information system (LIS), specifically designed for cytogenetic laboratories, that may interface with other systems. Finally, case reports, which may include a copy of the karyotype, are prepared and sent to the referring physician.

CASE REPORTS

The case report includes a description of the chromosomal finding in International System of Cytogenetic Nomenclature (ISCN) format with interpretations in common medical and lay terminology. The ISCN is a special descriptive language for reporting classical cytogenetic and FISH results. Its use ensures that geneticist worldwide can interpret case findings. When abnormalities are detected, suitable recommendations, such as genetic counseling, referral to specific types of specialists, or additional genetic testing for the patient or other at-risk family members, will appear on the laboratory report.

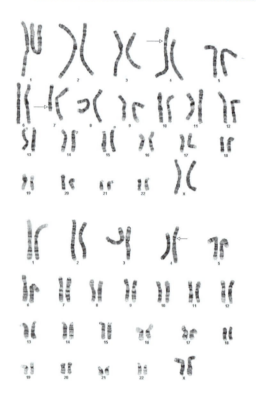

■ **FIGURE 14-1** A karyotype showing an organized arrangement of chromosomes from a single cell with chromosomes positioned according to size, centromere position and banding pattern. The karyotype of the individual at the top, prepared from a blood specimen, shows a balanced translocation of material between chromosome 4p and 7q. If the translocation breakpoints lie between transcribed genes, the individual will have a normal phenotype. However, depending on the amount of material and specific genes involved, carriers of balanced translocations may be at increased risk for having multiple spontaneous abortions and unbalanced affected live births. The karyotype at the bottom is from the translocation carriers' amniotic fluid specimen. The fetus received only one of the mother's translocation products so has a major imbalance of genetic materials. Risk for translocation carriers must be assessed individually since breaks and rejoining can occur at any location within the genome producing innumerable rearrangements. (Images courtesy of Gregory Mengden, Ph.D., Southwest Genetics, San Antonio, TX.)

ADVANTAGES AND LIMITATIONS

Classical cytogenetic analysis provides a broad-spectrum scan of the entire genome, but may fail to detect small abnormalities or classify all rearrangements in complex cases. In spite of this limitation, classical cytogenetics has established that a chromosome abnormality affects 1 in each 200 live births, contributing significantly to morbidity and disease. Classical cytogenetics is frequently more appropriate for initial genetic evaluations of individuals with particular genetic syndromes, for cancer specimens, or for periodic follow-up in cancer studies to monitor disease progression or response to therapy. FISH is more appropriate for determining the presence or absence of a specific sequence when the overall scan appears normal but the phenotype indicates an abnormality. FISH serves as a quick screen for major numerical abnormalities in prenatal or newborn analysis or as intermittent follow-up to monitor disease progression following cancer treatment. Combined, the two complementary techniques provide a powerful analysis system.

▶ FLUORESCENT IN SITU HYBRIDIZATION (FISH)

HISTORY

In 1969, Gall and Pardue published the method of in situ hybridization (ISH) using radioactive probes hybridized to cytological specimens. In 1981, Harper demonstrated that the method could be used for gene mapping by localizing the insulin gene to chromosome 11 band p15. Simultaneously, the safety hazards, lengthy hybridizations, and much of the cost associated with radioactivity were eliminated in the 1980s. First, Bauman pioneered fluorescent labeling of RNA probes in 1980. In 1986, Pinkel adapted the fluorescent technique to DNA probes, allowing direct detection that retains the same level of sensitivity achieved by the older isotopic method. Following this fluorescent improvement, cytogenetics laboratories immediately began isolating, cloning, and labeling probes to augment traditional cytogenetic techniques.

By the early 1990s, some commercially produced quality controlled probes began to be available with the menu increasing each year. Although the FDA has approved few probes for clinical use, more are approved each year. Most probes are still considered investigational, and their use on clinical specimen requires that a disclaimer statement be included on the laboratory report. Repeatedly, probes have been shown to be a valuable adjunct to classical cytogenetic analysis by increasing the sensitivity of abnormality detection several-fold. FISH permits visualization, localization, and determination of copy number of specific DNA sequences in either interphase nuclei or on metaphase chromosomes.

THEORY

The basic principles of all molecular techniques are the same and have been covered in detail in Chapters 12 and 13. Briefly, the target DNA inside an intact cell is immobilized to a support medium, the microscope slide. The target DNA and probe DNA are both denatured. The single stranded nucleic acid probe is allowed to hybridize to the single stranded nucleic acid target. Subsequently, the probe's hybridization site is visualized, or detected, by means of a fluorescent label. Unlike all other molecular techniques, in situ hybridization allows the morphological features of cells and chromosomes to remain intact since DNA is not extracted from its normal location. Consequently, the chromosome of origin, the position on the chromosome, and the linear relationship along the length of the chromosome of one probe to another can be visualized.

PROCEDURE

Specimen Requirements

Any intact nucleated cell is a potential target for FISH procedure. Partially degraded specimens, as is sometimes seen in spontaneous abortion materials, may prove difficult to analyze. The target cells are fixed and immobilized onto a glass slide where hybridization occurs. Although cultured specimens provide both metaphase chromosomes and interphase cells for observation, uncultured samples are submitted for analysis. Uncultured specimens, which include amniotic fluid, blood or bone marrow smears, cytospin preparations, touch preparations from solid tumors, thin tissue sections from paraffin embedded blocks and single cells from blastomeres, gametes, or first- or second-polar bodies, are frequently used. Using uncultured specimens greatly improves turnaround time, as cell cultures encompass a lengthy process.

Types of Probes

Probes are derived from one of three classes of DNA: satellite, unique sequence, or whole chromosomes (WC). Satellite and unique sequence probes may be used on metaphase chromosomes or on interphase nuclei. Whole chromosome probes (paints or WCPs) are derived from flow-sorted or microdissected chromo-

somes. Due to their diffuse nature, WCPs are routinely useful only on metaphase chromosomes. Individual small probes may be synthesized or grown in a vector (e.g., BAC or bacterial artificial chromosomes, YAC or yeast artificial chromosomes) then purified of host DNA and other contaminants.

Class I probes consists of repetitive or satellite sequence. The repetitive regions vary in sequence lengths and genome position. The most useful probes of this class are alpha (α)-satellite probes and telomere probes. The α-sequences are specific for most chromosomes making them very useful to count, or enumerate, the number of chromosomes present. The telomeric probes identify telomeres regardless of their location within the chromosome.

Alpha-satellite consists of a 171-base pair (bp) monomer repeated tandemly around the centromere of each human chromosome. The number of repeats is extremely variable between individuals. The majority of α-satellite repeats are identical, but approximately 3% are sufficiently polymorphic so that most chromosomes can be uniquely identified. Except for chromosome pairs 13 and 21 or 14 and 22, all chromosomes can be distinguished from each other using only α-satellite probes. Alpha satellite probes have been useful in enumeration of chromosomes in prenatal, neonatal, abortus, and cancer specimens. They also serve as internal controls for unique sequence and fusion or break-apart probes. However, rare polymorphisms which allow cross-hybridization must be kept in mind when planning experiments.

Telomeric repeats, conserved over species, consist of $(TTAGGG)_n$ sequences and are located at each end of all chromosomes. The numbers of repeating units are variable between individuals and decrease with age. An all-Telomere probe will identify all telomere sequences, even if they have been translocated into an interior chromosomal position. Individual chromosomes cannot be identified using only an all-Telomere probe.

Class II probes consists of unique sequences that may or may not code for genes and occur at only one locus. These probes are designed to detect microdeletions, microduplications, oncogenes, chimeric genes, translocation genes, or subtelomeric rearrangements. For example, recently both fusion and break-apart probes have been designed to detect translocations involved in specific cancers. Many of the original unique sequence probes were designed to aid in the diagnosis of microdeletion syndromes.

Chromosome arm specific subtelomeric probes have been helpful in identifying cryptic rearrangements that involve only very small regions of DNA near the ends of chromosomes. Subtelomeric regions are gene rich so even small imbalances of these regions produce noticeable deleterious phenotypes and mental retardation. Telomere probes may also serve as internal control probes for other unique sequence probes. Rearrangements of the telomeric regions often go undetected by standard cytogenetic techniques.

Class III probes consists of whole chromosome paints (WCPs). WCPs consist of mixtures of many unique and chromosome specific repetitive sequences distributed along the length of a single chromosome.

Slide Pretreatment

Regardless of variations in techniques due to different probe or cell types, quality (flatness) of specimens on the slide directly affects **hybridization** efficiency. To assure that slides have the potential to produce acceptable results, they are monitored during production by constant evaluation, using phase contrast microscopy. By phase evaluation, metaphase chromosomes must dry flat and appear dark gray and have smooth edges and be nonrefractile with little or no visible surrounding cytoplasm. Interphase nuclei should appear flattened and have little visible cytoplasm. Tight control of environmental humidity and temperature ensures cell suspension fixative evaporates at a rate that produces flattened cells without membrane rupture. Environmental conditions are carefully adjusted until acceptable slides are produced. Many laboratories use a humidity and temperature control chamber for slide preparation to ensure consistent results.

Some protocols require freshly prepared slides with little or no aging while other protocols use slides prepared several days before FISH is attempted. Slides can be stored at −20°C if they are not used the same day as prepared. Slides may be artificially "aged" by baking them in an oven at 60°C from 4 to 16 hours, if necessary. Generally, older slide preparations give weaker signals and may require amplification for detection. Some laboratories have greater success with slides less than two weeks old that were not artificially aged if the slides are treated in 2XSSC, pH 7.0 for 30 minutes at 37°C prior to denaturation. This appears to prevent overdenaturation of the DNA that inhibits hybridization. To ensure background banding when counterstaining with DAPI (4,6-*Di*amino-2-*P*henole-*I*ndole) freshly prepared slides may be made, aged overnight, and baked at 65°C for 4 hours before denaturation. Whichever condition is specified in the protocol should be followed rigidly as subsequent aspects of the procedure have been adjusted to work with those specified conditions.

Denature and Dehydrate

Hybridization can occur only if both target and probe DNA are denatured (made single-stranded or melted) and mixed on the slide under appropriate conditions. Probe and sample may be denatured independently or co-denatured after they are mixed on the slide. To denature target chromosomal DNA, place the specimen slide into a solution of 70% formamide in 2XSSC (300 mM NaCl, 30 mM sodium citrate), pH 7.0 at 73°C for 2 to 3 minutes. With this method, no more than two slides can be processed simultaneously because of temperature fluctuations with the addition of each slide. DNA may also be alkali denatured; however, few laboratories use this method. Neither underdenatured nor overdenatured DNA hybridizes probe efficiently. Underdenatured DNA does not allow access by the probe, and overdenaturation breaks DNA, allowing segments to be removed and unavailable for hybridization.

Immediately after **denaturation,** the slides are immersed in successive, cold (−20°C) 70%, 80%, and 95% ethanol rinses for 2 minutes each. The cold ethanol stops the denaturation, aids in maintaining the denatured state, and dehydrates the preparation. Slides should be probed the same day they are denatured.

If denatured separately from target, probes are placed into a hybridization buffer of 50% to 65% formamide in 2XSSC at 70°C for 5 minutes. The denatured probe is then stored immediately in a 4°C ice slurry bath to inhibit reannealing. Denatured probes should be used as soon as possible.

HYBRIDIZATION TO TARGET

To hybridize probe to target, denatured probe is placed onto the denatured target area using a micropipet. Avoiding air bubbles, place the coverslip over the target to spread the probe over the entire target area. Coverslip edges are usually sealed with rubber cement to prevent evaporation. Slides are then incubated at 37°C in a moist chamber from two hours to overnight depending on the probe type. After **hybridization,** the nonbound and nonspecific bound probe must be washed from the slide to allow visualizing a sharp signal at the target site.

The exact wash conditions are called "stringency" and differ for each different type of probe. **Stringency conditions** are determined primarily by base pair (bp) length and GC (guanine-cytosine) composition of the probe. Posthybridization wash stringency is controlled by salt concentration, pH, and temperature. Low-stringency washes fail to remove nonspecific bound probe, resulting in excessive background signals (noise) which may confuse interpretations. Additional washing with more stringent conditions will produce usable results. When initial wash conditions are too stringent, even specifically bound probe is removed, and no signal will be detected. In that case, the entire process will need to be repeated using an initial lower stringency wash.

Stringency conditions may have to be empirically determined for newly developed "home brew" probes or if one hapten is substituted for another when using indirectly labeled probes. Manufacturers provide suggested stringency conditions for commercially available directly labeled probes. When unsatisfactory results are obtained, it is important that only one stringency variable be changed with each repeated attempt. The easiest condition to change is temperature. Table 14-1✪ shows how to alter wash conditions.

Initially, laboratories process slides individually when the FISH test volume is small. However, when test volumes increase, semiautomated heat controlled blocks, similar to thermocyclers, allow simultaneous denaturation, hybridization, and incubation of target and probe on a hotplate like surface. Several slides can be processed simultaneously on this equipment, as long as reaction conditions are similar for all probes. This allows higher test volumes to be processed efficiently.

Label Probe with Fluorochromes

Probes must be tagged or labeled with a fluorochrome to render their location visible after hybridization to the target. Each labeling system has its own advantages and disadvantages that must be considered when selecting a probe. Labeling is possible as molecules may be covalently bonded directly to nucleotides that are then used to replace standard nucleotides in the probe. **Fluorochromes (fluors)** are attached to probes either directly or indirectly to

> ✱ **BOX 14-1 Changing Wash Conditions**
>
> Posthybridization wash conditions are altered to remove nonbound and nonspecific bound probe to produce sharp images of the probe hybridized to the target. Formamide controls the pH.

permit detection. If a fluorochrome molecule is attached directly to the nucleotide, the probe is directly labeled. If an intermediary reporter molecule is attached between the fluorochrome label and nucleotide, the probe is indirectly labeled. The intermediate molecules most used are haptens, either biotin or digoxigenin. Signals of indirectly labeled probes can be amplified by adding another layer of fluorochrome by an antigen-antibody complex.

Hapten or fluorochrome conjugated nucleotides are usually added to probes by nick-translation or random priming if the probe is grown in a vector or by end-labeling if the probe is synthetically synthesized (see Chapter 12). Using nick-translation with enzyme and nucleotide selection, one or more types of nucleotide (A, T, G, or C) can be replaced in the probe. Signals are stronger when the ratio of conjugated nucleotides in the probe is large, but the probe becomes more costly.

Directly Labeled Probes Fewer steps and reagents are required when direct labeled probes are used. Also, less background or nonspecific binding occur. However, directly labeled probes produce weaker signals that cannot be amplified. This is usually not a problem with the larger sized probes like alpha satellite or paints, but may be with many smaller unique sequence probes. Probes can be purchased with optional colored fluorochromes attached, so experiments can be designed to recognize each probe by a unique color.

Only a few individual signal colors can be viewed simultaneously with direct labeling. However, enough individual colors can be viewed to permit multiple simultaneous chromosome enumerations and good internal quality control protocols for deletion or rearrangement clarification.

Indirectly Labeled Probes When using indirectly labeled probes, the fluorochrome must be added to the specimen after the probe has hybridized to the target. If the probe signal is weak at detection, an additional round of intermediate hapten and fluor can be added, by an antigen-antibody complex, to amplify the signal. This is especially helpful when the probe size, as in many unique sequences, is very small or produces a

✪ TABLE 14-1

Posthybridization Wash Conditions

Increase Stringency	Decrease Stringency
Increase temperature	Decrease temperature
Increase formamide concentration	Decrease formamide concentration
Decrease salt concentration	Increase salt concentration

weak signal. Usually, no more than 2 to 3 rounds of amplification are possible as each round increases background noise. Signals may be captured and enhanced by computer imaging systems, if necessary.

Faded signals of indirectly labeled probes on slides that have been stored at −20°C for up to one year can be refreshed. The coverslip on the older specimen must be carefully removed, and a layer of fresh reporter molecules applied. Excess reporter molecules are washed away, fresh counterstain added, and the specimen re-coverslipped.

Fluorochromes (Fluors) and Counterstain

The hybridization site is detected by observing a signal from the fluorochromes, the label. Fluorochromes (fluorophores, fluors) are substances that emit electromagnetic radiation of a long wavelength, usually in the form of visible light, after they have absorbed energy from a source emitting shorter wavelengths of the spectrum. Many different fluorescent colors are available with some of the more common included in Table 14-2✪.

Application of counterstain to the probed specimen facilitates locating metaphase chromosomes or interphase nuclei when scanning at 10–40X magnification. Without counterstain, probe signals are difficult or even impossible to locate. Two counterstains, PI (propidium iodide) and DAPI (4,6-diamino-2-phenoleindole), are most commonly used. Both intercalate into the DNA spiral grooves and fluoresce when excited by the appropriate wavelengths. PI fluoresces red-

dish orange and DAPI fluoresces pale blue when bound to chromosomes or interphase nuclei. Care must be taken to use a counterstain that allows concurrent visualization of the probe. For example, the yellow of a fluorescein labeled probe will be difficult or impossible to see against an orange propidium iodide background. Yellow can be seen through blue, so DAPI is the counterstain of choice in this case.

Detection by Fluorescent Microscopy

Fluorescent microscopes are of two possible designs, either incident or transmitted, based on the position of the light source. Stronger signals are obtained by the incident design where the exciting light is positioned above the specimen stage with light passing through the objective lens to strike the object specimen. The portion of the light not absorbed by the specimen passes beyond the specimen and exits through the standard condenser location. It is helpful to remove the condenser and position a soft black, light-absorbing cloth (or other suitable surface) over the field stop to avoid reflected light. Alternatively, the condenser

✪ TABLE 14-2

Examples of Some Commonly Used Fluorochromes

Fluorochrome	Excitation (nm)	Emission (nm)	Color
Acridine orange	500	530	Reddish
Chromomycin A3*	436–460	470	Yellow
Coumarin	350	450	Blue
CY3	550	570	Red
CY5	650	680	Dark Red
DAPI*	345	425	Blue
Ethidium bromide (EB)	520	610	Red
Fluorescein FITC	490	525	Green
Hoechst 33258*	356	465	Blue
Propidium iodide (PI)*	520	610	Red
Rhodamine	540–560	580	Red
Texas Red	590	615	Red

can be lowered to reduce reflected light. This allows the emitted light of the fluorochromes to travel up through the objective to the eye or camera without interference. A commonly used light source is a high-pressure mercury vapor lamp. A 100–200 Watt lamp maximizes excitation so the smaller signals of unique sequence probes can be visualized.

Appropriate excitation and barrier filters must be inserted in the light path to produce sharp signals. The excitation filter is placed between the exciting light source and the specimen. Exciting wavelengths may be from the UV range (300–400 nm) of the electromagnetic spectrum into the visible blue-green range (400–500 nm). For optimum performance, the excitation filter transmits only a small range of wavelengths at the peak of absorption for the fluorochrome while the rest of the wavelengths are blocked. A matched filter, the barrier, is placed between the fluorochrome-stained specimen and the eye or camera. The barrier filter transmits only the fluorochrome's peak emitted wavelength and blocks all others producing a sharp image. Fluorescent filter sets are matched to optimize excitation and emitted signals of particular fluorochromes.

Recent design improvements in filter housing make it possible to switch rapidly from one matched filter set to another. Also, multi-bandpass filters, which allow simultaneous viewing of 2 to 3 fluors, are available. Each additional fluor viewed simultaneously reduces signal intensity, so weak signals may not be visible when viewed through these filters. The best viewing conditions occur with filter sets optimized for a single fluorochrome.

Each microscope manufacturer produces a continuous range of filter sets so all fluors can be viewed on any microscope. Fluorescent probes are labeled from the manufacturer with optimum excitation and emission ranges. Inspection of filter specifications will lead to selection of acceptable filters for use with each fluorochrome.

Analysis and Quality Control

The American College of Medical Genetics has published standards and Guidelines for Clinical Genetics Laboratories. Compliance is voluntary, but these guidelines closely agree with standards imposed by the College of American Pathology (CAP) who has deemed status with the Clinical Laboratory Improvement Act (CLIA) in regulating all genetics testing laboratories.

In order to ensure consistent and reliable daily clinical FISH results, several policies and practices should be instituted for probe validation and use:

- Blinded analysis of each specimen and external control specimen should be split between two competent technologists whose results normally agree within 5%.
- If there is suspicion of mosaicism, analysis should be performed on two independently processed specimen slides.
- Each laboratory must establish criteria for selecting cells for analysis (enumeration) for each probe and cell type. Different criteria may apply to different types of probes or specimens.
- The technologist must be familiar with characteristics of both probe and specimen. Especially for cancer specimens, technologists must recognize morphologically which cell types to include in the analysis.
- In general, interphase cells should have smooth margins, must not be broken, and must not overlap with other cells.
- Signals should be distinct, bright, and easily counted.
- There should be no cross-hybridization, fluorescent particles, or extraneous signals or "noise" in the background.
- Whole chromosomes paints are not interpretable in interphase cells, and analysis must be confined to metaphase cells.
- Both internal (known probe on target chromosome) and external controls (known negative and/or positive cell line) must be used for validation of probes on each cell type used clinically for establishing technologist proficiency and periodically to confirm proficiency.
- Standards are probe type specific, but in general, sensitivity and specificity of 98% are required.
- A positive control that most closely resembles the test situation with a known percentage of normal and abnormal cells should be included in each run.
- There must be documentation for number and type of signals (test and internal control signal) observed in each cell. Tallies will include cells with less than the expected number, the expected number, greater than the expected number of signals, and noncountable cells with signals. Approximately 90% of interphase cells should meet scoring criteria. *Exception:* The criteria used in gene amplification analysis may include a category where signals are so numerous they coalesce and are uncountable.
- Criteria for countable signals are necessary, especially in interphase cells. For example, cells with all compact signals are countable, but cells with split signals are not countable if the split is wider than

the signal. Criteria must include consideration of morphological difference in DNA appearance during different stages of the cell cycle.

■ Cells with no internal control signal or greater than the expected number of control signals are not countable, but should be included in the tallies as quality control (QC) indicators.

■ Counts from at least 50 and as many as 500 or more interphase cells may be necessary, depending on the diagnosis and probe type. However, counts from metaphase chromosomes may require only 5-20 cells, depending on diagnosis and probe type.

■ Nonreportable results should be repeated.

■ A minimum of two representative images (photographs or digital images) for each cell line should be maintained as part of the permanent record.

■ Results of individual's scores on test and controls must be tracked over time to assess test performance and trends.

■ All standard laboratory QC, such as testing of new reagents on control specimens before use on clinical specimens, apply.

It should be noted these regulations are currently under review. Many users have made negative comments regarding the practicality and necessity of some items.

Reporting

FISH reports must follow the rules and be written in International System of Cytogenetic Nomenclature (ISCN) language. A worldwide committee of experts reviews, updates, and periodically publishes the latest accepted version of this language. Its use ensures that interpretations will be understood worldwide. The language for reporting FISH includes whether the analysis was performed on metaphase (ish) or interphase cells (nuc ish), probe source (gene or locus symbol), the number of scored cells (5–500), and detailed hybridization results (X1, X2, etc.). A verbal interpretation, in layman's or non-geneticist's terms, is included in the report. Limitations, including those on manufacturer's product inserts, must be included on the report. Both normal and abnormal reportable results must be within ranges established and documented, with a 95% confidence level, from appropriate databases. Reports, in which analyte-specific reagents (ASRs) were used, must include a specific disclaimer statement provided by CLIA, but a clarifying interpretation from the laboratory may be included.

► CLINICAL APPLICATIONS

Applications of FISH have developed rapidly due to the ease in providing information for difficult cytogenetic analysis cases and the improvement in speed over traditional methods. One initial push for probe development was to map genes to particular chromosome or chromosome bands. FISH helped create an early gene map and is still used to localize isolated genes or DNA sequences and confirm sequence orientation. Another early use was for clarification of microdeletions that are often at or beyond resolution of the light microscope used for analysis of banded chromosomes. Additional uses include identification of marker chromosomes; identification of breakpoints in structural rearrangements; detection of cryptic translocations; numerical determination in prenatal, constitutional, and cancer specimens; identification of specific rearrangements or gene amplifications associated with cancer; monitoring engraftment in opposite sex bone marrow transplants; and in preimplantation genetic diagnosis. The clinical applications of FISH continue to be developed and refined.

CONTIGUOUS GENE SYNDROMES (MICRODELETIONS AND MICRODUPLICATIONS)

Contiguous gene syndromes have been defined as syndromes that result from a disruption of an adjoining cluster of genes. However, the individual genes within the cluster may appear as single gene disorders inherited in Mendelian fashion within families. Sometimes one to several contiguous genes in a small region may be disrupted so that several overlapping phenotypes may be produced in different patients, making diagnosis difficult. The majority of these syndromes were well characterized clinically before their cytogenetic etiology was determined. As laboratory techniques have improved, some syndromes have now been recognized clinically only after the detection of an identical chromosomal abnormality in several unrelated patients. There are currently approximately 30 contiguous gene syndromes with another one or two being added yearly. Table 14-3✿ lists some of the most common contiguous gene syndromes.

✪ TABLE 14-3

Some of the More Common Contiguous Gene Syndromes

Critical Region	Syndrome	Brief Clinical Features
del(4)(p16)	Wolf-Hirschorn	Craniofacial defects sometimes called "Greek Warrior Helmet." Pronounced growth and mental retardation.
del(5)(p15)	Cri-du-chat	Distinctive cry of infant sounds like a cat's meow, mental retardation, lack of speech, microcephaly, asymmetric growth.
del(1)(p36)	1p36 Deletion (Recognized only after cytogenetic identification of deletion)	Developmental and mental retardation, hypotonia, growth abnormalities, cranial and facial abnormalities, cardiac defects.
del(7)(p13)	Greig-Cephalopoly-syndactyly	Mental and developmental retardation, polysyndactyly, craniosynostosis.
del(7)(q11.2)	Williams	Cardiac defects, characteristic facies, very social personality, frequently increased musical abilities.
del(8)(q24)	Langer-Giedion	Facial and limb defects, mental retardation.
del(11)(p13)	Aniridia-Wilms tumor–Mental Retardation (WAGR)	Absence of the iris of the eye, mental retardation, genital development impaired, tumors of the kidney.
del(13)(q14)	Retinoblastoma	Tumors of the retina by age 2–3 years; bilateral if deletion inherited, unilateral if deletion acquired.
del(15)(q11-12)	Prader-Willi	Mild mental retardation, early feeding difficulties, small feet and hands, obsessive food consumption, early obesity.
del(15)(q11-12)	Angelman	Severe mental retardation, lack of speech, inappropriate laughter, "puppet-like" gait (ataxia).
del(16)(p13.3)	Alpha-Thalassemia with Mental Retardation	Characteristic facial features, mental retardation, alpha-thalassemia.
del(16)(p13.3)	Rubinstein-Taybi	Broad thumbs and great toe, mental retardation, characteristic facies includes beaked nose, short stature.
del(17)(p11.2)	Smith-Magenis	Mental retardation, short fingers, brachycephaly, midface hypoplasia, self-mutilation behaviors common.
dup(17)(p11.2)	Charot-Marie-Tooth 1A	Developmental delay, characteristic facies.
del(17)(p13.3)	Miller-Dieker	Lissencephaly, mental retardation, anomalies of heart, kidney and digestive track, failure to thrive with short life expectancy (<2 years).
del(20)(p11.23p12.2)	Alagille	Vertebral arch defects, pulmonary stenosis, chronic cholestasis, dysmorphic facial features.
del(22)(q11.2)	DiGeorge/Velocardio-facial	Abnormal or absent thymus and parathyroid, conotruncal heart defects, cleft palate, characteristic facies, hypocalcemia.
dup(22)(q11.2)	Cat-Eye	Coloboma, choanal atresia, learning disabilities, mental retardation.
del(X)(p22.3)	Xp22.3 Deletion (Kallman syndrome)	X-linked ichthyosis, mental retardation, epilepsy, ocular albinism.
del(Y)(q13)	Yq Chromosome Deletion	Idiopathic infertility, unilateral cryptochidism.

Individually, contiguous gene syndromes are rare de novo events. Most of the known disruptions are chromosomal microdeletions, all of which are thought to be underdiagnosed. One of the more recognized disruptions, a deletion of chromosome 22q11 region, accounts for at least 15% of all congenital heart defects. Collectively these syndromes contribute significantly to mental retardation, developmental delay, learning disabilities, and disease.

A significant percentage of individuals with a phenotype consistent with one of the contiguous gene syndromes have abnormalities not detectable by the best quality high-resolution chromosome analysis. High-resolution chromosome analysis has a resolution limit of

✳ **BOX 14-3**   **Detection of Microdeletion Syndrome**

The first microdeletion syndrome was detected cytogeneti-cally in 1982. Note the different phenotypes for deletion or duplication of the same material. According to current un-derstanding of formation of these nonrandom rearrange-ments, both duplication and deletion syndromes should exist for each disturbed genomic region. Probes to detect some of these syndromes are available commercially, and some are available only in the laboratory of the investiga-tor who isolated and cloned them.

approximately 2–3 Mb while FISH can routinely detect deletions in the range of 1–2 Mb (Figure 14-2■). In cases of very small deletions, a definitive diagnosis often can-not be made cytogenetically. For example, only about 70% of Prader-Willi syndrome patient's deletions can be detected by high-resolution cytogenetic techniques. Ap-propriate probes can detect deletions in an additional 25% of affected individuals. Not only is the detection rate increased, but also the time required to perform the diagnostic procedure is reduced.

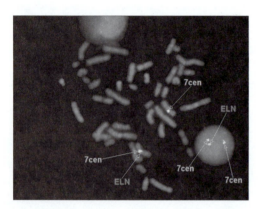

■ **FIGURE 14-2** A high-resolution chromosome analysis. Williams syndrome is diagnosed most easily using a unique locus specific sequence probe labeled here in red. The probe contains the sequence for the elastin gene which is deleted in Williams syndrome patients. The control probe, an alpha satellite sequence, is la-beled in green. The internal control probe verifies that both copies of chromosome seven, the chromosome on which the Williams syndrome critical region occurs, are present. All alpha satellite and some locus specific probes are large enough to be visible in both interphase cells and metaphase spreads. The target sequence deletion is indicated by the lack of a red signal on one chromosome seven and only one red signal with two green signals in the interphase cells. (Image courtesy of Gregory Mengden, Ph.D., Southwest Genetics, San Antonio, TX.)

Microdeletions of these specific regions occur more frequently than can be accounted for by chance. Re-cent investigations by Lupski have detected unique characteristics of the DNA architecture, low copy repeats (LCR), on both sides of the frequently deleted regions. LCR in close proximity contribute to misalign-ment during meiosis which predispose those regions to nonrandom unequal crossover events during meiosis. When genetic exchanges occur between the mis-aligned regions, the result is a small deletion in one chromosome and a small duplication of the same ma-terial in the homolog.

Lupski's work predicts that a complementary dupli-cation syndrome should exist for each of the recog-nized deletion syndromes. Recently, cytogenetics laboratories have begun to identify duplication syn-dromes for a few of these regions. Duplications of ge-netic material are generally better tolerated, producing milder but different phenotypes than do deletions of the same material. The generally milder phenotypes make it more difficult for physicians to recognize a syndrome and request genetic testing. Duplications for these very small regions are detectable only by FISH in interphase cells or by genomic microarrays. As the ge-netic etiologies of milder syndromic features are recog-nized and FISH techniques continue to improve, more duplication of these small regions will be identified.

A very small percentage of patients with a clinical diagnosis of some contiguous gene syndromes do not have deletions or duplications demonstrable with ei-ther chromosome analysis or FISH. For many of these individuals, a phenomena known as **uniparental di-somy (UPD)** has been demonstrated using molecular techniques described elsewhere in this text. UPD is the inheritance of both copies of a single chromosome from a single parent. This is a rare event, but has been confirmed for several different chromosomes in nu-merous individuals by several different laboratories.

Since the correct amount of DNA is present, UPD causes no deleterious effect in the individual unless the involved chromosome contains an imprinted region.

Imprinting is a modification of DNA that occurs during gametogenesis. Genes in imprinted regions are differentially expressed during the individual's lifetime. Some regions are imprinted during maternal meiosis, and other regions, sometimes adjacent to maternal imprints, are imprinted during paternal meiosis. Loss of imprinted regions on a chromosome from one parent due to UPD, or deletion, results in disease. In these rare cases of UPD, there is no deletion or duplication, and neither chromosome analysis nor FISH is diagnostic.

PRENATAL DIAGNOSIS

An amniotic fluid or chorionic villus specimens for prenatal analysis may be obtained from any woman who is at risk for having a child with a chromosome abnormality. The most frequent risk factor is age. As women age, their risk for **trisomy** 21 increases from approximately 1/2000 live births at age twenty to 1/12 live

births at age forty-seven years. The risk for all trisomies increases with maternal age, but none as dramatically as for trisomy 21. Collectively, 1/200 live born individuals has a chromosome abnormality. Some abnormalities have no phenotypic effect, but may affect reproduction, some produce only mild phenotypes, and some produce severe phenotypes with very early demise. Table 14-4✪ lists the most commonly encountered syndromes with numerical abnormalities observed in both prenatal and constitutional specimens.

A commercial probe cocktail, specific for chromosomes 13, 18, 21, X, and Y, each labeled with a different colored fluor, is used for rapid detection of numerical abnormalities for these chromosomes in uncultured prenatal specimens. Numerical aneuploidies of these chromosomes represent approximately 75% of all abnormalities currently detected prenatally by classical cytogenetic techniques. Cell culture is not required for FISH, so the results are available within a day or two of specimen receipt. Infrequent trisomies

✪ TABLE 14-4

The Most Common Numerical Chromosomal Syndromes

Karyotype	Syndrome	Features	Frequency
47,XX,+13 46,XY,t(13;15)	Trisomy 13 or Patau	Severe mental and developmental retardation, microcephaly, congenital heart, kidney and open scalp defects, cleft lip and palate, < 10% survival beyond 1 year	1/10,000–1/12,000 live births
47,XY,+18	Trisomy 18 or Edward	Severe mental and developmental retardation, low set ears, small mouth, index finger overlapping the middle and ring fingers, rocker-bottom feet, cleft lip and palate, mean survival 2.5 months	1/6,000–1/8,000 live births
47,XX,+21 46,XY,i(21;21) 46,XX,t(14;21)	Trisomy 21 or Down	Flat face, Brushfield spots, up slanting eyes, small ears, hands and feet, IQ usually 25–50, premature aging, 70% have heart defects, increased incidence of respiratory infections and leukemia, early Alzheimer.	1/650–1/700 live births
45,X 45,X/46,XX 46,X,i(Xq)	Turner	Lax skin on nape of neck, short stature, lymphodemia of feet and hands at birth, narrowing of aorta, amenorrhea, infertile, 98%–99% of conceptions result in spontaneous abortion	1/1000 live birth females
47,XXX 46,XX/47,XXX 48,XXXX 49,XXXXX	Multiple X	Most have normal phenotype, menstrual irregularities, taller than sibs, premature menopause; some are sterile, some have decreased IQs and impaired fine motor skills	1/1000 live birth females
47,XXY 48,XXXY	Klinefelter	Tall stature, sterile, and small genetalia; some have gynecomastia and various degrees of reduced IQs	1/1000 live birth males
47,XYY 48,XXYY 48,XYYY	XYY	Most have normal phenotype, tall stature, fertile with increased incidence of severe acne.	1/1000 live birth males

✳ BOX 14-4

Frequencies at live birth are lower than frequencies observed prenatally. Significant spontaneous abortion loss is observed for all categories between prenatal detection and term delivery. All trisomies are not the result of a free extra copy of the chromosome. For example, Robertson-

ian translocations, exchanges between D and G group chromosomes, are responsible for approximately 2–3% of affected live-birth Down syndrome individuals. Carriers of Robertsonian translocations have a significant increased risk of affected pregnancies.

for other chromosomes, such as 8, 9, and 22, are detected cytogenetically, but not by this kit. Most of the 25% of anomalies not detected consist of structural abnormalities that are distributed throughout the genome. Phenotypes are determined by the segments of the genome involved in the abnormality so the range observed varies from mild to lethal. Abnormalities the size of those seen in contiguous gene syndrome are rarely detected prenatally. This probe set does not detect any structural rearrangements involving any chromosome, including those involving the chromosomes detected by the cocktail. Nevertheless, the AneuVysion assay (enumeration of 13, 18, 21, X, and Y), approved by the FDA for prenatal diagnosis, has proven to be 99.8% concordant with standard cytogenetic techniques for the abnormalities it is designed to detect. Currently, classical cytogenetics remains the best genome scan readily available.

ACQUIRED ABNORMALITIES

Cancer is a genetic disease. Cancers studied so far appear to have some form of gene mutation as the critical initiating and progression factors. Some mutations can be seen as cytogenetic abnormalities, numerical or structural, while other mutations are observable only by molecular methods. Cytogenetics has guided discovery of genes important in carcinogenesis by identifying specific chromosomal regions nonrandomly disrupted in cancerous tissues.

The classic example of a chromosome abnormality diagnostic for a particular cancer is derivative chromosome 22, or der(22), of CML (chronic myelogenous leukemia; see Figure 14-3■). This abnormality was identified by classical cytogenetic techniques in 1960 by Nowell and Hungerford. The der(22) was later demonstrated to result from a translocation, t(9;22)(q34;q11), which juxtaposes the *abl* oncogene on chromosome 9 with the *bcr* (break cluster regions) sequence on chromosome 22. The translocation pro-

duces a chimeric gene that is always active and that produces an abnormal kinase. Normal kinases, important in controlling the cell cycle, are regulated by being turned on then turned off as needed. This translocation, or one of its modifications, is found in greater than 95% of CML cases. It is believed the remaining cases may have another disease that is masquerading as CML and may mimic other diagnostic characteristics.

Fusion and break-apart translocation probes have been designed to identify specific translocations which may be diagnostic or prognostic in cancer studies. **Fusion probes** were designed to identify genomic regions that have been moved close to each other by translocation. The first fusion probe developed detects the chimeric gene region of CML patients. Fusion probes consist of two probes that each spans a breakpoint on one of the involved chromosome. Each probe is labeled a different color. On the chimeric (translocated) chromosomal region a third color, due to blending of the two individual fluorescent colors brought together by the translocation, is detected. In normal cells or normal chromosomes, the two probes hybridize at distant locations and produce two distinct different colored signals. The opposite type of probe is a "break-apart" that detects segments which have moved away from each other. **Break-apart probes** span the critical breakpoints and are detected as an increase in the number of signals of a specific color.

Diagnostic probes detect the primary or initiating genetic change observed at the earliest cancer stage. As cancer progresses, additional secondary changes accu-

✳ BOX 14-5

The types of genes identified most often involved in carcinogenesis are oncogenes, tumor suppressor genes, and other genes important in cell cycle regulation such as cytokines.

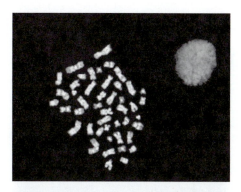

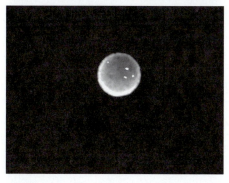

■ **FIGURE 14-3** The translocation characteristic of chronic myelogenous leukemia can be detected cytogenetically or by one of several probe types. The image above depicts a fusion probe used to detect the translocation. The probe for the nine critical region is labeled in red. The BCR region sequence is labeled in green. The two colors are placed side-by-side, resulting in a color change to yellow, when portions of both critical regions are translocated. Analysis can be performed on either chromosomes or interphase nuclei. (Images courtesy of Siddharth Adhvaryu, Ph.D. University of Texas Health Science Center at San Antonio, San Antonio, TX.)

mulate. Some changes are specific and some appear to be random. For instance, as CML progresses from the chronic to the acute stage, additional nonrandom cytogenetic changes occur. The specific secondary changes are +8, i(17q), +19, +21 or an additional der(22) with a variable order of appearance. These specific secondary changes may be accompanied by random changes. Probe cocktails are available which detect the specific secondary changes that appear before physical symptoms and other features of disease crisis are observed. Thus, these secondary changes are predictive of disease progression. After initial diagnostic staging by classical cytogenetics, either serial cytogenetic studies or serial FISH studies are critical in monitoring response to therapy and disease progression.

FISH gene amplification analysis on tumor materials correlates with results obtained by other molecular methods such as Southern blot, dot-blot, quantitative PCR, or expression arrays. Since FISH examines and evaluates individual cells, intratumoral heterogeneity, which cannot be detected by other techniques, is readily assessed. *Her2/neu* in breast cancer is an example of gene expression/amplification readily assayed with FISH from fine needle aspiration biopsy. *Her2/neu* expression status is predictive of response to chemotherapy, but its relation to hormonal therapy remains uncertain. Thus, FISH for *Her2/neu* provides information important to the patient and physician in making treatment decisions. The patient described in the case study would have had classical cytogenetic analysis of her initial tumor combined with some other molecular approach to define the abnormalities present. Treatment of her recurrent cancer with Herceptin might be followed by FISH for *Her2/neu* expression.

No other application of FISH is under development or experiencing more utilization than in diagnosis of both soft tissue and solid tissue cancers. Table 14-5✪ shows examples of probes developed to detect genes identified as important in the development of solid cancers. Table 14-6✪ lists samples of probes that have been developed to detect the most commonly observed cytogenetic abnormalities in leukemia and lymphoma. Methods that convert tests to automated or semiautomated procedures are appearing at a rapid pace, and probes specific for solid tumors or for hematopoietic tumors have been developed. These automated systems work best with disaggregated tissues where single cell solutions are firmly affixed to slides before denaturation and hybridization.

RESEARCH APPLICATIONS

The potential for FISH has been recognized and adopted for many applications throughout the clinical and research laboratory. Development of appropriate sequence specific probes has allowed detection and expression studies of viral, bacterial, and parasitic organisms. These FISH methods are often as fast and specific as PCR methods.

Isolated sequences, including genes, can be localized in the genome and the linear relationship of one sequence to another determined. The success or failure of experiments attempting to insert sequences into host organisms can be verified, and fragments, markers, and complex rearrangements of cancer or constitutional

✪ TABLE 14-5

Probes Important for Solid Tumor Assessment

Gene(s)	Location	Probe Type	Cancer
Epidermal Growth Factor Receptor Gene EGFR (HER-1/erb-B1)	7p12	EGFR/CEP Copy Number, Dual Color	Breast
HER-2/neu or c-erbB2 or HER-2	17q11.2-q12, 17q11.1-q11.1	Dual Color, Copy Number	Breast, Ovarian, Multiple
C-myc Oncogenes	8q24.12-q24.13	LSI C-MYC Amplification	Breast, Prostate, Multiple
ZNF217 Candidate Oncogenes	20q13	Copy Number or Amplification	Breast
Cyclin D1 locus (PRADI and CCND1)	11q13	Dual Color, Copy Number	Breast
RB1 Tumor Suppressor	3q14.3	Single Color	Retinoblastoma, Multiple
EGFR, C-myc, Chromosome 5, Chromosome 6	5p15.2, 6p11.1-q11, 7p12, 8q24	Copy Number, Multi Color	Lung
p53	17p13.1	Copy Number	Bladder; Multiple
C-myc	8p22,8q24, 12q24.13, 8p11.1-q11.1	Multi-color Probe Cocktail	Prostate
p16 Tumor Suppressor; Chromosome 9	9p21	Dual Color	Bladder, Multiple
Chromosomes 3, 7 and 17, p16 Tumor Suppressor	3p11.1-q11.1, 7p11-q11.1, 9p21, 17p11.1-q11.1	Multi-color Probe Cocktail, Copy Number	Bladder
Androgen Receptor Gene	Xq12		Prostate
N-myc Oncogene	2p224.1	Single Color, Copy Number	Multiple

materials can be identified, DNA damage from environmental exposures can be evaluated, and components of cell structures can be identified and gene expression measured. The list of uses continues to grow.

► ADVANTAGES AND LIMITATIONS OF THE FISH PROCEDURE

No one test modality can stand alone in all situations. Reaching an accurate diagnosis often involves analysis by several modes with a contribution to diagnostic results from each. In situations requiring determination of the presence or absence of a specific sequence, FISH clearly is the definitive diagnostic test. When using FISH, a specific question is asked about a specific region, and the result is a specific answer about that region. As with any technique, there are both advantages and limitations.

ADVANTAGES

- Results are available within 1-2 days.
- Results are generally specific and highly accurate for most applications.
- Probes are commercially available, labeled in a selection of fluors for almost all centromere, telomere, cancer gene rearrangements, and contiguous gene syndrome regions.
- Cell culture is not necessary, except when whole chromosome paints are used.
- Viable cells are not necessary.

LIMITATIONS

- Commercial probes are available for only the most commonly encountered unique sequence disorder regions. Family specific regions of interest, such as

✪ TABLE 14-6

Probes Important for Hematopoietic Disorder Assessment

Gene	Location	Probe Type	Cancer
AML1;ETO	t(8;21)(q22;q22)	Dual Color, Dual Fusion Translocation	AML
PML;RARA	t(15;17)(q22;q21.1)	Dual Color, Translocation	AML
RARA	17q21	Dual Color, Break Apart	AML
MLL	11q23	Dual Color, Break Apart	AML, ALL
MYH11;CBFB	inv(16)(p13q22) t(16;16)(p13;q23)	Dual Color, Break Apart	AML
ABL;BCR	t(9;22)(q34;q11.2)	Dual Color, Dual Fusion Translocation	AML, ALL, CML
ABL;BCR	t(9;22)(q34;q11.2)	Dual Color, Translocation	AML, ALL, CML
ABL;BCR	t(9;22)(q34;q11.2)	Dual Color, Single Fusion Translocation	AML, ALL, CML
D5S721/EGR1	Chromosome 5, 5q13	Dual Color	MDS
D7S522	Chromosome 7, 7q31	Dual Color	MDS
Centromeric	Chromosome 8	Single Color	AML, CML
D5S721/CSF1R	Chromosome 5, 5q33-q34	Dual Color	AML, MDS
D20S108	20q12	Single Color	AML, MDS
p16 Tumor Suppressor	9p21	Dual Color	ALL
TEL/AML1	t(12;21)(p13;q22)	Dual Color, Fusion	ALL
Chromosome 8 MYC/IGH	(8;14)(q24;q11)	Tri-color, Dual Fusion	ALL, NHL
p53	17p13.1	Single Color, Copy Number	CLL, NHL, MM
D13S25, D13S319	13q14.3	Single Color	CLL, MM
MYC	t(8;22)(q24;q11) t(2;8)(p11;q24)	Dual Color, Break Apart Rearrangement	ALL, NHL
IGH	14q32	Dual Color, Break Apart Rearrangement	NHL, MM

ALL = acute lymphocytic leukemia

NHL = non-hodgkin's lymphoma

MDS = myelodys plastic syndrome

CLL = chronic lymphocytic leukemia

AML = acute myelogenous leukemia

MM = multiple myeloma

CML = chronic myelogenous leukemia

private rearrangement breakpoints or rare deletion syndromes, may need to be isolated and cloned by the laboratory.

- The false positive rate is sometimes as high as 5-10% for detecting minimal residual disease of leukemia specimens that are characterized by monosomy.

- No information is obtained about the rest of the genome.

- Not applicable to degraded cells or DNA.

- An epi-fluorescent microscope equipped with appropriate filter sets and a digital imaging system is necessary.

▶ ADVANCED APPLICATIONS

The first six advanced applications mentioned require metaphase chromosomes prepared by conventional cytogenetic air-dried techniques. In addition to human

✻ BOX 14-6

Diagnostic work has progressed faster in hematological disorders than in solid tissues since soft tissues have been more amenable to culture than solid tissue cancers. The probes represented in Table 14-6 are only a small portion of what has been developed to detect the most commonly observed cytogenetic abnormalities in leukemia and lymphoma. New probes with greater sensitivity and specificity are constantly being released. Some genes play a role in the carcinogenesis of different cell lines and tissues and may appear in multiple probe panels.

cells, all have been applied to many types of animal cells, including multiple primates, rodents, birds, and fish, as well as plant cells. The last techniques require no chromosome preparations.

WHOLE CHROMOSOME PAINTS

The technique of "painting" a single entire chromosome a color has been available since the late 1980s. By the early 1990s, commercially available whole chromosome painting probes for each human chromosome, labeled with either orange or green, were available. By the mid 1990s paints specific for single chromosome arms or single region of one arm became available. Whole chromosome paints (WCPs) are based on sequences unique to each chromosome and include both repetitive and single copy sequences. Shared repetitive sequences are not included in painting probes and are suppressed with excess unlabeled complementary sequences, example, Cot 1. Consequently, telomeres and centromeric regions do not fluoresce. Due to the diffuse nature of DNA during interphase, WCPs cannot generally be interpreted in interphase cells and are useful only on metaphase spreads. WCPs detect chromosomal regions from a specific chromosome regardless of their rearranged location in the genome. Paints are very useful in clarifying complex rearrangements such as those often seen in cancer specimens.

ALL-TELOMERE FISH

Since many deleterious rearrangements have been detected that involve only the tips of chromosomes, which are hard to detect with classic cytogenetic techniques, a method allowing each telomere to be investigated in a single experiment was needed. The *Telomere Probe Kit* contains a slide with 24 grids, each grid prespotted with chromosome specific differentially labeled subtelomere probe. Analysis of metaphase chromosomes must be performed in each of the 24 grids to ensure no chromosome has a cryptic rearranged telomere. Using this kit, rearrangements of subtelomeric regions are often detected in children with mental retardation or learning disabilities of unknown etiology, especially when associated with minor physical anomalies such at those seen in the face, ears, hands, or feet.

MULTICOLOR FISH

M-FISH (multifluor or multiplex) uses five different colored fluorochromes combined in various proportions to produce 31 combinations of color. These combinations are sufficient to uniquely and simultaneously identify each human chromosome, 22 autosome pairs plus X and Y. Each whole chromosome probe is labeled with a unique combination of the five fluors. The cytogenetic specimen is probed with a cocktail containing all 24 whole chromosome probes. The colors produced by combinatorial labeling are not sufficiently unique to identify each visually with the naked eye. Computer imaging and color interpretation are necessary. In M-FISH, a complex series of narrow band-pass excitation and emission filters sequentially image the individual whole chromosome probes. Dedicated software assigns a classification color for each chromosome that is distinguishable to the human eye, and combines the separate images into one. The combined image is displayed on the computer screen and can be printed. M-FISH has been used to identify complex rearrangements of constitutional specimens, markers of unknown origin, and small rearrangements. Resolution limitations usually prevent observation of rearrangements smaller than 2–3 Mb.

SPECTRAL KARYOTYPING

Like M-FISH, multicolor spectral karyotyping (SKY) involves the use of combinatorial labeling to produce 24 distinctively colored whole chromosome paints to uniquely identify each human chromosome. SKY differs from M-FISH in its image acquisition process. In SKY, discrimination of the spectral profile at each pixel of an image requires Fourier spectroscopy with charged coupled device imaging and specialized software. The assigned classification colors of the unique spectral signature of each chromosome is captured in a single image and projected onto the computer screen for viewing or printing. SKY has been used to identify chromosomal material of unknown origin, including small markers, complex rearrangements from cancer and constitutional material, amplified genes as represented by double minute chromosomes and homogeneously staining regions, and small translocations. Resolution limitations usually prevent detection of the smallest abnormalities such as those seen in the contiguous gene syndromes.

COLOR BANDING OR RX-FISH

Two fluorescent color-banding techniques are possible. In the first, two sets of subregional specific probes labeled in either red or green fluorochromes produce a color pattern of approximately 110 bands per haploid when hybridized to human chromosomes. The pattern is sufficient to uniquely identify all human chromosomes, but there are insufficient bands to identify other than large anomalies.

A second methods uses probes derived from gibbon flow sorted chromosomes. Gibbons, either *Hylobates concolor* or *Hylobates syndactylus,* are among the great apes closely related to humans with a sequence homology of approximately 98%. Since evolutionary divergence of humans and gibbons, several chromosomal rearrangements have occurred. Using a combinatorial labeling technique with dyes Cy3, Cy5 and FITC, 7 distinct colored bands are produced when gibbon whole chromosome probe is hybridized to human chromosomes. A fluorescent microscope equipped with a quad band-pass filter and a digital imaging system is necessary to view the color-banding pattern. This technique has been useful in some clinical cases by identifying breakpoints of both solid and soft tissue cancers, identifying the origin of marker chromosomes and intrachromosomal rearrangements in constitutional cases. However, the technique usually produces 100 bands or less so that most small deletions, inversions, and translocations are not detected.

COMPARATIVE GENOME HYBRIDIZATION

CGH compares a normal human genome (control-1) to a test human genome (target), such as a tumor specimen. CGH has the advantage of not requiring culture or metaphase cells from the target. Many tumors have been refractory to growth in vitro so standard cytogenetic analysis has been difficult or impossible. The entire extracted genomic DNA of both target and control are fractionated and each labeled with a different color, such as green fluorescein isothyocyanate (FITC) for the control and red tetramethylthodamine isothiocyanate (TRITC) for the target. Denatured and labeled control and target DNA are mixed in equal quantities and probed to a normal denatured control-2 metaphase chromosome preparation which is fixed to a slide. The control-1 and target compete for hybridization sites on the metaphase chromosomes of control-2. If both probes are present in equal amounts, a blending of the two colors will be seen. An extra copy of a sequence in the target will show the target's probe color at that sequence on the control-2 metaphase. A deleted sequence in the target will show control-1's probe color at that sequence on the metaphase. This quantitative two-color FISH technique is very powerful in identifying complex unbalanced rearrangements often present in tumors or constitutional studies. CGH has also identified gene amplifications and marker chromosomes. CGH has become the method of choice for analysis of tissues difficult to culture or from which quality banded metaphases cannot be prepared.

MICROARRAYS

Genomic microarrays are in development and limited use by many researchers and are beginning to be available commercially. Indications are that genomic microarrays may eventually provide whole genome scans that will detect very small deletions and duplications exceeding current high-resolution cytogenetic techniques. Genomic arrays are a modification of CGH in which small clones of selected regions of normal control DNA are spotted in duplicate in a random pattern onto prepared glass slides. Digested and differentially color-labeled specimen (target) and normal DNA (control) are mixed in equal amounts and hybridized to the slide. Following hybridization, computer interpretation of the spectrum for each hybridization on the slide shows the expected, a duplicated or a deleted amount of DNA as compared with the normal control. A computer collates the information for each spot and draws a graph indicating the amount of DNA in each region of every chromosome represented on the array.

Microarrays are proving to be useful for identifying duplications and deletions of both constitutional and acquired disorders. Rearrangements, such as balanced translocations or inversions, are not detected. Also arrays are being developed to span large genes such as cystic fibrosis or muscular dystrophy. Other anticipated chips would assay for common cancer genes or the known contiguous gene syndromes. These "cytogenetic chips" could increase the resolution of chromosome analysis in prenatal diagnosis to include not only numerical abnormalities but also all recognized contiguous gene syndromes. Genomic microarray technology is equivalent to performing hundreds to thousands of FISH experiments simultaneously on the same specimen. The potential for genomic microarrays is enormous.

SUMMARY

FISH is a rapidly evolving and expanding molecular cytogenetic technique for determining the presence or absence of specific sequences of DNA. It may be used alone or in combination with classic cytogenetic techniques. Unlike all other molecular techniques, in situ hybridization techniques such as FISH allow the morphological features of cells and chromosomes to remain intact since DNA is not extracted from its normal location. Most probes for FISH, however, are still considered to be investigational by the FDA, and their use on clinical specimen requires that a disclaimer statement be included on the laboratory report.

Probe availability will gradually improve as more and more regions are cloned and made commercially available. Results are available in one to two days, and greatly enhance classic cytogenetic resolution when applied appropriately. FISH promises to become a major test modality in the clinical cytogenetic laboratory.

POINTS TO REMEMBER

▶ Classical cytogenetics is frequently more appropriate for initial genetic evaluations of individuals with particular genetic syndromes, for cancer specimens, or for periodic follow-up in cancer studies to monitor disease progression or response to therapy.

▶ FISH is more appropriate for determining the presence or absence of a specific sequence when the overall scan appears normal, but the phenotype indicates an abnormality, as a quick screen for major numerical abnormalities in prenatal or newborn analysis, or as intermittent follow-up to monitor disease progression following cancer treatment.

▶ Probes are derived from one of three classes of DNA: satellite, unique sequence, or whole chromosomes.

▶ Probes must be tagged or labeled with a fluorochrome to render their location visible after hybridization to the target.

▶ The case report includes a description of the chromosomal finding in International System of Cytogenetic Nomenclature (ISCN) format with interpretations in common medical and lay terminology.

LEARNING ASSESSMENT QUESTIONS

1. What is a label?
   a. a molecule, such as a hapten, attached to a probe
   b. DAPI
   c. a molecule attached to a probe which allows visualization
   d. a short segment of DNA

2. An appropriate specimen type for FISH is:
   a. a microthin slice of bone.
   b. a suspension of adult red blood cells.
   c. filtered urine or spinal fluid.
   d. an unspun amniotic fluid specimen.

3. What is hybridization?
   a. overnight treatment at 37°C
   b. covalent binding of a fluorochrome to a bound probe

   c. bonding of complementary bases
   d. melting or making DNA single stranded

4. The component on the fluorescent microscope that limits the wavelengths of light that strikes the fluorochrome is a(n):
   a. excitation filter.
   b. objective lens.
   c. emission filter.
   d. condenser.

5. After hybridization excessive or nonspecific bound probe is removed by:
   a. incubation in 2X SSC at 37°C for one hour.
   b. serial washes in buffer at pH 7.0.
   c. observing stringent wash conditions of pH, temperature, and salt.

d. serial five-minute slide washings in tap water until sharp signals are observed.

6. Whole chromosome paints are:
   a. useful in detecting complex rearrangements in interphase nuclei.
   b. restricted to metaphase chromosomes analysis.
   c. useful in detecting microdeletions.
   d. the basis of microarray technology.

7. Advantages of indirect labeled probes do not include:
   a. less expense to purchase than direct labeled probes.
   b. amplification if the signal is weak.
   c. labeling with a choice of fluors.
   d. fewer protocol steps.

8. Counterstains:
   a. aid in locating probe signals.
   b. increase contrast between similar colored fluor signals.
   c. soften the image for easier viewing.
   d. mask background fluorescence.

9. FISH advantages include all the following except:
   a. viable cells are not necessary as long as membranes are intact.
   b. control probes for each chromosome are commercially available.
   c. cell culture is generally not necessary except for whole chromosome paints.
   d. provision of a quick (two to three day) genome wide scan.

10. Routine uses for FISH have not included which of the following applications?
    a. detection of microdeletions or cryptic translocations in individuals with multiple anomalies
    b. single base pair mutation analysis of single gene disorders
    c. identification of marker chromosomes
    d. determine gene amplification status in solid tumors

11. The ISCN (International System of Cytogenetic Nomenclature) description of a FISH result does not include:
    a. source or name of probe.
    b. number of each type of signals observed.
    c. color of probe signals.
    d. whether analysis was performed using interphase or metaphase cells.

12. A fluorochrome that emits a blue signal is:
    a. fluorescein.
    b. DAPI.
    c. rhodamine.
    d. propidium iodide.

13. The major disadvantage of FISH as compared with cytogenetics testing is:
    a. longer turnaround times.
    b. the requirement of cell culture.
    c. that color blind individuals cannot perform analysis or interpret results.
    d. only present or absent from the genome and not location is indicated.

14. FISH has diagnostic application in all the following except:
    a. paternity identification.
    b. preimplantation genetics for numerical abnormalities or familial rearrangements.
    c. monitoring response to chemotherapy.
    d. microdeletion syndrome.

15. Analysis of fusion probes requires which of the following parameters?
    a. dual color labeling and evaluation by two technologists
    b. evaluation by two technologists on two different slide preparations
    c. evaluation of 500 cells from two slides if analysis by only one technologist
    d. single color labeling and evaluation by one technologists

REFERENCES

American College of Medical Genetics. 2002. *Standards and Guidelines for Clinical Genetics Laboratories,* 3rd ed. Bethesda, MD. Also at www.faseb.org/genetics/acmg.

American College of Medical Genetics/American Society of Human Genetics Statement. 2002. Technical and clinical assessment of fluorescence in situ hybridization: An ACMG/ASHG position statement. I. Technical considerations, *Gen in Medicine* 2:356–61.

American Society of Human Genetics/American College of Medical Genetics Test and Technology Transfer Committee. 1996. Diagnostic testing for Prader-Willi and Angelman syndromes: Report

of the ASHG/ACMG Test and Technology Transfer Committee. *Am J Hum Genet* 58:1085–88.

Ballif, B. C., C. D. Kashork, and L. G. Shaffer. 2000. The promise and pitfalls of telomere region-specific probes. *Am J Hum Genet* 67:1356–59.

Barch, M., T. Knutsen, and J. Spurbeck, eds. 1997. *The AGT Cytogenetics Laboratory Manual,* 3rd. ed. Lippincott-Raven Publishers, New York, pp. 557–95.

Bauman, J. G. J., J. Wiegant, P. Borst, and P. van Duijn. 1980. A new method for fluorescence microscopial localization of specific

DNA sequences by in situ hybridization of fluorochrome-labeled RNA. *Exp Cell Res* 128:485–90.

Bischoff, F. Z., D. E. Lewis, D. D. Nguyen et al. 1998. Prenatal diagnosis with use of fetal cells isolated from maternal blood: Five-color fluorescent in situ hybridization analysis on flow-sorted cells for chromosomes X, Y, 13, 18, and 21. *Am J Obstet Gynecol* 179:203–9.

Block, A. W. 1999. Cancer cytogenetics. In: *The Principles of Clinical Cytogenetics*, ed. (S. L. Gersen and M. B. Keagle), Humana Press, Totowa, NJ, pp. 345–420.

Brewer, C., S. Holloway, P. Sawalnyski, A. Schinzel, and D. Fitzpartick. 1998. A chromosomal deletion map of human malformations. *Am J Hum Genet* 63:1153–59.

Bruder, C. E., C. Hirvela, L. Tapia-Paez et al. 2001. High resolution deletion analysis of constitutional DNA from neurofibromatosis type 2 (NF2) patients using microarray-CGH. *Hum Mol Genet* 10:271–82.

Callen, D. F., H. Eyre, M. Y. Yip, J. Freemantle, and E. A. Haan. 1992. Molecular cytogenetic and clinical studies of 42 patients with marker chromosomes. *Am J Med Genet* 43:709–15.

Cheung, V. G., M. Morley, F. Aguilar et al. 1999. Making and reading microarrays. *Nat Genet* 21:15–19.

Cheung, V. G., N. Nowak, W. Jang et al. 2001. Integration of cytogenetic landmarks into the draft sequence of the human genome. *Nature* 409:953–58.

Christensen, B., T. Bryndorf, J. Philip, X. Xing, and W. Hansen. 1993. Prenatal diagnosis by in situ hybridization on uncultured amniocytes. Reduced Sensitivity and potential risk of misdiagnosis in blood stained samples. *Prenat Diagn* 13:581–87.

Colleaux, L., M. Rio, S. Heuertz et al. 2001. A novel automated strategy for screening cryptic telomeric rearrangements in children with idiopathic mental retardation. *Eur J Hum Genet* 9:319–27.

Cooper, M. L., J. B. Redman, D. E. Mensing, and S. W. Cheung. 1988. Prenatal detection of chromosome aneuploidies in uncultured amniocytes by FISH: Advantages and limitations. *Am J Hum Genet* 63: A161.

Cremer, T., J. Landegent, A. Bruckner et al. 1986. Detection of chromosome aberrations in the human interphase nucleus by visualization of specific target DNAs with radioactive and non-radioactive in situ hybridization techniques: Diagnosis of trisomy 18 with probe L1.84. *Hum Genet* 74:346–52.

Cremer, T., P. Lichter, J. Borden, D. C. Ward, and L. Manuelidis. 1988. Detection of chromosome aberrations in metaphase and interphase tumor cells by in situ hybridization using chromosome-specific library probes. *Hum Genet* 80:235–46.

Crolla, J. A. 1998. FISH and molecular studies of autosomal supernumerary marker chromosomes excluding those derived from chromosome 15, II. Review of literature. *Am J Med Genet* 75:367–81.

Dauwerse, J. G., J. Wiegant, A. K. Raap, M. H. Breuning, and G. J. B. van Ommen. 1992. Multiple colors by fluorescence in situ hybridization using ratio-labeled DNA probes create a molecular karyotype. *Hum Mol Genet* 1:593–98.

De la Chapelle, A., R. Herva, M. Koivisto, and P. Aula. 1981. A deletion in chromosome 22 can cause DiGeorge syndrome. *Hum Genet* 57:253–56.

Devriendt, K., J-P. Fryns, and G. Mortier. 1998. The annual incidence of DiGeorge/velocardiofacial syndrome. *J Med Genet* 35:789–90.

Dewald, G., R. Stallard, A. Alsadi, et al. 2000. A multicenter investigation with D-FISH BCR/ABL1 probes. *Cancer Genet Cytogenet* 116:97–104.

Dewald, G. W., W. A. Wyatt, A. L. Juneau, et al. 1998. Highly sensitive fluorescence in situ hybridization method to detect double BCR/ABL fusion and monitor response to therapy in chronic myeloid leukemia. *Blood* 91:3357–65.

Driscoll, D. A., J. Salvin, and B. Sellinger. 1993. Prevalence of 22q11 microdeletion in DiGeorge and velocardiofacial syndromes: Implications for genetic counseling and prenatal diagnosis. *J Med Genet* 30:813–17.

Du Montcel, S. T., H. Mendizabal, S. Ayme, A. Levy, and N. Philip. 1996. Prevalence of 22q11 microdeletion. *J Med Genet* 33:719.

Eils, R., S. Uhring, K. Saracogulu et al. 1998. An optimized, fully automated system for fast and accurate identification of chromosome rearrangements by multiplex-FISH (M-FISH). *Cytogenet Cell Genet* 82:160–71.

Estabrook, L. L., M. Sapeta, C. Lytle et al. 1999. Prenatal interphase FISH using the AneuVysion probe set in over 10,000 samples. *Am J Hum Genet* 65(suppl):A162

Evsikov, S. and Y. Verlinsky. 1998. Mosaicism in inner cell mass of human blastocysts. *Hum Reprod* 13:3151–55.

Fan, Y. S. ed. 2002. *Molecular Cytogenetics: Protocols and Applications*. Humana Press, Totowa, NJ.

Fan, Y. S. and S. A. Farrell. 1994. Prenatal diagnosis of interstitial deletion of 17(p11.1p11.2) (Smite-Magenis syndrome). *Am J Med Genet* 49:253–54.

Flint, J., A. O. M. Wilkie, V. J. Buckle. 1995. The detection of subtelomeric chromosomal rearrangements in idiopathic mental retardation. *Nat Genet* 9:132–40.

Gall, J. G. and M. L. Pardue. 1969. Molecular hybridization of radioactive DNA to the DNA of cytological preparations. *Proc Natl Acad Sci USA* 64:600–604.

Giraudeau, F., D. Aubert, I. Young et al. 1997. Molecular-cytogenetic detection of a deletion of 1p36.3. *J Med Genet* 34:314–17.

Gohlke, B. C., K. Haug, M. Funkami, et al. 2000. Interstitial deletion in Xp22.2 is associated with X-linked ichthyosis, mental retardation, and epilepsy. *J Med Genet* 37: 600–602.

Guan, X. Y., P. S. Meltzer, and J. M. Trent. 1994. Rapid construction of whole chromosome painting probes by chromosome microdissection. *Genomics* 22:101–7.

Guan, X. Y., J. M. Trent, and P. S. Meltzer. 1993. Generation of band-specific painting probes from a single microdissected chromosome. *Human Molecular Genet* 2:1117–21.

Guan, X. Y., H. Zhang, M. Bittner et al. 1996. Chromosome arm painting probes. *Nature Genet* 12:10–11.

Harper, M. E., A. Ullrich, and G. F. Saunders. 1981. Localization of the human insulin gene to the distal end of the short arm of chromosome 11. *Proc Natl Acad Sci* USA 78:4458–60.

Hoang, M. P., A. A. Sahin, N. G. Ordonez, and N. Sneige. 2000. HER-2/neu gene amplification compared with HER-2/neu protein overexpression and interobserver reproducibility in invasive breast carcinoma. *Am J Clin Pathol* 113:852–59.

International Working Group on Preimplantation Genetics. 2001. 10th anniversary of preimplantation genetic diagnosis. *J Assist Repro Genet* 18:66–72.

Jalal, S. M., M. E. Saw, N. M. Lindor, K. J. Thompson, and G. S. Sekon. 2001. Detection of diagnostically critical, often hidden, anomalies in complex karyotypes of hematologic disorders by multicolor FISH. *Brit Jour Hemat* 112:4, 9750–79.

Jocobson, C. and D. Duggan. 2002. Increasing cytogenetic resolution with array technologies. *J Assoc of Gen Tech* 28:128–33.

Juyal, R. C., F. L. Figuera, F. L. Gauge et al. 1996. Molecular analyses of 17p11.2 deletions in 62 Smith-Magenis syndrome patients. *Am J Hum Genet* 58:998–1007.

Kallioniemi, A., L-P. Kallioniemi, J. Piper et al. 1994. Detection and mapping of amplified DNA sequences in breast cancer by comparative genomic hybridization. *Proc Natl Acad Sci USA* 91:2156–60.

Kallioniemi, A., L-P. Kallioniemi, and D. Sauder. 1992. Comparative genomic hybridization for molecular cytogenetic analysis of solid tumors. *Science* 258:818–21.

Kao, F. T. and J. W. Yu. 1991. Chromosome microdissection and cloning in human genome and genetic disease analysis. *Proc Natl Acad Sci USA* 88:1844–48.

Knight, S. J. L. and J. Flint. 2000. Perfect endings: A review of subtelomeric probes and their use in clinical diagnosis. *J Med Genet* 37:401–9.

Knight, S. J. L., S. W. Horsley, R. Regan et al. 1997. Development and clinical application of an innovative fluorescence in situ hybridization technique which detects submicroscopic rearrangements involving telomeres. *Eur J Hum Genet* 5:1–8.

Knight, S. J., D. M. Lese, K. S. Precht et al. 2000. An optimized set of human telomere clones for studying telomere integrity and architecture. *Am J Hum Genet* 67:320–32.

Klinger, K., G. Landes, D. Shook et al. 1992. Rapid detection of chromosome aneuploidies in uncultured amniocytes by using fluorescence in situ hybridization (FISH). *Am J Hum Genet* 51:55–65.

Koehler, U., F. Bigoni, J. Wienberg, and R. Stanyon. 1995. Genomic reorganization in the concolor gibbon (Hylobates concolor) revealed by chromosome painting. *Genomics* 20:287–92.

Konkin, D., B. Farago, G. Williams, and A. Dawson. 2001. Variant Philadelphia chromosomes. *J Assoc of Gen Technol* 27:44–46.

Knutsen, T. and T. Ried. 2000. SKY: A comprehensive diagnostic and research tool. A review of the first 300 published cases. *J Assoc Genet Tech* 26: 3–15.

Knutsen, T., T. Veldman, H. P. Nash et al. 1997. Spectral imaging: Chromosomes in color. *Applied Cytogenetics* 23:26–32.

Kuwano, A., S. A. Ledbetter, W. B. Dobyns, B. S. Emanuel, and D. H. Ledbetter. 1991. Detection of deletions and cryptic translocations in Miller-Dieker syndrome by in situ hybridization. *Am J Hum Genet* 49:707–14.

Law, M. and S. M. Jalal. 2000. M-FISH technique: How to set up and analyze. *J Assoc Genet Tech* 26:51–53.

Lawce, H. 2000. Vysis GenoSensor Microarray: Report of a demonstration. *J Assoc of Gen Tech* 28:150.

Ledbetter, D. H. 1992. Cryptic translocations and telomere integrity. *Am J Hum Genet* 51:451–56.

Lee, C., D. Gisselsson, C. Jin et al. 2001. Limitations of chromosome classification by multicolor karyotyping. *Am J Hum Genet* 68:1043–47.

Lewin, P., P. Kleinfinger, A. Bazin, H. Mossafa, and S. Szpiro-Tapia. 2001. Defining the efficiency of fluorescence in situ hybridization on uncultured amniocytes on a retrospective cohort of 27,407 prenatal diagnoses. *Prenat Diagn* 20:1–6.

Lichter, P., T. Cremer, J. Borden, L. Maneulidis, and D. C. Ward. 1988. Delineation of individual human chromosomes in metaphase and interphase cells by in situ suppression hybridization using recombinant DNA libraries. *Hum Genet* 80:224–34.

Liyanage, M., A. Coleman, S. du Manoir et al. 1996. Multicolor spectral karyotyping of mouse chromosomes. *Nature Genet* 14:312–14.

Lowery, M. C. 2000. *Application of FISH Technology on Paraffin-Embedded Tissue, Procedural Tips and Trouble-Shooting Guide,* ed. Vysis. Downers Grove, IL.

Ludecke, H. J., G. Senger, U. Claussen, and B. Horsthemke. 1989. Cloning defined regions of the human genome by microdissection of banded chromosomes and enzymatic amplification. *Nature* 338:348–50.

Lupski, J. R. 1998. Genomic disorders: Structural features of the genome can lead to DNA rearrangements and human disease traits. *Trends Genet* 14:417–22.

Marquez, C., J. Cohen, and S. Munne. 1998. Chromosome identification in human oocytes and polar bodies by spectral karyotyping. *Cytogenet Cell Genet* 81:254–58.

Mitelman, F., ed. 1995. An International System for Human Cytogenetic Nomenclature, published in collaboration with *Cytogenet. Cell Genet.* Karger, Basel, Switzerland.

Muller, S., P. C. O'Brien, M. A. Ferguson-Smith, and J. Weinberg. 1998. Cross-species color segmenting: A novel tool in human karyotype analysis. *Cytometry* 33:445–52.

Muller, S., M. Rocchi, M. A. Ferguson-Smith, and J. Weinberg. 1997. Toward a multicolor chromosome bar code for the entire human karyotype by fluorescence in situ hybridization. *Hum Genet* 100:271–78.

Munne, S., T. Dailey, K. M. Sultan, J. Grifo, and J. Cohen. 1995. The use of first polar bodies for preimplantation diagnosis of aneuploidy. *Hum Reprod* 10:1014–20.

Munne, S., M. C. Magli, M. Bahce et al. 1988. Preimplantation diagnosis of the aneuploidies most commonly found in spontaneous abortions and live births: XY, 13, 14, 15, 16, 18, 21, 22. *Prenat Diagn* 18:459–66.

National Institutes of Health, Institute of Molecular Medicine Collaboration. 1996. A complete set of human telomeric probes and their clinical application. *Nat Genet* 14:86–89.

NCCLS. 2002. *Fluorescence In Situ Hybridization (FISH) Methods for Medical Genetics, Approved Guideline, MM7-P,* Vol. 21, No. 6.

Nederlof, P. M., D. Robinson, R. Akuknesha et al. 1989. Three color fluorescence in situ hybridization for the simultaneous detection of multiple nucleic acid sequences. *Cytometry* 10:20–27.

Oosterwijk, J. C., W. E. Mesker, M. C. Wuwerkerk-van Velzen et al. 1998. Development of a preparation and staining method for fetal erythroblasts in maternal blood: Simulteneous immunocytochemical staining and FISH analysis. *Cytometry* 32:170–77.

Pinkel, D., J. Landegent, C. Collins et al. 1988. Fluorescence in situ hybridization with human chromosome-specific libraries: Detection of trisomy 21 and translocations of chromosome 4. *Proc Natl Acad Sci USA* 85:9138–42.

Pinkel, D., R. Segraves, D. Suder et al. 1997. High resolution analysis of DNA copy number variation using comparative genomic hybridization to microarrays. *Nat Genet* 20:207–11.

Pinkel, D., T. Straume, and J. W. Gray. 1986. Cytogenetic analysis using quantitative, high-sensitivity fluorescence hybridization. *Proc Natl Acad Sci* USA 83:2934–38.

Reid, T., A. Baldini, T. C. Rand, and D. C. Ward. 1992. Simultaneous visualization of seven different DNA probes using combinatorial fluorescence and digital imaging microscopy. *Proc Natl Acad Sci USA* 89:1388–92.

Reid, T., G. Landes, W. Dackowski, K. Klinger, and D. C. Ward. 1992. Multicolor fluorescence in situ hybridization for the simultaneous detection of probe sets for chromosomes 13, 18, 21, X, and Y in un-cultured amniotic cells. *Hum Mol Genet* 1:307–13.

Reid, T., M. Liyanage, S. du Manoir 1997. Tumor cytogenetics re-visited: Comparative genomic hybridization and spectral kary-otyping. *J Mol Med* 75:801–14.

Riegel, M., A. Baumer, M. Jamar et al. 2001. Submicroscopic termi-nal deletions and duplications in retarded patients with unclassi-fied malformation syndromes. *Hum Genet* 109:286–94.

Schaffer, L. G., N. Agan, J. D. Goldberg et al. 2001. American Col-lege of Medical Genetics Statement on Diagnostic Testing for Uni-parental Disomy. *Gen in Med* 3:3 206–11.

Schaffer, L. G., D. H. Ledbetter, and J. R. Lupski. 2000. Molecular cytogenetics of contiguous gene syndromes: Mechanisms and consequences of gene dosage imbalance. In Charles R. Scriver, William S. Sly, Arthur L. Beaudet and David Valle, *The Metabolic and Molecular Basis of Inherited Diseases,* New York, McGraw-Hill, pp. 1291–324.

Schrock, E., S. du Manoir, T. Veldman et al. 1996. Multicolor spec-tral karyotyping of human chromosomes. *Science* 273:494–97.

Schwartz, D., T. W. Depinet, J. Leana-Cox et al. 1997. Sex chromo-some markers: Characterization using fluorescence in situ hy-bridization and review of literature. *Am J Med Genet* 71:1–7.

Shapira, S. K. 1998. An update on chromosome deletion and mi-crodeletion syndromes. *Current Opinion in Pediatrics.* 10:622–27.

Shapira, S. K., C. McCaskill, H. Northrup et al. 1997. Chromo-some 1p36 deletions: The clinical phenotype and molecular char-acterization of a common newly delineated syndrome. *Am J Hum Genet* 61:642–50.

Shapiro, D. N., M. B. Valentine, S. T. Rowe et al. 1993. Detection of N-myc gene amplification by fluorescence in situ hybridization: Diagnostic utility for neuroblastoma. *Am J Pathol* 142:1339–46.

Shuster, M., U. Bockmuhl, and S. M. Gollin. 1997. Early experi-ences with SKY: A primer for the practicing cytogenetic technolo-gist. *Applied Cytogenetics* 23:33–37.

Smith, R. F. 1990. *Microscopy and Photomicrography: A Working Manual.* CRC Press, Inc., Baca Raton, FL.

Speicher, M. R., S. Gwyn Ballard, and D. C. Ward. 1996. Karyotyp-ing human chromosomes by combinatorial multi-fluor FISH. *Nat Genet* 12:368–75.

Spritzen, R. J. Velocardiofacial syndrome and DiGeorge sequence. *J Med Genet* 31:423–24.

Spurbeck, J. L., A. R. Zinsmeister, K. J. Meyer, and S. M. Jalal. 1996. Dynamics of chromosome spreading. *Am J Med Genet* 61:387–93.

Strovel, J. W., K. D. Lee, C. Punzalan, and S. Schwartz. 1992. Pre-natal diagnosis by direct analysis of uncultured amniotic fluid and chorionic villus cells using interphase fluorescence in situ hy-bridization (FISH). *Am J Hum Genet* 51:A12.

Swillen, A., A. Vogels, K. Devriendt, and J. P. Fryns. 2000. Chro-mosome 22q11 deletion syndrome: Update and review of the clinical features, cognitive-behavioral spectrum, and psychiatric complications. *Am J Med Genet* 97:128–35.

Tajiri, T., K. Shono, Y. Fujii et al. 1999. Highly sensitive analysis for N-myc amplification in nueroblastoma based on fluorescence in situ hybridization. *J Pediatr Surg* 34:1615–19.

Tardy, E. P. and A. Toth. 1997. Cross-hybridization of the chromo-some 13/21 alpha satellite DNA to chromosome 22 or a rare poly-morphism? *Prenat Diagn* 17:487–88.

Tepperberg, J., M. J. Pettenati, P. N. Rao et al. 2001. Prenatal diag-nosis using interphase fluorescence in situ hybridization (FISH): 2-year multi-center retrospective study and review of the literature. *Prenat Diagn* 21:2993–301.

Thangavelu, M., P. X. Chen, and E. Pergament. 1998. Hybridiza-tion of chromosome 18 alpha-satellite DNA to chromosome 22. *Prenat Diagn* 18:922–25.

Tkachuk, D. C., D. Pinkel, W. L. Kuo, H. U. Weier, and J. W. Gray. 1991. Clinical applications of fluorescence in situ hybridization. *GATA* 8:67–74.

Trask, B. and D. Pinkel. 1990. Fluorescence in situ hybridization with DNA probes. *Methods Cell Biol* 33:383–400.

Trask, B. J. 1991. Fluorescence in situ hybridization: applications in cytogenetics and gene mapping, *Trends in Gen* 7:282A–282F.

Veldman, T., C. Vignon, E. Schrock, J. D. Rowley, and T. Ried. 1997. Hidden chromosome abnormalities in hematological malignancies detected by multicolor spectral karyotyping. *Nat Genet* 15:406–10.

Verlinsky, Y., N. Ginsberg, M. Chmura et al. 1995. Cross-hybridization of the chromosome 13/21 alpha satellite DNA probe to chromosome 22 in the prenatal screening of common chromosomal aneuploidies by FISH. *Prenat Diagn* 15:831–34.

Verlinsky, Y., J. Cieslak, V. Ivankhnenko et al. 1998. Prevention of age-related aneuploidies by polar body testing of oocytes. *J Assist Repro Genet* 16:165–69.

Verma, R. S. and S. Luke. 1992. Variations in alphoid DNA se-quences escape detection of aneuploidy at interphase by FISH technique. *Genomics* 14:113–16.

Vierbach, R., H. Engels, U. Gamerdinger, and M. Hansmann. 1998. Delineation of supernumerary marker chromosomes in 38 patients. *Am J Med Genet* 76:351–59.

Wang, J. C., M. B. Passage, P. H. Yen, L. J. Shapiro, and T. K. Mo-handas. 1991. Uniparental heterodisomy for chromosome 14 in a phenotypically abnormal familial balanced 13/14 translocation carrier. *Am J Hum Genet* 48:1069–74.

Warburton, D. 1991. De novo balanced chromosome rearrange-ments and extra marker chromosomes identified at prenatal diag-nosis: Clinical significance and distribution of breakpoints. *Am J Hum Genet* 49:995–1013.

Ward, B. E., S. L. Gersen, M. P. Carelli et al. 1993. Rapid prenatal diagnosis of chromosomal aneuploidies by fluorescence in situ hybridization: Clinical experience with 4,500 specimens. *Am J Hum Genet* 52:854–65.

Weier, H. U. G. and J. W. Gray. 1992. A degenerate alpha satellite probe, detecting a centromeric deletion on chromosome 21 in an apparently normal human male, shows limitations of the use of satellite DNA probes for interphase ploidy analysis. *Anal Cell Pathol* 4:81–86.

Williams, J. III, L. Yu, B. T. Wang et al. 1995. Prenatal diagnosis of human XX males: Confirmation of X-Y interchange by fluores-cence in situ hybridization. *Applied Cytogenetics* 21:5–8

Winsor, E. J., S. Dyack, E. M. Wood-Burgess, and G. Ryan. 1999. Risk of false-positive prenatal diagnosis using interphase FISH test-ing: Hybridization of alpha-satellite X probe to chromosome 19. *Prenat Diagn* 19:832–36.

Zhao, L., K. Hayes, and A. Glassman. 2000. Enhanced detection of chromosomal abnormalities with the use of RxFISH multicolor banding technique. *Cancer Genet Cytogenet* 118:108–11.

15

Histocompatibility Laboratory Techniques and Applications

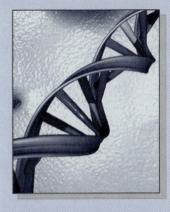

■ CHAPTER CHECKLIST

After reading and studying this chapter, the reader should be able to:

1. Compare and contrast different HLA test techniques.
2. Discuss the HLA tests required for different types of transplants.
3. Describe the advantages of DNA typing over other methods.
4. List the precautions to be taken when performing DNA testing.
5. Discuss DNA test methods for determining engraftment following bone marrow/progenitor cell transplants.
6. Compare and contrast the accreditation requirements/personnel requirements between an HLA lab and a clinical laboratory.

Ⓔ CASE IN POINT

A 5-year-old girl with acute lymphocytic leukemia (ALL) is identified as a candidate for a bone marrow transplant. Her three siblings and her parents are drawn for HLA typing to determine compatibility. Both parents and two siblings are a one-haplotype match. Her younger brother is a two-haplotype match, or HLA identical. High-resolution HLA typing at the DR locus using PCR confirmed that brother and sister are HLA identical. Posttransplant marrow engraftment was determined, and prognosis for complete recovery was good.

ISSUES TO CONSIDER:

After reading the patient's case history, consider

- The purpose and clinical application of histocompatibility testing
- Tests performed to determine histocompatibility
- The purpose of high-resolution HLA typing
- Means to determine bone marrow engraftment
- Posttransfusion prognosis for this patient based on the identified donor

IMPORTANT TERMS

Allelic ladder	Haplotype	Nested
Allogeneic	Histocompatibility (HLA) testing	Oligonucleotide probe/primer
Capillary gel electrophoresis	Hybridize	Polyacrylamide gel
Chimera (chimersim)	Informative locus	electrophoresis
Complement dependent	Intron	Polymerase chain reaction
microtoxicity (CDC) test	Mixed lymphocyte culture	(PCR)
Dendritic cells	(MLC)	Polymorphic
Ethidium bromide (EB)	Mixed lymphocyte reaction	Progenitor cell
Exon	(MLR)	Splits
Graft versus host disease	Multiparous	Stem cell
(GVHD)	Multiplex PCR	

▶ INTRODUCTION

Following transplant, an immune response can be cellular (generated by antigen mismatches between donor and recipient) or humoral (generated by recipient antibodies to antigens on the donor MHC). Transplant rejection can be initiated by the immune cells of the recipient or by immunocompetent cells on the donor tissue that are transferred to the recipient during transplantation. The purpose of **histocompatibility (HLA) testing** is to assess tissue compatibility between a transplant donor and potential recipient prior to transplant. An example of a clinical application of HLA testing is described in the opening case study. The siblings and the parents of the five-year-old girl were tested to determine tissue compatibility and to find the most suitable donor.

This area of the laboratory evolved as a result of observations in animal studies that demonstrated that:

■ Grafts between genetically identical animals are accepted.

■ Grafts between genetically identical animals are rejected at a speed dependent on where the genetic differences lie.

■ The ability to accept a graft is dependent on the recipient sharing all of the donor's HLA genes.

The results of HLA testing, in conjunction with surgical intervention to prepare and obtain the organ, and immunosuppression of the patient are closely coordinated in order to maximize the chances of long-term survival of the tissue graft posttransplant. Together, these three factors serve as predictors of transplant success.

The basic tests performed in the Histocompatibility laboratory are (1) HLA typing of the potential recipient and donor(s), (2) haplotype determination (bone marrow/ progenitor cell transplants only), (3) evaluation of patient sera for HLA antibodies, and (4) crossmatching potential recipients against a donor to determine compatibility. The testing performed prior to transplantation depends on the type of transplant (e.g., solid organ versus bone marrow/hematopoietic **stem cell** or **progenitor cell**).

Ensuring a compatible donor for each recipient is a complex process requiring collaboration between the medical staff, the HLA laboratory, and the transplant coordinators. Histocompatibility testing utilizes specialized procedures necessitating dedicated reagents and complex quality control. Interpretation of test results requires extensive experience and knowledge. Generally HLA laboratories are located in medical centers with solid organ or progenitor cell transplant programs. Although accreditation can be obtained through the College of American Pathologists (CAP), the recognized regulatory agency for HLA laboratories is the American Society of Histocompatibility and Immunogenetics (ASHI). There are two federal agencies providing oversite in the transplant arena, the United Network for Organ Sharing (UNOS) (solid organ transplants) and the Foundation for the Accreditation of Cellular Therapy (FACT, formerly the Foundation for the Accreditation of Hematopoietic Cell Therapy or FAHCT) (bone marrow/progenitor transplants). While UNOS has given deemed status to CAP as well as to ASHI, FACT requires that all transplant-related work-ups be performed in ASHI accredited laboratories. This chapter presents different HLA test techniques and the HLA tests performed for different types of transplants. The advantages of molecular-based methods over other techniques are discussed. Last, accreditation and personnel requirements for HLA laboratories are presented.

► HISTORICAL OVERVIEW

The major breakthrough in histocompatibility testing was the introduction, and then miniaturization, of the **complement dependent cytotoxicity (CDC) test** in the 1960s. Today serological assays based on CDC remain the basic and most fundamental tests in HLA laboratories. Initially the CDC test utilized sera from **multiparous** women to identify antigens present on the surface of lymphocytes. The switch to antisera containing monoclonal antibodies helped to standardize the test and to enhance its reproducibility. In the 1970s, cellular assay measuring the incompatibility at Class II loci, the **mixed lymphocyte reaction (MLR)/mixed lymphocyte culture (MLC),** was introduced. The 1990s ushered in the age of DNA. Initial data from work utilizing molecular methods indicated that HLA loci were much more **polymorphic** than demonstrated by serologic analysis. Today DNA-based testing is standard for Class II typing and is quickly supplanting serological methods for Class I typing. CDC remains the test of choice for antibody identification and crossmatching. There are three types of HLA test techniques in use today. These are serological, cellular, and molecular. Depending on the laboratory, each may be utilized to different degrees. Table 15-1✪ shows HLA test techniques and their clinical applications.

► SEROLOGICAL TECHNIQUES

Serology is used to type a recipient or donor for Class I and Class II antigens, evaluate patient serum for HLA antibodies, and crossmatch potential recipients against a donor to determine compatibility (Table 15-1). All serological methods, except for flow cytometry, are variations of CDC. Because Class I and Class II antigens are present on different cell types, various isolation techniques may be required to obtain the appropriate cells for testing. (Table 15-2✪).

SPECIMEN COLLECTION, TRANSPORTATION, AND STORAGE

Blood should always be collected in sterile tubes to prevent contamination. Serologic and cellular assays use viable cells. Thus, labs must employ strict guidelines to ensure optimal sample collection, transportation, and storage. Table 15-3✪ lists the requirements for different types of HLA testing. The sample should arrive in the laboratory within 24 to 48 hours after drawing to ensure viability. Because of ease of isolation and its high HLA antigen expression, the lymphocyte is the cell of choice in serologic studies. The specimen of choice in live patients is peripheral blood because it contains a high number of lymphocytes (~50–90%

✪ TABLE 15-1

HLA Test Techniques and Their Applications

Procedure	Test Method	Types of Transplant
Serology	CDC	
	■ Class I and Class II HLA typing	Renal and nonrenal solid organ
	■ Antibody screen or percent reactive antibody (PRA)	
	■ Antihuman globulin augmented CDC	
	■ T cell specific crossmatch	
	■ B cell specific crossmatch	
	Flow cytometry	
Cellular	MLC (MLR)	Bone marrow/progenitor cell
Molecular	PCR	Bone marrow/Progenitor cell
	■ Class I and Class II HLA typing	
	■ Short tandem repeat (STR) testing assessing engraftment	

✪ TABLE 15-2

Sample Flow Using Serological Methods

Serological HLA Test Scheme

Cell separation

Mononuclear (monocyte) cell removal (optional)

Enrich the cell suspension for the lymphocyte population of choice (optional)

- Differential adherence in nylon wool columns
- Differential lysis of non-B or non-T cells with monoclonal antibody and complement
- Positive selection on magnetic beads with T or B cell specific monoclonal antibody

Serological procedures

- HLA typing using CDC with supravital staining or two-color fluorescence detection
- Serum screening for antibodies (percent reactive antibody or PRA)
- Donor-specific T and B cell cross matches (CDC or flow cytometry)

T lymphocytes, 5–20% B lymphocytes) and is easy to obtain. However, lymph nodes (75% T lymphocytes, 25% B lymphocytes) and spleen (50% T lymphocytes, 50% B lymphocytes) are also acceptable.

Peripheral blood should be collected in either sodium heparin or acid citrate dextrose (ACD) anticoagulant. Sodium heparin and ACD maintain cell viability for up to 72 hours at room temperature with optimal

cell recovery occurring at 48 hours after collection. Cell viability can be affected by factors such as exposure to temperature extremes, failure to maintain aseptic technique during collection, failure to provide supportive media after collection, and patient treatment regimens. Phlebotomy techniques should minimize cell lysis and shearing because cell fragmentation may interfere with cell separation and cause background interference af-

✪ TABLE 15-3

Specimen Requirements for Different Types of HLA Testing

Protocol	Anticoagulant of Choice	Optimal Storage Time and Temperature	Assay	Use
Serologic Assays (cells)	Sodium heparin (phenol free) or ACD	<48 hours at room temperature	Complement dependent cytotoxicity (CDC)	■ Class I and II typing ■ Antibody screening ■ Crossmatch
Serologic Assays (cells)	Sodium heparin (phenol free) or EDTA	<24 hours at room temperature	Flow cytometry	Complement-independent crossmatch for patients undergoing a 2nd or 3rd transplant
Serologic Assays (serum)	None	<72 hours at 4°C or >72 hours at −20 to −70°C	CDC	■ Antibody screening ■ Crossmatch
Cellular Assays	Sodium heparin (phenol free)	<48 hours at room temperature	Mixed lymphocyte response (MLR)/Mixed lymphocyte culture (MLC)	Class II (D region) compatibility
DNA-Based Assays	EDTA or ACD	<48 hours at room temperature or up to 5 days at 4°C	Typing	■ Class I and II typing ■ Allele sequencing ■ Engraftment in BMT patients

(Adapted from *ASHI Lab Manual*, 3rd ed. 1994)

fecting test interpretation. The amount of blood collected depends on the tests to be performed and the patient's absolute lymphocyte count. Approximately $20–60 \times 10^6$ lymphocytes are needed to perform Class I and Class II HLA typing by serology. Since individuals with a normal white blood cell have about 1×10^6 lymphs per 1 ml of blood, 20–60 ml of blood is required to perform serological typing. This volume varies by patient, and is affected by patient age, gender, drug, alcohol or tobacco use, presence of infection, and any other condition that may alter the number, types, and proportion of white blood cells in the circulation.

Blood anticoagulated in lithium heparin is acceptable only if it is processed immediately since this anticoagulant is toxic to white blood cells upon prolonged exposure. Partially clotted blood may be used if the blood is less than a few hours old and has been kept at room temperature. Sodium oxalate, or ethylenediaminetetraacetic acid (EDTA), should not be used because these anticoagulants chelate (remove) divalent cations (e.g., calcium) from the blood. This interferes with complement activation in the CDC assays. Blood for cross-matching should be collected in plain red top tubes, with no gel. It is recommended to store all anticoagulated samples at room temperature prior to processing since refrigeration decreases cell viability. After separation from cells, serum samples should be kept at 2–8°C until testing and at −70°C for long-term storage.

The specimen of choice from a cadaveric donor is lymph nodes, which can be obtained quickly by surgical procedures. These samples contain nearly 100% lymphocytes. If the lymph nodes are inadequate, spleen may be used. Since both of these tissues (particularly the spleen) have a high number of fragile B cells, it is recommended that they be transported in cell culture medium with antibiotics to ensure viability and to minimize the chances of bacterial contamination. Although not an optimal sample from cadavers, periph-

eral blood can, and is, used in many cases because of the ease of transportation and lack of preservation requirements. The best sample for cell isolation depends on donor status (alive or dead) and the type of assay (e.g., HLA typing versus crossmatch).

LYMPHOCYTE PREPARATION

Techniques for the isolation of lymphocytes, the first step in serological testing, are based on separation by cell size or density or the ability to phagocitize and adhere to surfaces. Density gradient centrifugation, the most common method, employs Ficoll-Hypaque (FH) to separate mononuclear cells from the other formed elements in the blood. Ficoll is a high molecular weight sucrose polymer that enhances rouleaux formation of red blood cells. Hypaque is an organic compound that increases the density of the solution. After being layered over FH, the formed elements separate relative to their specific gravity compared with FH when centrifuged at low speed $(400 \times g)$ (see Table 15-4). Figure 15-1 shows the schematic diagram of the separation of formed elements in peripheral blood after centrifugation with (FH). After centrifugation, the interface layer (containing mononuclear cells such as lymphocytes and monocytes) is removed and washed three times and/or recentrifuged to remove contaminating platelets. Cell recovery can be affected by layering too much blood onto the FH (causing contamination), rough specimen handling, jerky centrifugation, or rapid breaking of the centrifuge.

Pure mononuclear cells obtained from density gradient centrifugation can be used for Class I HLA typing and for MLC. However, since monocytes can ingest the detection dye and cause a false positive HLA typing result, some labs prefer to further separate lymphocytes from monocytes. These additional methods capitalize on the monocyte's tendency to phagocytize and/or to adhere to glass or plastic. For example, one technique

✪ TABLE 15-4

Separation of Formed Elements in Peripheral Blood after Centrifugation with FH

Specific Gravity (RT)	Formed Element	Position in Tube
<1.025	Cellular debris	Plasma fraction
1.025–1.035	Platelets	Plasma fraction
1.070–1.080	Lymphocytes and monocytes	Interface
1.077	FH	Below the Interface
1.080–1.090	Granulocytes	Bottom
1.085–1.115	Red blood cells	Bottom

Centrifugation

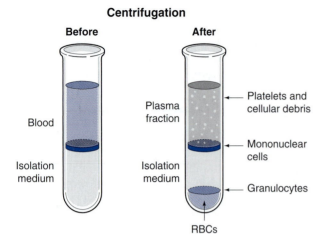

■ FIGURE 15-1 Schematic of the separation of formed elements in peripheral blood after centrifugation with FH.

calls for mixing the mononuclear cell suspension with iron filings. Monocytes in the suspension phagocytize the filings, and when centrifuged, the weight of the iron forces these cells to the bottom of the tube with the lymphocytes remaining at the interface. Commercial preparations for cell separation are also available. Lympho-Kwik™ isolation medium uses a cocktail of specific monoclonal antibodies to lyse nonlymphocytic cells. Since the predominant lymphocyte (~ 80%) in the peripheral blood is the T cell, the suspensions prepared by methods separating lymphocytes from

mononuclear cells are primarily composed of T lymphocytes. These techniques are adequate for recovering cells for use in Class I studies.

Class II HLA antigens are present primarily on the surface of B lymphocytes and to a lesser degree on the surface of activated T lymphocytes. Typing tests for Class II HLA antigens (e.g., HLA-DR and HLA-DQ) require suspensions enriched for B cells. Several methods, as shown in Box 15-1✳, are utilized to separate T- from B-lymphocytes.

After isolation, the cells are tested for viability by mixing an aliquot with a supravital dye such as trypan blue. When the pattern of staining is examined under the microscope, at least 95% of the lymphocytes must have ingested the dye (indicating viability) to ensure reliable HLA test results. In suspensions with viabilities less than 95%, recovery can be improved by resuspending the suspension over FH. Upon centrifugation, nonviable and marginally viable cells will leak, absorb the dense FH medium and sink, leaving less cells at the interface but a cell population that is primarily viable.

HLA TESTING: COMPLEMENT DEPENDENT CYTOTOXICITY ASSAY

The CDC is the basic serological test procedure. This two-stage assay is used for the following purposes:

■ Type cells for Class I and Class II HLA antigens

■ Screen sera for antibodies

✳ BOX 15-1 Separation of T cells and B cells

1) Sheep red blood cell rosetting is a simple and inexpensive technique based on antigen expression. T lymphocytes have a receptor for a cell surface antigen, CD2, which is present in high density on sheep red blood cells. When T lymphs and sheep cells are mixed, the CD2 receptor on the T cell surface binds the sheep cells. When greater than three sheep red blood cells bind to a T lymphocyte, the buoyant density of the T cell decreases, causing the T cell/RBC rosette to pass through a FH gradient when the solution is centrifuged. Non-rosetting (B) cells will collect at the FH interface. Further addition of a hypotonic solution will lyse the sheep red blood cells and allow collection of a suspension rich in T cells.

2) Magnetic microsphere is another method. In the magnetic microsphere method, two tubes are set up. In each tube, cells are mixed with superparamagnetic beads coated with monoclonal antibodies directed against antigens present on the surface of either T (e.g., CD8, CD4, or CD3) or B (e.g., CD 19 or 20) lymphocytes. The T or B

cells in the tube bind with the antigen specific monoclonal antibody coated beads. A magnet is then used to pull the beads (plus their attached cells) against the side of the tube. The supernatant containing the other cell type is decanted, leaving a cell population enriched for either T or B cells. Magnetic beads are easy to use, fast (less than 15 minutes), inexpensive, and can be used with several types of patient samples. They provide high-quality cell suspensions, particularly for Class II typing.

3) Differential adherence involves passing mononuclear cells over a solid surface such as nylon wool. B cells and monocytes adhere to the wool while T cells do not. After incubation, the column is washed, and the T-cell enriched wash solution is collected while the B cells and monocytes remain stuck to the wool. Agitating the column and then washing it with cold media induces a temperature change that dislodges the B cells from the column. Subsequent washing yields a solution enriched for B lymphocytes while the monocytes remain rigidly attached to the wool.

- Donor-specific T and B cell crossmatching
- For reagent quality control (QC)

Although the lymphocyte is the cell of choice, the test can be performed using any nucleated cell type expressing adequate quantities of appropriate Class I and Class II molecules. The CDC test is based on complement dependent antibody mediated cell lysis. Best results are obtained using suspensions enriched for T or B lymphocytes when performing Class I and Class II typing, respectively.

HLA Typing

In the CDC test, patient cells are tested against a panel of known HLA antisera. Figure 15-2■ shows the schematic diagram of the CDC assay. Typically, an aliquot of cells is added to each well of a 96-well typing tray with each well containing a different antiserum (A). Figure 15-3■ shows a histocompatibility technologist pipeting sample into a 96-well typing tray. If the antigen on the cell surface corresponds to the antibody in the sera, the antibody will bind to the cell. A source of complement, usually fresh frozen rabbit serum, (B) is added after an incubation period. If the complement attaches to the bound antibody and activates the complement cascade, the cell membrane will be damaged, affecting the cell's ability to retain or exclude supravital or fluorescent dyes (C) that facilitate distinction between intact and injured cells. Formalin is added (D) to preserve the cells after staining. Cell lysis is determined (E).

In the two-color fluorescent procedure, damaged cells (those having the antigen specific for the antibody present) will take up **ethidium bromide (EB)** dye and appear orange under the microscope. Undamaged cells (those not having the antigen specific for the antibody) will take up carbonylmethyl fluorescein diacetate (CFDA) or acridine orange, (AO) dye and show a green color. The overall color reaction in each well is scored as 1 or 2 (green color = no damage, antigen not present, negative test), 4 (equivocable), or 6 or

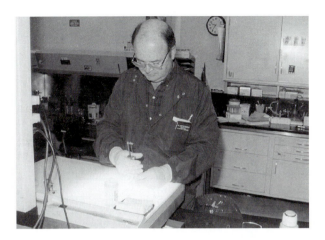

■ **FIGURE 15-3** Histocompatibility technologist pipetting sample into a 96-well typing tray.

8 (orange color = damage, antigen present, positive test) (Figure 15-4■ and Table 15-5✪). Each score is equivalent to a predetermined percent lysis. If greater than 50% of the cells take up the dye, the reaction is considered positive (6 or 8). The antigen specificity is deduced from pattern of injury (positive, negative) in the wells. Because of the cross-reactivity between HLA reagents, the cells in at least two wells in the 96-well tray will react with the same antibody. In order to assign an HLA type, the patient's cells must react with both wells. Trays purchased from some commercial vendors provide computer programs that assist in antigen identification.

Panel Reactive Antibody

The PRA assay also utilizes the CDC method. However, here the process is reversed from that used in HLA typing with patient *serum* being tested against a panel of lymphocytes with well-defined HLA specificities. The PRA assay serves several purposes: (1) to prospectively identify the presence of antibodies in a patient's serum

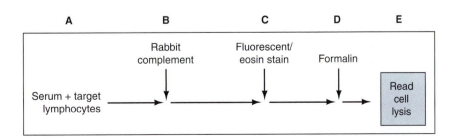

■ **FIGURE 15-2** Schematic of the CDC assay. (From: Lorentzen, D.F. 2002. HLA Testing in the Clinical Setting. University of Wisconsin Hospital and Clinics, Madison, WI used with permission.)

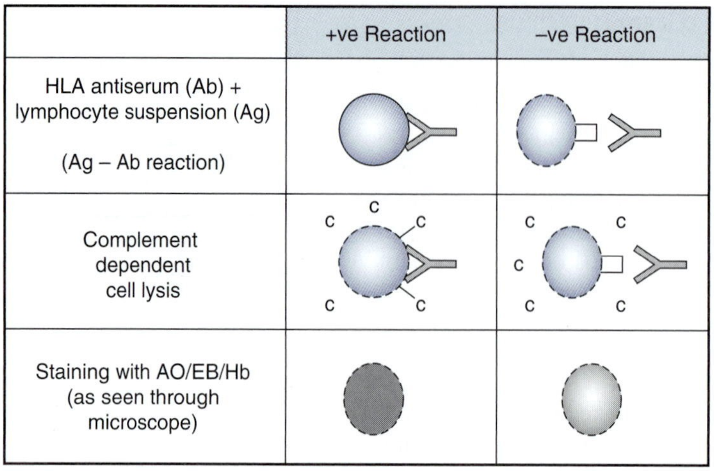

	+ve Reaction	−ve Reaction
HLA antiserum (Ab) + lymphocyte suspension (Ag) (Ag − Ab reaction)		
Complement dependent cell lysis		
Staining with AO/EB/Hb (as seen through microscope)		

■ **FIGURE 15-4** Interpretation of a Positive and Negative CDC Reaction Using the Two-color Fluorescent Procedure. (From: Page, G., *Tissue typing for beginners*).

(as the result of transfusion, pregnancy, or prior transplant); (2) to identify the HLA specificity of the antibody (and thus predict the HLA antibodies to be avoided when donors are selected); and (3) to identify patients with irrelevant antibodies such as IgM autoantibodies (enabling appropriate techniques to be selected to avoid false positive readings at the time of the donor-specific crossmatch). Cells from a sufficient number of individuals must be used to include the appropriate HLA types to as sign an antibody specificity. The panel of HLA antigens must also be appropriate for the population being tested. The PRA assay is per-

formed on renal, heart, and lung transplant patients. Liver transplant patients are usually tested retrospectively. Bone marrow/progenitor cell transplant recipients are not tested for PRA under most circumstances.

The PRA assay is initially done when the patient is identified as a candidate for transplant. Subsequent samples are collected monthly to track the presence of antibody/antibody titer. To ensure that results from different specimens are comparable, the screening panels should remain the same over time. Once tested, PRA samples are stored at −70°C and protected from CO_2 and evaporation. The stored serum can be used later to assess compatibility with a prospective donor in the donor-specific crossmatch.

A positive PRA is not necessarily a contraindication to transplant. However, if the PRA is greater than 60% (i.e., serum from the patient having a positive reaction to specificities found in at least 60% of panel), odds favor a positive T cell crossmatch. Studies show that these patients have a decreased chance of compatibility with an unrelated donor. ELISA based and flow cytometry methods can also be used to perform the PRA.

Donor-Specific Crossmatch

The donor-specific crossmatch (XM) is performed immediately prior to transplant. In this test, donor lymphocytes are tested against the potential recipient's most current serum sample. The purpose of the donor-specific crossmatch is to detect antibodies in the serum of the potential recipient targeted against antigens present on donor cells that may cause hyperacute rejection. Table 15-6✿ shows several factors to consider when performing the donor-specific XM.

✪ TABLE 15-5

Scoring scheme for the CDC test

Score	% Cell Death	Result
1	0–10	Negative
2	11–20	Negative
4	21–50	Weakly positive (equivocal). Helpful information in these cases includes (1) data on the behavior of other antisera of similar specificity, (2) the general reaction of antiserum against other cells, and (3) the circumstances for which the test is performed
6	51–80	Positive
8	81–100	Strongly Positive
0	Unreadable	

Each field is scored as 1, 2, 4, 6, or 8.

✪ TABLE 15-6

Factors to Consider in the Donor-Specific XM

Factor/Step	Step	Reason
Serum sample selection	Use current sample drawn within 48 hours of transplant if patient has preexisting HLA Class II antibodies or within 7 days prior to transplant if no antibodies have been identified.	■ Antibodies peak after a sensitizing event (e.g., blood transfusion, graft rejection, pregnancy). ■ A + XM with remote peak serum does not predict a poor outcome.
Wash steps (Amos)	Removal of unbound serum before the addition of complement.	Increases sensitivity; removes potential anticomplementary factors in patient's serum
Augmentation by AHG	Added after wash steps and prior to addition of complement.	■ AHG cross-links C1q and enhances its affinity for the cell. ■ Involves significant lab quality control. Commercial AHG reagents are not quality controlled for use in CDC augmentation.
Immunoglobulin class	If the autocrossmatch is positive, treat serum with **dithiothreitol (DTT).** If negative after treatment, antibodies were IgM.	IgM class antibodies are usually autologous and have no effect on graft rejection when observed in dialysis patients or those with autoimmune disease, receiving antihypertensive or antiarrythmic medications

Several modifications have enhanced the ability of the basic CDC technique to detect low levels of HLA antibody. In the Amos modification, one to three washes are performed following the initial cell-serum incubation. The washes remove aggregated immunoglobulin from the serum that may activate complement prematurely and make it unavailable for binding to cell membranes. Another modification to increase sensitivity, performed after the three Amos wash steps and prior to the addition of complement, is the addition of an anti-human globulin (AHG) (usually goat-antihuman κ) to each well. After a short incubation of one to two minutes, the rabbit complement is added as usual. The AHG increases the likelihood of complement binding and subsequent cell injury when HLA antibodies are below the detectable level of the standard crossmatch.

The AHG-augmented CDC T cell XM detects HLA Class I antibodies. It is performed using the potential recipient's most current serum sample and T lymphocytes isolated from the donor. If the T cell XM is positive, the transplant is contraindicated.

An AHG-augmented CDC T cell XM is always performed prior to kidney and pancreas transplantation. It is not performed prior to heart transplantation because of the limited organ preservation time unless the patient has a known antibody. The role of crossmatching in bone marrow and liver transplants is not well defined. Many studies have failed to demonstrate an adverse effect of a positive donor-specific XM in liver transplantation.

The AHG-augmented CDC B cell XM detects antibodies to HLA-DR and HLA-DQ Class II antigens; HLA-A, HLA-B, HLA-C Class I antibodies of weak specificity; and non-HLA specific antibodies (e.g., autoantibodies). It is performed on sensitized patients using B lymphocytes isolated from the donor. These cells have a higher density of Class II molecules and are more sensitive to complement dependent assays than T cells. This test includes a 37°C incubation period using autologous cells. A positive B cell-specific XM is not a contraindication to transplant but is a risk factor, especially in patients previously transplanted. Studies have indicated that DR-specific and high-titer B cell antibodies promote graft rejection. This test is affected by the assay sensitivity, serum sample selected, class of immunoglobulin in the patient's serum, and the presence of autoantibodies. It may involve adsorbing recipient serum with platelets to remove Class I antibody prior to the XM since many renal patients have mixed Class I and Class II antibodies. Platelets are used for adsorption because they express Class I but not Class II antigen. Table 15-7✪ lists sources of error commonly encountered in HLA typing and XM reactions.

FLOW CYTOMETRY

Specimen Preparation

Like other serological assays, flow cytometry testing requires viable cells for testing. Optimally, the viability of the sample received should be greater than 80%. For each potential recipient tested, six tubes are set up for the first recipient serum sample and two tubes for each additional serum sample (see Table 15-8✪ for tube setup). Donor cells, isolated from peripheral blood, lymph nodes, or spleen, are added to each tube. Four

✪ TABLE 15-7

Sources of Error in HLA Typing and Crossmatch Reactions

Potential Source of Error	Problem	Resolution
Mixing	Incorrect mixing of cells, serum, complement or eosin may cause false negative results.	Ensure adequate mixing.
Contamination	Carryover into the next well by the microsyringe needle.	Add positive control to wells last.
Complement	Variable activity of different lots of rabbit antisera as a source of complement.	Do not use human and guinea pig serum. Rabbit is best because it provides other factors that reacts with human cells.
		Test each lot of complement for activity and cytotoxicity. Titrate serum against several cells with appropriate +/− antisera.
Antisera	Tendency for false positive or false negative reactions or reactions with other antigens or a CREG.	Use fully characterized antisera.
Fixation step	False negative results.	After adding stain fixative, wait 30–40 minutes before reading to allow complete settling of cells. Injured cells settle more slowly.
Premature coverslipping	Tray cannot be read on day of testing.	Put uncoverslipped tray in the refrigerator overnight. Do not coverslip until tray ready to read. This minimizes formation of air bubbles which obscures readings.
Positive and negative controls	Control sera should mimic test sera in all characteristics except antibody specificity.	Use approved negative and positive controls. Appropriate negative control is pooled human serum from nontransfused males containing no lymphocytotoxic antibodies by sensitive assays such as flow cytometry. Approved positive control is a Class I tray mixture of HLA antisera (e.g., Bw4 plus Bw6) that reacts with all cells.
Phase adjustments	Phase microscope not adjusted properly.	
False negative reactions	■ Failure to add reagents (antiserum, complement) ■ Reagent no longer active ■ Ambient temperature too low ■ Inadequate mixing of reagents during incubation ■ Anticomplementary activity in antiserum or rabbit serum ■ Contamination by platelets or granulocytes	
False positive reactions	■ Nonviable cell preparations ■ Toxic materials in reagents (complement and buffers) ■ Incubation temperature too high ■ Incubation period too long ■ pH, isotonicity problem in reagents ■ Carryover of positive antiserum into adjacent negative well	
Technical variations	Dye quenches.	Choice of dye and delayed reading.

(Adapted from ASHI Lab Manual, 3rd ed. 1994)

tubes serve as controls, and at least two, depending on the number of recipient samples to be tested, are patient sera. The cells/serum are incubated for 30 minutes at 4°C to allow any HLA Class I or Class II antibodies in the recipient serum to bind to the corresponding antigen on the surface of the donor cells. After washing, fluorescein isothiocyanate (FITC) labeled anti-IgG is added to each tube and serves to bind

✪ TABLE 15-8

Setup of Tubes for a Flow Cytometry Crossmatch

Tube #	1° Antibody/Serum	2° Antibody
1	Negative control tube NHS or autologous serum	FITC IgG + CD3 PE
2	Negative control tube NHS or autologous serum	FITC IgG + CD20 PE
3	PBS	FITC IgG + CD3 PE
4	PBS	FITC IgG + CD20 PE
5	Patient sample #1	FITC IgG + CD3 PE
6	Patient sample #1	FITC IgG + CD20 PE

NHS: Non-human serum such as 2% fetal calf serum; PBS = phosphate buffered saline; FITC = fluorescein isothiocyanate; PE = phycoerythrin; CD3 = monoclonal antibody specific for T cells; CD 20 = monoclonal antibody specific for B cells

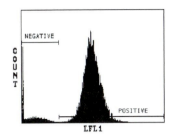

■ **FIGURE 15-5** This histogram shows a negative control and a positive specimen superimposed on each other. If the shift in the cell population is greater than 10 channels from the negative control, it is considered to be positive.

to any human IgG antibody present on the surface of the cells. Next, phycoerythrin (PE) labeled monoclonal antibodies anti-CD3 (targeting T cells) or anti-CD 20 (targeting B cells) is added to the appropriate tube. These fluorescent dye markers serve to identify T (FITC, green fluorescence) or B (PE, red fluorescence) cells. After dye staining, the cells are resuspended in 2% paraformaldehyde to stabilize the antibody-cell relationships. They can be stored up to one week at 4°C before testing on the flow cytometer.

Analysis

When performing flow cytometry analysis, cells previously resuspended in 2% paraformaldehyde are brought to room temperature prior to testing. Cells are aspirated into the flow cytometry instrument and forced to pass single file through a fluid stream after laser excitation of the attached fluorophore. Analysis by flow cytometry involves simultaneously measuring light scatter at small and large angles (reflecting cell size and granularity or cell type) and fluorescence emission (reflecting the binding of fluorescently tagged monoclonal antibodies). Results are printed on a histogram, which must be interpreted by the technologist or a pathologist as shown in Figure 15-5■.

A cell showing FITC (green) fluorescence identifies it as a donor cell which has bound antibody present in the patient serum. Simultaneous red fluorescence indicates that antibody has bound to either a T cell or to a B cell, depending on the PE labeled monoclonal anti-

body that was added to the tube. A HLA Class I antibody will react with B and T cells while a HLA Class II antibody reacts with B cells only. Other cell types, such as monocytes and platelets, can also be studied by flow cytometry by changing the PE labeled monoclonal antibody used to mark the cells (Figure 15-6■).

Using Flow Cytometry in HLA Testing

The most common use of flow cytometry in HLA testing is the donor-specific XM. Studies indicate that a patient with a negative AHG-CDC that is positive by flow cytometry XM is at risk for an increased number of rejection episodes and possibly early graft failure. Both the flow cytometry XM and the AHG-CDC XM use a reagent specific for human immunoglobulin to assist in the detection of HLA-directed antibodies in the patient's serum. However, flow cytometry has been shown to have a sensitivity 10 to 50 times that of the AHG-CDC assay, and it is not dependent on complement activation to obtain a result. Flow cytometry laboratories are found primarily in medical centers associated with busy transplant programs. The instrument required for these studies is expensive (approximately $100,000), and testing requires the purchase of costly monoclonal antibody reagents with short expiration dates. Like HLA, flow cytometry is a highly specialized area requiring dedicated training to interpret the histogram patterns.

► CELLULAR TECHNIQUES

ONE WAY MIXED LYMPHOCYTE REACTION/MIXED LYMPHOCYTE CULTURE

The mixed lymphocyte culture (MLC), also called the mixed lymphocyte reaction (MLR), can provide information about cellular recognition that may not be determined by serologic or DNA-based typing methods. A

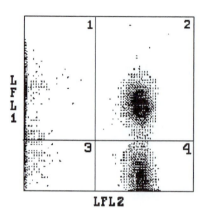

■ **FIGURE 15-6** This is a histogram of a T-cell crossmatch showing a negative control and a positive specimen superimposed on each other. Region 1 shows cells that have antibody, but are T-cells. Region 2 shows T-cells with antibody. This is the positive reaction. Region 3 shows non-T-cells with no antibody. Region 4 shows T-cells that have no antibody. This is the negative control. Therefore, regions 3 & 4 are negative and regions 1 & 2 are positive.

"cellular crossmatch" measures the ability of a patient's lymphocytes to recognize and respond to foreign HLA Class II antigens on the cell population from another (**allogeneic**) individual. Prior to testing, a mononuclear cell population (termed the "stimulator") is treated with mitomycin C or is irradiated to inhibit DNA synthesis. When treated and untreated cells are mixed together in a 1:1 ratio, T cells in the untreated population will "respond" to any Class II differences between itself and the non-T cells (e.g., B lymphocytes, monocytes, **dendritic cells**) in the treated (stimulator) population by proliferating. In the process of proliferation, the newly synthesized DNA in the untreated cells will uptake tritiated thymidine. Uptake is measured over a six-day period. High levels of platelets and granulocytes can inhibit the MLC. Each laboratory must define what constitutes a weak versus a strong response. Generally, a response of <15%–20% indicates a similar specificity. The MLC uses pure mononuclear cell suspensions in the stimulator population because monocytes and B lymphocytes are effective in promoting cell proliferation.

► MOLECULAR TECHNIQUES IN HLA

Molecular techniques have transformed histocompatibility testing. The ability to discriminate between HLA alleles at the most basic level has clarified and expanded our understanding of MHC and its importance in the success of tissue transplantation/immunoresponsiveness. Because of the high reproducibility of **polymerase chain reaction (PCR)**-based assays between laboratories (>99%), DNA testing is beginning to replace serology for both Class I and Class II HLA typing. Compared with serological typing methods, DNA techniques are specific, flexible, robust, and reproducible. For example, two cross-reactive groups or **splits** have been associated with HLA-DR6, a Class II antigen (DR13 and DR14) using serological methods. Molecular typing, on the other hand, has established the existence of more than 60 alleles of DR13 and more than 40 alleles of DR14, for a total of more than 100 possible alleles associated with the Class II HLA-DR6 antigen. Further, this testing indicates that as many as 25% of serologically typed DR results may be incorrect. Studies indicate that the predictability for DNA-based tissue matching may be better than that of the MLC. This is especially important in progenitor cell/bone marrow transplantation where **graft versus host disease (GVHD)** is one of the major complications or causes of death. DNA-based methodology is utilized in three areas of the HLA lab: HLA typing, gene sequencing, and engraftment monitoring following bone marrow/progenitor cell transplant.

ADVANTAGES OF DNA-BASED TESTING

Unlike serology, DNA-based HLA does not require isolation of viable lymphocytes, is not influenced by the health of the patient, and the reagents utilized are not limited by lot-to-lot specificity. The primary DNA reagent, a synthetic **oligonucleotide probe/primer,** has a definitive nucleotide sequence that allows manufacture according to a standardized protocol almost immediately after new alleles are discovered. These probe/primer combinations are unique for a certain allele, assuring no cross-reactivity between antigen groups as seen in serology. Depending on the probe/primer design, DNA testing can identify alleles that are indistinguishable using serologic typing. Testing can be carried out at several levels of resolution with ready analysis at the allele level (as opposed to the protein level, the identification level of serology). For example, whereas serologic typing identifies the DR4 protein, DNA typing identifies over 40 DR4 allelic variations of this protein. Molecular testing also eliminates the "blanks" identified in serology, resulting from homozygosity at a particular locus or from lack of the sera containing the appropriate antibodies to type the allele.

Molecular HLA techniques begin with PCR to amplify the gene region of interest. Two main typing methods are used. These are PCR-sequence specific oligonucleotide probes (PCR-SSOP) and PCR-sequence specific oligonucleotide primers (PCR-SSP). Typing by these techniques can be defined as "low resolution" or "high resolution." Low-resolution typing identifies the HLA group present (e.g., DR1 or DR4) and equates to serology. It is used primarily in progenitor cell/bone marrow transplantation for the initial typing of prospective related or unrelated donors. High-resolution typing specifically defines the HLA subtype (allele) for that group (e.g., DRB1*0102 or DRB1*0401). Once a donor is identified at the low-resolution level, as demonstrated by the case presented at the beginning of this chapter, higher resolution typing is performed to ensure identity at the allele level. This is particularly important when parents are not available to determine haplotypes or when parents share HLA antigens. Table 15-9✪ shows the events that take place in HLA testing using molecular-based methods.

SPECIMEN COLLECTION AND DNA EXTRACTION

Since DNA is available by extraction from any nucleated cell and DNA testing does not require viable cells, specimens collected for molecular assays do not have to be transported immediately. After collection in ACD or EDTA, peripheral blood DNA remains intact for up to five days when stored at room temperature and up to two weeks when refrigerated at 2–8°C. However, a freshly drawn sample is best since the DNA degrades with time. Anticoagulants containing heparin should

---

✪ TABLE 15-9

Sample Flow Using Molecular-Based Methods

Molecular HLA Test Scheme

Separation of buffy coat from whole blood

Lysis of red blood cells

Extraction of DNA from white blood cells

Hydration of DNA pellet

Amplification of HLA alleles using PCR and various HLA-specific primers or probes (PCR-SSOP or PCR-SSP)

Detection of amplified fragments

- ■ Electrophoresis and ethidium bromide staining
  1. Interpretation of gels
  2. Correlation of electrophoretic bands with HLA antigens
- ■ Enzyme/Chemiluminescence (light)/fluorescence

Correlation of results via manual or computer assisted programs

---

not be used since heparin inhibits the PCR. Assuming a normal white blood cell count, a 200 μl aliquot of peripheral blood is usually sufficient for isolating the 6–10 μg of DNA necessary for one full typing. Using the buffy coat versus peripheral blood to extract DNA increases the number of white blood cells available for DNA extraction and increases the final yield of DNA. With the availability of commercial kits, the DNA extraction procedure takes less than one hour. Once extracted, the concentration of DNA in the extracted sample is measured by spectrophotometry at the absorbance wavelengths 260 nm and 280 nm. For optimal results, the DNA 260/280 ratio of the extracted DNA should be greater than 1.4 and have a purity of greater than 80%. A ratio of less than 1.5 indicates protein contamination, which could affect amplification. In these cases, reextraction is recommended. Once extracted, the DNA can be stored in buffer or sterile water and is stable indefinitely at −70°C. Reagents used in DNA testing should be stored at −70°C in a non–frost free freezer. This avoids numerous freeze-thaw cycles over time, which degrades the DNA primers and inactivates the enzymes in the kit.

POLYMERASE CHAIN REACTION

PCR is an in vitro procedure that mimics the process of DNA replication (Figure 15-7■). The components of the PCR are patient DNA, dNTP or nucleotides (adenine, thymine, guanine, or cytosine denoted generically as NTP), *Taq* DNA polymerase, specific primer sets

The Polymerase Chain Reaction

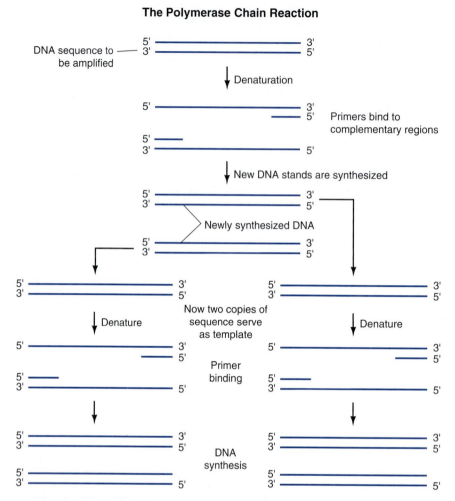

After two cycles, four copies of original sequence are available to serve as templates
for synthesis of additional strands during the next cycle.

■ **FIGURE 15-7** Polymerase chain reaction (PCR). Short, 15–20 base pair oligonucleotide primer sequences complementary to the 3′ end of the region of interest on
each DNA strand bind to the denatured DNA and serve as a starting point for DNA
synthesis. *Taq* DNA polymerase catalyzes the addition of nucleotides to the end of
the primers. The nucleotide added to the end of the primer is dictated by the sequence order on the original strand. (Wisecarver, 1997. Used by permission, American Society of Clinical Pathology).

that flank the region of interest, Mg+, and buffer. The
reagents and DNA are combined to make the total
volume 10 to 100 μl per tube, depending on the procedure. The PCR reaction tubes are placed in an instrument called a thermal cycler, where the reaction takes
place. For each PCR, an average of 30 cycles is performed, with each cycle doubling exponentially the
amount of DNA product present in each tube. A cycle
consists of three steps: denaturation, annealing, and
extension. In the denaturation step, the DNA is heated
to approximately 95°C. At this temperature, the hydro-

gen bonds holding the double-stranded DNA helix together break and the strands separate. In the second
step, the temperature is cooled to 55–70°C. At this
temperature, primers flanking the region to be amplified anneal (attach) to the complementary sequences
on the patient's DNA if they are present. In the third
step, primer extension, the temperature is raised to
72°C. The reaction is catalyzed by a thermostable DNA
polymerase enzyme (*Taq* DNA polymerase) that is resistant to the high temperatures needed for denaturation. The enzyme attaches to the DNA and guides the

addition of nucleotides onto the end of the primer to extend its length. The nucleotide (adenine, thymine, guanine, or cytosine) added onto the 3′ end of the primer is determined by the nucleotide at the corresponding position on the patient DNA strand. By repeating this three-step cycle 20 to 40 times, millions of copies of a specific HLA sequence are generated, enough to be detected colorimetrically or by electrophoresis. The primer sets used in PCR correspond to the polymorphic regions (e.g., α2–α3 region of the Class I gene or the β1 region of the DRB1 gene) of the DNA that distinguish specific alleles.

PCR-SEQUENCE SPECIFIC OLIGONUCLEOTIDE PRIMERS

PCR-SSP takes advantage of unique HLA polymorphisms to specifically amplify alleles with sequences complimentary to a given primer pair. This method of HLA typing uses PCR to amplify genomic (patient) DNA using formulations of allele or group specific primer sets contained in a 96-well thermal tray. Results are visualized by electrophoresis. PCR-SSP is a qualitative procedure. Interpretation of the electrophoretic gel is based on the presence or absence of an amplified fragment of a specific size on an electrophoretic gel in conjunction with the presence of an internal control. This technique is used for typing small numbers of samples within a short period of time and is usually employed in small- and medium-sized HLA laboratories. Commercial kits are available that are designed to provide low- to medium-resolution of the HLA Class I A, B, and C and Class II DRβ, and DQβ loci. The alleles amplified are described in *Tissue Antigens,* 2001, by the International Nomenclature Committee of WHO. Most heterozygous combinations can be determined using this method.

In the PCR-SSP reaction, patient DNA is added to a tube containing buffer, distilled water, and *Taq* DNA polymerase. A portion of this mixture is aliquoted to each of the 96 wells on the tray. Each well contains prealiquoted HLA allele-specific primers and internal control primers (Table 15-10✪).

Following PCR, the fragments are electrophoresed on a 2% agarose gel which is stained with EB and then placed on a UV transilluminator for visualization. Fragment migration is seen as bands migrating to specific positions on the gel depending on their size. For each well, the internal control and HLA-amplified fragment (if amplification occurred) migrate to different, nonoverlapping positions on the gel. The control band may be missing or appear weaker in the presence of allele-specific amplification but must be seen in the absence of allele-specific amplification to ensure that the PCR has been successful. If no internal control or allele-specific band is detected in a particular well, then that well is considered a failed reaction and must be repeated. A PCR marker with known size fragments is placed in the last lane of each row on the gel to estimate the base pair position of the bands. Each tray includes a negative control in the very last lane. The negative control sample is an aliquot of distilled water

✪ TABLE 15-10

Typical Set up of a 96-Well Typing Tray for HLA-DNA Testing

Patient Name												
	1	2	3	4	5	6	7	8	9	10	11	12
A	lane 1	lane 9	lane 17	lane 25	lane 33	lane 41	lane 49	lane 57	lane 65	lane 73	lane 81	lane 89
B	lane 2	lane 10	lane 18	lane 26	lane 34	lane 42	lane 50	lane 58	lane 66	lane 74	lane 82	lane 90
C	lane 3	lane 11	lane 19	lane 27	lane 35	lane 43	lane 51	lane 59	lane 67	lane 75	lane 83	lane 91
D	lane 4	lane 12	lane 20	lane 28	lane 36	lane 44	lane 52	lane 60	lane 68	lane 76	lane 84	lane 92
E	lane 5	lane 13	lane 21	lane 29	lane 37	lane 45	lane 53	lane 61	lane 69	lane 77	lane 85	lane 93
F	lane 6	lane 14	lane 22	lane 30	lane 38	lane 46	lane 54	lane 62	lane 70	lane 78	lane 86	lane 94
G	lane 7	lane 15	lane 23	lane 31	lane 39	lane 47	lane 55	lane 63	lane 71	lane 79	lane 87	lane 95
H	lane 8	lane 16	lane 24	lane 32	lane 40	lane 48	lane 56	lane 64	lane 72	lane 80	lane 88	lane 96

Each well contains a different allele-specific primer pair. All reagents (including the allele-specific primers flanking the region of interest) except patient DNA and *Taq* DNA polymerase are prealiquoted into the wells. Once PCR is accomplished, the contents of the wells are transferred to the designated lane of a 2% agarose gel for electrophoresis.

left in an open tube in the processing area while the test is being set up. The primer sets in the negative control well detect the presence of contaminating genomic DNA. If a band is present in the negative control lane on electrophoresis, it indicates contamination, voiding the test results. DNA contamination is also suspected if, upon interpretation, there are more than two alleles per locus, there is unexpected inheritance found in the haplotype determinations, or if the high-resolution typing differs from low-resolution or serologic typing. Cases have been reported in which DNA typing differs from previous serological typing. In these instances, DNA is generally considered the reference method.

Interpretation is performed by visual inspection of a gel photograph (Figure 15-8■). In the presence of a control band, the absence of a band at the appropriate base pair location for a particular primer is a negative reaction, and a band at the appropriate base pair location is a positive reaction. Unused primers may form a diffuse band comigrating with the dye front. This primer dimer effect appears below the area where specific product is found, usually below 80 base pairs, and should be ignored. A worksheet/computer program is provided by the manufacturer to assist the technolo-

gist in determining which allele, or group of alleles, the respective primers identify. Two independent interpretations of the data should be performed. Each typing is read and interpreted by the technologist performing the test. A second technologist or the supervisor reinterprets the typing to assure the validity of the results. If the two interpretations do not agree and cannot be resolved, the typing should be repeated. Where possible, ambiguities are resolved through family studies and **haplotype** inheritance. Typings that cannot be resolved may be sent to the tray manufacturer for allele-specific typing or sequencing, and are usually performed at no charge.

PCR-SEQUENCE SPECIFIC OLIGONUCLEOTIDE PROBES

This technique is accurate, reliable, and specific. It is used when many samples are typed in large batches and generally utilizes commercial kits. The SSOP method can be forward or reverse based. In the forward-based SSOP method (Figure 15-9■), PCR-amplified DNA from multiple patients is attached to a solid support and then denatured. When an HLA allele-specific oligonucleotide probe is exposed to the solid sup-

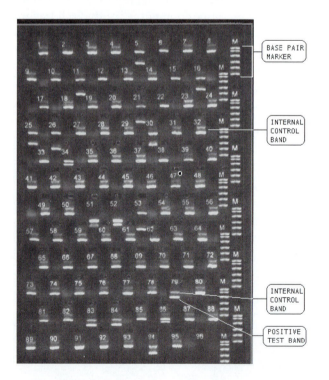

■ FIGURE 15-8 PCR-SSP electrophoretic gel.

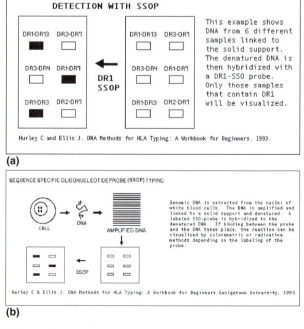

■ FIGURE 15-9 (a) Schematic of forward based PCR-SSOP. (b) Detection with forward based PCR-SSOP. (Source: Hurley and Ellis, 1993. Used by permission).

port, the probe will anneal (**hybridize**) to the patient DNA fragment if the complementary sequence is present. Prior to hybridization, the probe was tagged with an enzyme (e.g., alkaline phosphatase) or light (chemiluminescent) producing compound. The addition of a substrate yields a colored compound. The pattern of color (or light) indicates which patients were positive or negative for that particular allele. In the reverse format (Figure 15-10■), different oligonucleotide probes are immobilized to the solid support. One patient's DNA labeled with, for example, biotin, is mixed with the immobilized probes. Addition of avidin labeled with a fluorescent or enzyme tag allows visualization of hybridization. The pattern of hybridization is indicative of the HLA alleles present.

SEQUENCE BASED TYPING

SBT is a method that directly determines the nucleic acid sequence of the HLA alleles carried by an individual. SBT is a manual, labor intensive procedure accomplished on PCR products. It is performed primarily on those patients needing bone marrow/progenitor cell transplants who do not have a complete/highly matched related donor. When a matched, unrelated volunteer donor is identified by the National Marrow Donor Program (NMDP) or other regional registries, the first step is HLA typing by serologic or low-resolution DNA methods of HLA-A, B, and C locus antigens followed by high-resolution HLA-DRB1 allotyping of each potential donor. Since as many as one-third to one-half of the HLA-phenotypically matched unrelated donors actually have HLA disparity at one or more alleles, Class I SBT is recommended prior to final donor selection. One method utilized in SBT is the BigDye™

(PE-Applied Biosystems, Foster City, CA) protocol. Here, genomic DNA isolated from peripheral blood collected in either ACD or EDTA prior to administration of platelet or red cell transfusions is used. In the first step, PCR and HLA locus-specific primers amplify a 2,000 base pair region of DNA template representing **exons** 1 to 5. Each of the PCR products is then reamplified using individual **nested** primers that flank exons 2, 3, and 4. Sequencing is performed on an automated ABI Prism 377 DNA Sequencer (PE-Applied Biosystems, Foster City, CA) using a proprietary fluorescence sequencing chemistry. The data from forward- and reverse-based sequencing reactions for each exon are edited, assembled into a linear sequence, and analyzed with a variety of additional software to assign the HLA Class I alleles for each HLA locus.

SHORT TANDEM REPEAT TESTING TO DETERMINE BONE MARROW ENGRAFTMENT

STR is a qualitative/semiquantitative procedure performed post–bone marrow/progenitor cell transplant to determine the degree of donor engraftment, as in the case presented, and to evaluate the presence/absence of disease/relapse. STR testing distinguishes recipient from donor cells.

Tandemly repeated DNA nucleotide sequences are widespread throughout the human genome. Because they are extremely polymorphic (variable) from one person to another, they are useful genetic markers with applications primarily in gene mapping, linkage analysis, and human identity testing. Tandemly repeated DNA sequences can be classified into two groups based on the size of the repeat region. Minisatellites (also called variable number of tandem repeats or VNTRs) have a core of repeats of 9–80 base pairs. Microsatellites (short tandem repeats or STRs) have a core of repeats of 2–7 base pairs and can be found every 6–15 kb along the DNA, generally in **introns** and untranslated areas. Each time the VNTR/STR repeat sequence is encountered, the number of copies varies. Thus, each chromosome has hundreds of VNTR or STR sites with each site having two alleles and each allele having a different number of tandem repeats. Because of less variability within the repeat region and a shorter repeat unit, STR loci have been adapted for use in assessing bone marrow/progenitor cell engraftment.

The first step in STR testing is to find an **informative locus.** Informative markers, through differences in band size and distribution, allow a unique donor and recipient pattern to be determined. To that end, peripheral blood from the donor and

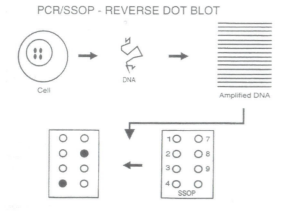

■ FIGURE 15-10 Schematic of reverse based PCR-SSOP.

recipient are collected prior to transplant. The extracted DNA is amplified by PCR using sets of primers corresponding to multiple STR loci. If the donor and recipient are related, they will share many STR alleles, and multiple loci may have to be tested in order to find one that is informative. However, studies show that when primer sets for common STR loci are used, one of these is usually informative in approximately 90% of the cases. This process may be simplified by using **multiplex PCR.** Following PCR, the STR alleles can be separated by size via denaturing **polyacrylamide gel electrophoresis** or **capillary gel electrophoresis** after labeling the PCR products by radioactive (rare today) or nonradioactive (fluorescence or by silver staining the gel) methods. Qualitative STR methods detect only the presence of recipient cells. Determination of engraftment requires quantitation of the STR alleles present. In order to do this, both the recipient and donor must have at least one unique STR allele. Quantitatation can be accomplished on stained electrophoretic gels by densitometry of the bands or though the analysis of fluorescently labeled PCR products by computer software on an automated DNA analyzer.

Engraftment is determined by comparing the band patterns of the recipient pre- and posttransplant to that of the donor. Complete engraftment is determined if only donor STR alleles are detected. A mixed **chimera** is present if recipient and donor alleles are detected. Relapse is associated with the presence of mainly recipient STR alleles, after having mainly donor alleles for a time.

The significance of detecting both donor and recipient patterns is dependent on the time interval from transplant. A mixture of both types is possible within the first two weeks after transplantation. However, this finding one-year posttransplantation would represent graft rejection and/or disease recurrence. This often depends on the original disease and type of marrow conditioning used at the outset. Correlation with clinical status and consideration of the interval between bone marrow transplantation and testing is necessary for proper interpretation of results (Figures 15-11■ and 15-12■).

DNA methods have proven to be accurate, reliable, and much more precise than serological methods for HLA analysis. They provide the application of methods accurate enough to ensure transplant success. However, at this time, molecular techniques are primarily manual and thus labor intensive, time consuming, and expensive. Future challenges are to fully utilize this technology while making it cost effective for routine employment in the HLA laboratory.

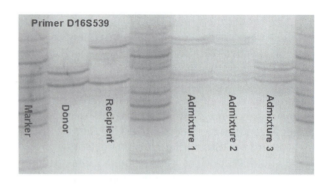

■ FIGURE 15-11 Example of a silver stained gel following electrophoresis for STR analysis. The informative locus is on chromosome 16 and the primer used is D16S539. From left, the allelic ladder (lane 1), donor pre-transplant (lane 2), recipient pre-transplant (lane 3), allelic ladder (lane 4), admixture 1, 0% donor (lane 5), admixture 2, 20% donor (lane 6), admixture 3, 95% donor (lane 7), allelic marker (lane 8) (From CAP survey ME-C 2000).

▶ HLA LABORATORIES

TYPES OF HLA LABORATORIES

Due in great part to the work of the International Histocompatibility Workshops, the first HLA-typing laboratories were established in the late 1960s and early 1970s to support kidney or developing bone marrow transplantation programs. In the late 1970s, as techniques for identifying HLA antibodies and HLA-typing became more reliable HLA laboratories were established in blood banks and regional blood procurement centers to support the growing need for HLA-matched platelets in major transfusion centers. Other facets of HLA testing, such as disease association and paternity testing, began to emerge in the 1980s. Today histocompatibility laboratories are found within three main environments: blood bank laboratories (independent or hospital based), separate entities within a larger clinical or commercial laboratory, or independent laboratories supporting only transplantation programs. They can be broken down into four categories based on the complexity and repertoire of testing provided (Table 15-11✪).

ACCREDITATION/REGULATORY AGENCIES

In 1988 Congress passed the Clinical Laboratory Improvement Ammendments (CLIA) which established standards for laboratory testing to ensure accurate and reliable patient test results regardless of where the test was performed. All laboratories in the United States (except Washington and New York, which are exempt)

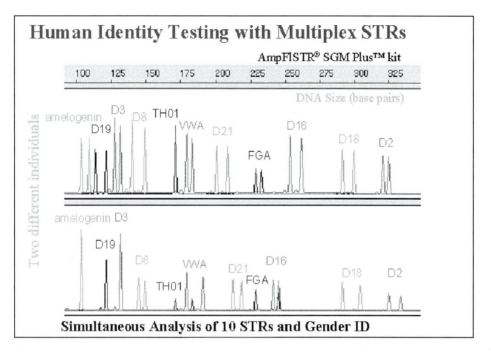

■ FIGURE 15-12 Example of a multiplex PCR in STR testing using the ABI 310 (PE-Applied Biosystems, Foster City, CA). This methodology utilizes 10 loci that are analyzed for informativeness in one PCR reaction. Products are separated electrophoretically in a single lane on a polyacrylamide gel. As fluorescently labeled PCR products migrate through the gel, fluorescence information is converted into alleles with base-pair sizes and peak areas corresponding to the fluorescent bands. Percentages of mixed populations are determined by relative peak areas. Depending on the genotype, allele, and locus, as low as 2.5% of the minor cell component can be detected. The differences in the peak height can be calculated to determine percentage of donor present. This picture compares the peaks in the donor and patient pretransplant.

must obtain a CLIA certificate from the Centers for Medicare & Medicaid Services (CMS, previously known as the Health Care Financing Administration or HCFA). CMS certification is based on the complexity of testing performed and mandates routine proficiency testing. All histocompatibility laboratories are considered high-complexity testing laboratories under CLIA. Laboratories can choose to be surveyed by CMS or by a private accrediting organization. Approved accrediting organizations under CLIA for histocompatibility laboratories include the American Association of Blood Banks (AABB), the American Society for Histocompatibility and Immunogenetics (ASHI), and the College of American Pathologists (CAP). These agencies use or incorporate the CLIA 1988 requirements into the standards used for inspection. The accrediting agent used depends on the environment in which the HLA lab is found. For example, the AABB inspects and accredits blood banks with HLA-related activities usually compatibility testing for single donor HLA-matched platelets. CAP inspects

and accredits all aspects of the clinical laboratory. Their HLA laboratory checklist is more extensive than the AABB. The most comprehensive inspection and accreditation process for HLA labs is performed by ASHI, which exclusively inspects and accredits HLA laboratories. Up until 2005, all HLA labs supporting transplantation programs had to have ASHI accreditation. UNOS gave ASHI deemed status to inspect and accredit HLA labs, and in 2005, CAP was also awarded deemed status. The Foundation for the Accreditation of Cellular Therapy (FACT), which accredits many of the major bone marrow transplantation programs, also requires support labs to be ASHI accredited.

The accreditation process begins with application and inspection. External laboratory professionals perform an on-site inspection. The inspection entails evaluation of every aspect of the laboratory. Inspectors start at the beginning with general policies, qualifications and competence of personnel, safety, and facilities. They cover the entire testing process from the

✪ TABLE 15-11

Categories of Testing in the Different Types of HLA Laboratories

Laboratory Category	Testing	Application	Comment
HLA Typing Only	HLA typing only	Disease association studies Paternity testing Typing volunteer bone marrow (BM) donors for unrelated BM transplant programs	Usually component of a larger commercial lab providing a wide range of clinical lab testing
Support for Transfusion Centers	HLA typing HLA antibody (ab) screening Ab ID on patient sera	Supports the need for single donor HLA-matched platelets	Often established in blood banks or transfusion services
Support for Transplantation Programs	Serological, molecular and cellular techniques	Solid organ and/or bone marrow transplantation programs	Most complex and labor-intensive level of testing
	HLA typing (serology/DNA) HLA ab screening and ID Crossmatching by cytotoxic and/or flow cytometry Adsorption techniques for removal of IgM ab that interfere with the crossmatch procedure	Solid organ transplant programs	Provides 24 hour/7 days a week service
	HLA typing by DNA (low and high resolution) Haplotype determinations in family studies Cellular techniques (MLC) Engraftment monitoring (STR)	Bone marrow transplant programs	
Major Research and Training Programs	Any test outlines in support for transplantation programs Sequence-based typing (SBT)	Support large transplantation programs Leading participants in International Workshops	Associated with universities with large R & D components
	DNA-sequencing to determine the presence of new HLA alleles	Principal source of new doctoral personnel entering the HLA field	

specimen collection, the procedures used, quality assurance and quality control, interpretation, and reporting of the results and final disposition of the specimens. After passing the initial inspection, the laboratory is awarded accreditation for a two-year period. At midcycle, the laboratory is required to perform a self-inspection and submit a package for review. Laboratories that cannot pass the on-site inspection are given a period of 30 days to correct the deficiencies cited. If the deficiencies can be corrected within the allotted time, the laboratory is accredited. Laboratories that cannot correct the deficiencies are placed in probationary status and cannot report laboratory results.

At the time all deficiencies are corrected, the lab may reapply for accreditation and start the process over. Every two years, an on-site inspection is performed to renew the accreditation.

PERSONNEL

Compliance with federal regulations means having a staff that is qualified and competent enough to accomplish the tasks required. Table 15-12✪ outlines the qualifications for HLA laboratory personnel under CLIA. ASHI, in collaboration with UNOS, has begun to

✪ TABLE 15-12

Qualifications for HLA laboratory personnel under CLIA

HLA Laboratory Personnel	Qualifications	Comment
Laboratory Director	■ Licensed doctor of medicine, doctor of osteopathy, or doctor of podiatry, or doctoral degree in a biological or clinical laboratory science from an accredited institution ■ 4 years of lab training/experience in histocompatibility or 2 years of lab training/experience in general immunology plus 2 years of lab training/experience in histocompatibility	
Technical Supervisor	Same as laboratory director	
General Supervisor	■ Bachelor's degree ■ 3 years experience in human HLA testing under the supervision of a qualified director or ■ In lieu of a bachelor's degree, 5 years of supervised experience ■ Certification as a histocompatibility specialist, CHS (ABHI), is desirable	Provides day-to-day supervision of testing personnel and reporting of test results
Testing personnel ■ Histocompatibility technologist	■ 1 year of supervised experience in human HLA testing, regardless of academic degree/other training, experience ■ Certification as CHS or CHT (ABHI) is desirable	
■ Histocompatibility technician	< 1 year of supervised experience in human HLA testing, regardless of academic degree or other training and experience	
Clinical consultant	Must meet same qualifications as a laboratory director	Functions in the absence of an on-site director

establish curricula for training laboratory directors and HLA specialists. The American Board of Histocompatibility and Immunogenetics (ABHI) is a certifying board offering voluntary credentialing examinations in the field of histocompatibility and immunogenetics. ABHI provides certification and promotes continuing education for histocompatibility and immunogenetics professionals. The Board is sponsored by ASHI. ABHI offers four levels of certification: (1) Certified Histocompatibility Associate: CHA(ABHI), (2) Certified Histocompatibility Technologist: CHT(ABHI), (3) Certified Histocompatibility Specialist: CHS(ABHI), and (4) Diplomate of the ABHI: D(ABHI).

There are no formal training programs for histocompatibility technologists. Most medical technology programs have little or no training in histocompatibility testing and clinical immunology. As a result, individual laboratories are responsible for training their own technologists. Training varies from lab to lab depending on the extent of their HLA requirements. In a lab that supports a solid organ transplantation pro-

gram, it may take six months for the technologist to be competent to perform all the testing required to be in an on-call position with no direct supervision.

Continuing education of personnel is an integral part of a good laboratory operation. Opportunities for continuing education in histocompatibility are limited but available. ASHI and the South-Eastern Organ Procurement Foundation (SEOPF) conduct regional meetings and workshops. SEOPF offers a one-week course at both the basic and specialist level. In addition, ASHI holds an annual meeting containing both scientific and educational programs.

QUALITY ASSURANCE/ QUALITY CONTROL

QA and QC have always been important components of laboratory medicine. In the past, laboratories focused on the analysis part of the testing procedure, including calibration, intrarun controls, interrun controls, internal QC, and external QC. Today, however, lab consolidation and the demands of managed care have forced laboratory managers to look at other models of quality assurance in an effort to reduce costs. Total quality management (TQM), continuous quality improvement (CQI), and other QA management paradigms track the entire testing process, and they have been found to be quite effective in controlling laboratory costs. The vast majority of lab managers now recognize that regular review of preanalytical procedures and reporting methods (postanalytical) is essential in order to produce high-quality results. Today, QC is just one part of the QA program. QC is defined is "a planned system of activities whose purpose is to provide a quality product" while QA refers to "a planned system of activities whose purpose is to provide assurance that the QC program is actually effective."

QA in the histocompatibility laboratory is an entire system of procedures, communications, expectations, and results. The system begins when the physician talks to the patient and determines that HLA testing needs to be done and ends when the results are back in the hands of the physician so that he/she may use the information to make decisions regarding the patient. Figure 15-13■ shows the quality assurance cycle for histocompatibility testing. An HLA lab includes all the components of the familiar clinical laboratory. Every process that is monitored and controlled in the clinical laboratory from specimen collection to turnaround time is also moniteted in the HLA laboratory.

In the area of QC, the HLA laboratory is unique in that reagents not only need special handling, but also require special testing, sometimes prior to selection and/or purchase. Each new lot of complement, antiglobulin reagent, and protein supplement must be tested before purchase. Most suppliers will give complementary samples so the testing process can be done prior to lot selection.

■ Protein supplements must be tested against the antibody-screening panel to ensure that they lack HLA antibodies before being used as a control or supplement.

■ Antiglobulin reagents used in the enhanced crossmatch must be tested to select the optimal dilution that will increase sensitivity over the level seen in the cytotoxicity test without antiglobulin. Several lots should be tested to find one that will be sensitive but not strong enough to cause cytotoxicity in the negative control.

■ Complement is the probably the most important reagent to QC since every cytotoxic reaction depends on it. Several lots should be titered to determine the optimal lot number and dilution to be

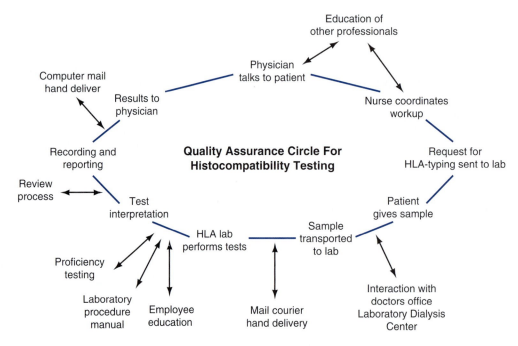

■ **FIGURE 15-13** Quality Assurance (QA) Circle for Histocompatibility Testing (SEOPF, 2001. Used with permission).

used. Each lot is tested with known antisera, both positive and negative, and known cells. The complement titration is performed by making serial dilutions of both the complement and the antisera. These dilutions are tested against each other to determine the cut-off for a strong positive reaction and still have a clean negative reaction.

As in all clinical laboratories, the HLA laboratory must participate in external proficiency testing. CAP, ASHI, SEOPF, and University of California at Los Angeles (UCLA) Tissue Typing DNA laboratory provide approved samples for proficiency testing. These samples cover most facets of HLA testing, including serological and molecular typing, antibody detection and identification, and crossmatching. CAP and ASHI also now include samples for engraftment monitoring. To monitor the tests, for which there are no proficiency samples available, such as the MLC, HLA labs must exchange samples with another accredited lab at least twice a year. In addition to external testing, ASHI requires HLA laboratory personnel to test a blind specimen at least once per year for each method that is performed.

SUMMARY

Histocompatibility testing is performed to evaluate tissue compatibility between a transplantation donor and potential recipient before transplantation occurs. The following tests are performed in the histocompatibility laboratory:

- HLA typing of the potential recipient and donor
- Haplotype determination
- Evaluation of patient sera for HLA antibodies
- Crossmatching potential recipients against donor

Serological, cellular, and molecular techniques are used in HLA testing depending on the resources of the testing laboratory. Each technique has its clinical applications and may be applied to different degrees.

All histocompatibility laboratories are deemed high-complexity testing laboratories under CLIA and therefore must be surveyed by CMS or by an accrediting organization. QA is an integral system in place in HLA labs to assure that every step in the process is monitored and quality controlled.

POINTS TO REMEMBER

▶ Different HLA test techniques and clinical application of histocompatibility testing.

▶ Advantages of molecular HLA typing over other methods.

▶ Methods for determining engraftment following bone marrow/progenitor cell transplant.

LEARNING ASSESSMENT QUESTIONS

1. A major breakthrough in histocompatibility testing was the introduction and miniaturization of the:
   a. mixed lymphocyte culture.
   b. complement dependent cytotoxicity test.
   c. polymerase chain reaction.
   d. mixed lymphocyte reaction.

2. All *serological* techniques used in histocompatibility testing are based on the CDC except:
   a. flow cytometry cross-match.
   b. HLA-antibody detection.
   c. HLA-Class I typing.
   d. HLA-Class II typing.

3. The cellular target of choice for histocompatibility testing is the:
   a. red blood cell.
   b. lymphocyte.

   c. epithelial cell.
   d. platelet.

4. The high level of specificity in molecular HLA-typing is very important in progenitor cell/bone marrow transplantation because of:
   a. hyperacute rejection of the graft.
   b. chronic rejection of the graft.
   c. engraftment monitoring following transplant.
   d. graft versus host disease.

5. Tandemly repeated DNA nucleotide sequences are useful as genetic markers because:
   a. they are extremely polymorphic.
   b. they can be classified into two groups based on size (VNTR and STR).
   c. they are found throughout the human genome.
   d. it is extremely difficult to find an informative locus.

REFERENCES

American Board of Histocompatibility and Immunogenetics (ABHI). Lenexa, Kansas, 2002. www.ashi-hla.org/abhi.

American Society for Histocompatibility and Immunogenetics (ASHI). Mt. Laurel, New Jersey, 2001. www.ashi-hla.org.

Bach, F. H. and D. B. Amos. 1967. HU-1: Major histocompatibility locus in man. *Science* 156:1506-1508.

Bennington, J. L. 1984. *Dictionary of Laboratory Medicine and Technology.* W. B. Saunders, Philadelphia.

Centers for Medicare and Medicaid Services. 2001. www.hcfa.gov.

Code of Federal Regulations. Title 42, Vol. 3, Part 493—Laboratory Requirements. Revised October 1, 2000.

Foundation for the Accreditation of Cellular Therapy (FACT). 2001. *Standards for Hematopoietic Progenitor Cell Collection, Processing & Transplantation,* 2d ed. Omaha, NE.

Henry, J. B., ed. 2001. *Clinical Diagnosis and Management by Laboratory Methods.* W. B. Saunders, Philadelphia, PA, pp. 927–48.

Histocompatibility Testing: Report of a Conference and Workshop. 1965. National Academy of Sciences—National Research Council, Washington, DC.

Hurley, C. K. and J. M. Ellis. 1993. *DNA Methods for HLA Typing. A Workbook for Beginners.* Version 2. Georgetown University, Washington, DC.

KuKuruga, D. and A. B. Eisenbrey. 1993. Role of molecular tools in tissue transplantation. *Lab Med* 24:589–95.

National Academy of Sciences—National Research Council. 1965. *Histocompatibility Testing: Report of a Conference and Workshop.* Washington, DC.

Page, G. (translated by Norman, P.). 1998. Tissue typing for beginners. (Gareth.page@gstt.sthames.nhs.uk). www.dlnet.vt.edu/view Metadata.jsp?OLOID=DLNET.

Perkins, H. A. 1997. HLA typing fro transplantation of stem cells from unrelated donors. *Lab Med* 28:451–56.

Phelan, D. L., E. M. Mickelson, H. S. Noreen et al. 1994. *American Society for Histocompatibility and Immunogenetics Laboratory Manual,* 3d ed. American Society for Histocompatibility and Immunogenetics, Lenexa, KS.

Rodey, G. E. 1991. *HLA beyond Tears.* De Novo, Inc., Atlanta, GA.

Roitt, I., J. Brostoff, and D. Male. 1989. *Immunology,* 2d ed. C. V. Mosley Company, St. Louis, MO.

Shapiro, H. M. 1993. *Practical Flow Cytometry,* 2d ed. John Wiley and Sons, New York.

South-Eastern Organ Procurement Foundation (SEOPF). Richmond, Virginia, 2001. www.seopf.org.

Spangler F. M. S., R&D Specialist, ARUP Institute for Clinical & Experimental Pathology.

Standards for Hematopoietic Progenitor Cell Collection, Processing & Transplantation, 2d ed. 2001. Foundation For The Accreditation Of Cellular Therapy (Fact), Omaha, Nebraska, 2001.

Tissue Typing Reference Manual. 1993 South-Eastern Organ Procurement Foundation (SEOPF), Richmond, VA.

United Network for Organ Sharing. Richmond, VA, 2001. www.unos.org.

United Network for Organ Sharing (UNOS). Bylaws, Appendix B—Attachment 1. Standards for Histocompatibility Testing. Richmond, VA, 2001. www.unos.org.

Van Deerlin, V. and D. G. B. Leonard. 2000. Bone marrow engraftment analysis after allogeneic bone marrow transplantation. *Clin Lab Med* 20:197–225.

Verdonck, L. F., E. C. Bosboom-Kalsbeek, W. T. M. van Blokland. et al. 1998. Microsatellite analysis for donor and recipient chimerism after bone marrow transplantation. *British Journal of Haemotology* 102:208–210.

Wisecarver, J. 1997. Amplification of DNA sequences. *Lab Med* 28:191–96.

Glossary

▶ A

Accuracy – A measurement of how close an answer is to the true value.

Acquired genetic mutation – A change in the genetic material that is neither inherited nor passed to offspring.

Acquired immunodeficiency syndrome (AIDS) – Clinical syndrome associated with HIV infection characterized by CD4+ T cell depletion, rare cancers, wasting, and opportunistic infections.

Activation unit – The complement components that combine to form the C3 convertase molecule.

Acute phase reactant (acute phase proteins) – Serum proteins produced by the liver in response to infection, inflammation, or tissue injury. Includes substances such as C-reactive protein (CRP), fibrinogen, haptoglobin, alpha1-antitrypsin.

Adaptive immunity – An immune response elicited by a specific stimulus from a foreign molecule that causes antigen recognition by B, T_H, and/or T_C cells. Results in proliferation and differentiation of the stimulated cells into effector cells and memory cells; immunity resulting from a previous encounter of the host with an antigenic stimuli; also known as acquired immunity; mediated by lymphocytes and characterized by specificity and memory.

Adenosine deaminase – Enzyme in the salvage pathway of purine degradation that catalyzes deamination of adenosine to inosine.

Agglutination reaction – The aggregation and clumping together of particles to form latticelike antigen-antibody precipitates usually visible to the naked eye.

Allele – One or more alternate forms of the same gene at the same site on the chromosome (e.g., blood types can be O, A, B, or AB).

Allelic ladder – Standard markers consisting of amplified fragments of the same lengths as several or known alleles for the locus.

Allergen – An antigen that induces a Type I hypersensitivity response.

Allergic rhinitis – Inflammation of the mucous membranes of the nose, eyes, eustachian tubes, middle ear, sinuses, and pharynx. Inflammation of the mucous membranes is attributed to a complex interaction of inflammatory mediators but ultimately is triggered by an immunoglobulin E (IgE)–mediated response to an extrinsic protein.

Alloepitope – Antigenic determinant from another individual of the same species.

Allotype – A genetic variant of proteins within a species encoded by alternative alleles at a single locus. Generally used to describe alternative structures within an immunoglobulin that vary from individual to individual without affecting the isotype or function of the immunoglobulin.

Allogenic – From the same species but not the same genotype.

Alpha satellite – A repetitive class of DNA found around the centromeres of humans.

Alternate pathway – Antibody-independent complement pathway triggered by microbial antigens.

Amplification – An increase in the number of copies of a sequence of DNA.

Amplification loop – A portion of the alternate complement pathway that involves a positive feedback loop and results in production of C3 convertase.

Analyte – Target molecule of a diagnostic test. In immunoassays the analyte can be either antibody or antigen—the component of a specimen or organism that is to be measured or demonstrated. In the diagnostic immunology or serology laboratory, the analyte is usually an antibody specific to an antigen of interest.

Analytic sensitivity – Measuring the smallest amount of an analyte or a specific disease.

Analytic specificity – The ability to detect only the analyte for which the test is designed.

Anaphylaxis – A systemic, potentially life-threatening Type I hypersensitivity reaction.

Anaphylotoxin – A fragment produced during the complement cascade that is responsible for release of histamine from basophils and mast cells. Results in physiological changes such as smooth muscle contraction and increased vascular permeability.

Anergy – A state in which there is nonresponsiveness to antigens.

Ankylosing spondylitis (AS) – *See* Spondyloarthropathies.

Anneal – Base-pairing of complementary nucleotides to form a double-stranded nucleic acid molecule.

Antibody – An immunoglobulin molecule characterized by specific amino acid sequence produced by the host as a result of a specific antigenic stimulation; a gamma globulin protein produced by plasma cells in response to a specific epitope. Antibodies bind to the epitope that stimulated their production and enhance removal of foreign antigens by processes, including phagocytosis and complement lysis.

Anticodon – Portion of tRNA that binds to the mRNA codon; complementary bases on tRNA that bind to the triplet codon of mRNA base triplet; three nitrogenous bases in the DNA sequence code for an amino acid codon; three bases on mRNA complementary to the base triplet in DNA deoxyribonucleic acid (DNA); nucleic acid polymer containing genetic sequences digest; collection of short sequences of DNA following digestion with restriction enzymes.

Antigen – Any substance that produces sensitivity and initiates an immune response from the host when it comes in contact or introduced to the host cell; a molecule that exhibits reactivity with an immunologic effector such as an antibody or T cell receptor.

Antigen-antibody complex – Formed by the specific binding of the antigenic determinant portion of antigen to the homologous antigen binding site on antibody.

Antigen binding site – Region of the antibody formed at the variable end of the heavy and light chains that is specific for an epitope.

Antigen dependent – An immune response or maturation event that is elicited by specific antigen.

Antigenic determinant – Also called an epitope. It is the specific sequence on an antigen with which an antibody reacts; portion of an antigen that is recognized and bound by the antigen binding site of antibody.

Antigen independent – An immune response or maturation event that is not specific to a particular antigen, but can be stimulated by any foreign material or by growth factors.

Antigen presenting cell (APC) – A phagocytic cell (monocyte/macrophage, dendritic cell, Langerhans cell, and other similar cells) that produces MHC Class II molecules and expresses MHC II on its cell membrane with polypeptide in a binding cleft.

Anti-idiotypic antibody – An antibody that reacts with the individual structural determinant (idiotope) on the variable region of other antibodies.

Antinuclear antibody – Autoantibody directed against antigens found in the nucleus of a cell (DNA, RNA, nuclear histones).

Antinuclear antibody test – Screening test (either fluorescent or enzyme linked immunoassay) for the presence antinuclear antibodies. The different patterns are indicative of the different types of antibodies.

Apoptosis – Programmed cell death.

Arthus reaction – Localized skin reaction caused by Type III (complex-mediated) hypersensitivity.

Ataxia telangiectasia – Autosomal recessive disorder characterized by abnormal gait, vascular malformations, neurologic deficits, increased incidence of tumors, and immunodeficiency.

Atopy – Term that refers to clinical manifestations of Type I hypersensitivity reactions.

Attenuation – The process of diminishing the virulence of a strain of a microbial organism; diminution of virulence of a pathogen.

Autoantibody – An immunoglobulin that is stimulated by a self-antigen and reacts with that antigen.

Autoimmune disease – Condition in which the reaction of the immune system to a self-antigen results in damage to, or destruction of, tissue and organs.

Autoimmune hepatitis – Organ-specific autoimmune disease characterized by lymphocytic infiltration of the liver and development of anti–smooth muscle antibodies.

Autoimmunity – Inappropriate response by the immune system to self.

Autologous – From the same individual.

Autosome – One of the chromosomes not involved in sex determination. Humans have 22 pairs of autosomes and one pair of sex chromosomes (the X and Y chromosomes) for a total of 46.

 B

Background – Extraneous staining or nonspecific probe signals.

Bacterial artificial chromosome (BAC) – A vector, developed from the naturally occurring F-factor, used to clone DNA fragment of 100–300 kb in *Escherichia coli*.

Base triplet – Three nitrogenous bases which in the DNA sequence code for an amino acid.

Bare lymphocyte syndrome – Class II MHC deficiency.

B cell (B lymphocyte) – A lymphocyte subset with surface immunoglobulin that can differentiate into plasma cells that secrete antibody in response to specific antigen stimulation.

B cell receptor (BCR) – Surface IgM and IgD on the mature B cell that recognize and bind to one specific antigen.

Benign – Not malignant.

Beta satellite – A repetitive class of DNA found near the centromeres in human.

Birth defect – An abnormality present at birth which can be inherited or due nongenetic conditions. Defects can be either physical or biochemical.

Branched DNA (bDNA) detection – A signal amplification assay used to detect and quantify target nucleic acid. The nucleic acid itself is not amplified by this technique.

Bruton's agammaglobulinemia – Congenital immunodeficiency also known as X-linked agammaglobulinemia.

▶ C

CD – Acronym for cluster of differentiation. Utilized in the nomenclature for leukocyte antigens.

CD3 complex deficiency – Immunodeficiency resulting from impaired expression of one or more of the proteins within the CD3 complex.

CD5+ cells – Cells expressing CD5.

C4 binding protein (C4bp) – Complement regulator protein that is a cofactor for Factor I. Combines with and inactivates C4b, therefore preventing C2 binding.

C1 inhibitor (C1INH) – Serine protease inhibitor that dissociates the C1qrs molecule and thus inactivates the molecule.

C3 convertase – The complement complex capable of cleaving C3. Individual components will vary among the three complement pathways.

Cancer – Unregulated, unabated cellular growth. Cancer cells are freed of normal restraint and migrate to other parts of the body. Cancer may be fatal.

Capillary gel electrophoresis – Adaptation of traditional gel electrophoresis that uses narrow-bore fused-silica capillaries containing polymers in a solution that acts as a molecular sieve to separate a complex array of large and small molecules. Injection into the capillary is accomplished by immersing the end of the capillary into a sample vial and applying pressure, either vacuum or voltage. Laser technology utilizing fluorescence is used to detect the samples as they exit the capillary.

Carrier state – A condition in which an individual or animal harbors a potentially pathogenic organism of infectious agent without the host showing signs of the disease but serves as source of infection to susceptible individuals.

Carcinogen – Substance capable of inducing tumor formation.

Carcinoma – Cancer originating in epithelial tissue.

Cell-mediated immunity – A subset of adaptive immunity mediated primarily by T lymphocytes producing cytokines that influence the behavior of other cells or that act as cytotoxic cells.

Cell surface marker – Molecule on the membrane of a cell that is defined by an antibody.

Central tolerance – Self-tolerance generated in the bone marrow or thymus; prevents self-reactive clones of lymphocytes from emerging.

Cellular transformation – Change in a cell from a benign to a malignant phenotype.

Centromere – A specialized structure of the chromosome to which spindle fibers attach during cell division.

Chediak-Higashi syndrome – Defective lysosomal function due to a mutation in a gene leading to increased fusion of lysosomal granules.

Chemotactic factor – A substance that activates cells to migrate in a specific direction (toward antigen).

Chemotaxis – Movement of cells in response to chemical stimulant.

CH_{50} assay – A diagnostic serological test to assess the function of the entire classical complement pathway.

Chimera/chimerism – Presence in an individual of cells of a different genetic origin; two or more cell lines.

Chromosome – An organized arrangement of cellular DNA that facilitates replication and cell division. The chromosome structure consists primarily of DNA, proteins, and RNA.

Chromosome band – A region that can be distinguished from adjacent regions by virtue of differential staining.

Chromosome painting – *See* Whole chromosome paint.

Chromosome region p – The abbreviation for the short arm of the chromosome which is always placed in the uppermost position when constructing the karyotype.

Chromosome region q – The abbreviation for the long arm of the chromosome which is always placed in the lowermost position when constructing the karyotype.

Chronic granulomatous disease (CGD) – Immunodeficiency resulting from mutations in the genes encoding components of phagocytic oxidase.

Classical pathway – The antibody dependent complement pathway.

Clinical accuracy – The overall ability of a test to both rule in and rule out an analyte or specific disease.

Clinical sensitivity – The percent test positivity in a population of affected patients where,

$$\frac{\text{Number of true positive results}}{\text{Number or true positive plus false negative results}} \times 100$$

Clinical specificity – The percent of negative test results in a population without the specified disease where,

$$\frac{\text{Number of true negative results}}{\text{Number of true negative plus false positive results}} \times 100$$

Clinical staging – A means of categorizing the extent of tumor dissemination based on the clinical presentation, usually for purposes of selecting appropriate treatment regimens. Each type of cancer has a unique staging system.

Clonal deletion – The process by which immature lymphocytes that bind to self-antigen are eliminated, resulting in self-tolerance.

Clone – A population of cells derived from a single precursor.

Cluster determinant (CD) – An antigen differentiating marker on the surface of white blood cells.

Coagglutination – Similar to agglutination reactions but with the addition of antibody-coated *Staphylococcus aureus*. The cocci are sensitized by binding large amounts of human antibody to the target antigen. This effectively creates a particle that is capable of binding thousands of antigens and will result in visible precipitate in a test sample containing the correct antibody.

Codominant – Full expression of both alleles of a gene pair in the heterozygote without either being influenced by the other.

Codon – Three bases on mRNA complementary to the base triplet in deoxyribonucleic acid (DNA): nucleic acid polymer containing genetic sequences digest: collection of short sequences of DNA following digestion with restriction enzymes.

Colonization – The presence of microorganisms, both potentially pathogenic and nonpathogenic microbial species, at a particular site.

Commensalism – A relationship between different species (host and organism) wherein one (organism) benefits from the other (host) without causing harm. The host species does not benefit from the relationship or organism.

Common variable immunodeficiency (CVID) – Defect in B cell activation, resulting in variable reductions in multiple Ig isotypes.

Comparative genome hybridization – The technique of comparing one genome to another.

Complement – Group of serum proteins involved in the immune response. Activation results in cell lysis or deposits of immunologically active fragments on cells.

Complement dependent microcytotoxicity test (CDC) – Assay used in histocompatibility testing that is based on cytolysis mediated by specific antibody in the presence of complement.

Complementary DNA (cDNA) – The synthesis of DNA enzymatically from RNA transcript by reverse transcription.

Complement fixation test – Serological test using an antigen-antibody complex to bind complement.

Complement receptor – Cell surface molecules that react with fragments of C3.

Complement regulatory proteins – Group of soluble and cell-bound molecules that control complement activation.

Concomitant immunity – Immunity generated in response to an actively growing primary tumor that prevents the outgrowth of a subsequently implanted identical second tumor.

Congenital – A trait present at birth which may be genetic or nongenetic. *See* Birth defect.

Conserved sequence – A sequence of DNA bases that has remained unchanged throughout evolution.

Contact dermatitis – Eczematous skin reaction caused by contact with certain chemicals or metals and mediated by Type IV hypersensitivity.

Constant region – The portion of the antibody molecule residing within the constant domains of both the heavy and light chains that is responsible for the isotype of the molecule (kappa or lambda for light chains and alpha, gamma, etc. for

heavy chains). These areas of the molecule are identical from cell to cell.

Costimulatory signal – Interaction of B7 with CD28 required for T cell activation.

C-reactive protein (CRP) – An acute phase reactant that increases in inflammation.

CREST syndrome – A form of scleroderma with calcinosis, Raynaud's syndrome, esophageal dysmotility, sclerodactyly, and telangietasis.

Crithidia luciliae test – Indirect immunofluorescent test for confirmation of anti-dsDNA antibodies. The organism used is a hemoflagellate that has a high concentration of dsDNA in the kinetoplast. Fluorescence of the kinetoplast is indicative of anti-dsDNA antibodies in the patient's serum.

Crossing over – The normal process of exchange of genetic material between the maternal and paternal homologs during meiosis; the exchange of genetic material between homologous chromosomes during the first meiotic division resulting in new combinations of genes. Also referred to as recombination.

Cross-reacting antigens – Molecules that may react to the same antibody. They may possess the same antigenic determinant even though they are not the same antigen.

Cross-reactive antibody – An antibody that recognizes not only a specific antigen but also other peptides with similar structures

Counterstain – Background stain to enable finding the item of interest, for example, chromosomes or cells.

Cyclic neutropenia – Immunodeficiency disorder characterized by periodic decreases in neutrophil numbers accompanied by increased incidence of bacterial infection.

Cytogenetics – The study of the physical appearance and behavioral characteristics of chromosomes.

Cytokines – A generic term for soluble molecules which mediate interactions between cells. Interferon γ and tumor necrosis factor (TNF) are cytokines; a soluble molecule that is elaborated from one cell type and attaches to receptors on another cell type, serving to allow communication between cells.

Cytotoxic T lymphocyte (CTL) – CD8+ subset of T lymphocytes.

 D

Decay accelerating factor (DAF) – Also known as CD55 and present on peripheral blood cells including erythrocytes. A membrane-bound complement regulator protein that dissociates C3 convertases in both the classical and alternate pathway.

Dendritic cells – Subset of monocytes; principle stimulator in MHC.

ds-DNA – Double stranded DNA.

Degradability – The potential of a molecule to be broken down into its component parts. For example, a protein is capable of being degraded into polypeptides.

Delayed hypersensitivity – T cell-mediated (Type IV) hypersensitivity reaction that occurs 24–72 hours after contact with an antigen.

Deletion – Loss of genetic material from a chromosome that often leads to biochemical or structural abnormality.

Denaturation – Separation or melting of the two DNA strands.

Denature/denaturation (as it relates to nucleic acids) – The separation of double-stranded nucleic acids into individual strands.

Deoxynucleotide phosphate – Abbreviated as "dNTP." Deoxynucleotide phosphates are individual DNA bases used in amplification reactions by DNA polymerase to synthesize new strands of DNA.

Deoxyribonucleic acid (DNA) – Molecule that contains the nucleotide sequence that codes for genes.

Diapedesis – The passage of inflammatory cells and other formed elements in the blood through the endothelial walls of the blood vessel.

DiGeorge syndrome – Genetic disorder associated with thymic aplasia, cardiac abnormalities, and immunodeficiency.

DNA polymerase – An enzyme, usually from the thermophilic bacterium *Thermus aquaticus* (called *Taq*) that will synthesize strands of DNA from a DNA template in amplification reactions in a $5' - 3'$ direction; enzyme responsible for replication of DNA.

Dnase – Enzyme that breaks down DNA.

Differentiation – The changing of the cell from one form to another to allow a different function after antigenic stimulation.

Direct labeling – A method of labeling probes in which the label is attached directly to the base.

Discoid lupus – A dermatitis seen in cutaneous lupus and not associated with the type of skin involvement seen in SLE.

Dithiothreitol (DTT) – Chemical inactivating agglutinating IgM antibodies by dissociating 19S IgM molecules into 7S subunits. IgG antibodies are not affected by this treatment.

Dohle bodies – Found within the cytoplasm of neutrophils and eosinophiles, these are oval aggregate structures of endoplasmic reticulum. These bodies stain light gray with Romanowsky stain and are associated with severe bacterial infection and toxic states, pregnancy, burns, cancer, and aplastic anemia.

Domains – Basic units of the linear structure of antibody and the T cell receptor (TCR) defined by disulfide bonds.

Dot plot – A graphical representation of data the shows the frequency of events for two characteristics. For example, the frequency of cells positive or negative for staining with two monoclonal antibodies.

Downstream – Sequences that are located in the 3' direction from some reference point.

 E

Electrochemiluminescence – A technique that detects antigen-antibody binding by exposing an attached electrochemically sensitive label to an electrode. This initiates an energy transfer reaction which concludes in the release of light measurable by a photodetector.

Electrophoresis – A method that is used to separate biomolecules (DNA, RNA, protein) through a matrix based on shape, size, and/or charge.

Endocytosis – The process of engulfing a particle by a cell (e.g., macrophage), resulting from the cell membrane surrounding the particle and pinching off to form a vacuole.

Endogenous – Originating within the organism.

Endonuclease – A cellular enzyme that cleaves DNA.

Enhancer – Regulatory sequence outside of the promoter that binds transcription factors.

Epitope – Minimal structural unit that can be recognized by a T or B cell receptor. Also called antigenic determinant; a specific site on an antigen that is recognized by the antigen binding site of antibody. *See* Antigenic determinant.

Epitope spreading – A process whereby epitopes distinct from and non-cross-reactive with an inducing epitope become major targets of an ongoing immune response. It has been best characterized as an exacerbating factor in CD4+ T cell-dependent autoimmune disease models and is believed to occur via presentation of antigens liberated by tissue destruction initiated by CD4+ T cells specific for a primary epitope.

Ethidium bromide – Dye that fluoresces when exposed to ultraviolet light; it intercalcates between DNA base pairs and is commonly used to locate DNA fragments in electrophoretic gels; dye that intercalates into nucleic acids and can be used to stain both DNA and RNA. The dye fluoresces orange when it is irridiated by UV light.

Eukaryote – Cells or organisms bounded by a membrane and containing well developed cellular components. All organisms other than blue-green algae, viruses, and bacteria are eukaryotes.

Exogenous – Originating outside of the organism.

Exon – Portion of a gene that is transcribed.

F

Factor B – A complement protein that is part of the alternate pathway; combines during complement C3 "tickover" to form C3 convertase.

Factor H – A complement regulator protein that acts with Factor I to cleave C3b.

Factor I – A complement regulator that functions to cleave C3b and C4b into inactive molecules.

False positive value – A positive result that is determined to be negative when compared with clinical outcome, a known standard or gold standard test.

False negative value – A negative result that is determined to be negative when compared with clinical outcome; a known standard or gold standard test.

Flow cytometer – An instrument used for the enumeration and characterization of cells in suspension. Cells are analyzed on a single cell basis, in a precise and rapid fashion. This instrument is typically used to identify cells labeled with fluorescent monoclonal antibodies to enumerate specific cell types.

Forbidden clone theory – The increased incidence of autoimmune disease in the elderly. In the normal individual, Ts (suppressor) cells tend to prevent activation of nontolerant clones of lymphocytes. Loss of a given antigen-specific T cell subset could result in the activation of nontolerant clones and formation of autoimmune disease.

Foreignness – The degree of difference between host and an invading molecule. The more difference (foreignness), the better the immune response.

Forward scatter – Light that scatter along the axis of the laser beam. It is reflective of cell size.

Fluorescent in situ hybridization (FISH) – The use of fluorescent labeled DNA probes to detect hybridization sites on metaphase chromosomes or the extended DNA fibers during interphase.

Fluorochrome – A molecule or compound that absorbs short spectral wavelengths followed by immediate emission of longer spectral wavelengths and heat. A molecule that absorbs light of one wavelength and emits light of a higher wavelength (different color).

▶ G

Gene – A sequence of chromosomal DNA that encodes the information for protein or polypeptide synthesis; the basic unit of hereditary information consisting of a linear sequence of nucleotides that code for a product; unit factor of inheritance.

Gene amplification – A presence of multiple copies of a specific sequence; often observed in tumor cells.

Gene rearrangement – A permanent change in the germline DNA that provides specificity to the antigen binding site of the antibody or T cell receptor.

Genetic map – A map of the relative position of genes or sequences on chromosomes. Position can be determined by FISH or frequency of transmission with other measurable positions. The distance between positions is measured in cM (centimorgans).

Genetic testing – Analysis of genetic material to determine predisposition to a particular condition or to diagnose a genetic disease.

Genomic DNA – The entire complement of an organism's DNA which is usually measured in the number of base pairs.

Germline – The DNA as it exists in the cell upon cell generation.

Gold standard – The best available approximation of the truth, either a clinical diagnosis or a reference test method.

Goodpasture's syndrome – Autoimmune disease characterized by autoantibodies reacting with glomerular and alveolar basement membrane collagen (type IV), resulting in renal and pulmonary damage.

Graft versus host disease (GVHD) – Immunologic attack on the recipient by immunologically competent donor cells that recognize incompatible recipient antigens.

Granulomas – Large clusters of activated macrophages, delayed type hypersensitivity T cells, and multinucleated cells that form in the chronic inflammatory response associated with Type IV hypersensitivity in attempt to wall off sites of persistent infection.

Graves' disease – An autoimmune disease in which the interaction of antibodies to the receptor for thyroid-stimulating hormone results in hyperthyroidism due to increased stimulation of the thyroid.

▶ H

Haplotype – A set of genetic determinants located on a single chromosome; complex of linked genes that resides on one of a pair of homologous chromosomes and that segregates en bloc; half of a genotype.

Hashimoto's thyroiditis – An autoimmune disease involving lymphocytic infiltration and production of autoantibodies to thyroglobulin and thyroid peroxidase, resulting in destruction of the thyroid gland and hypothyroidism.

Heavy chain – In an immunoglobulin, this is the chain that provides the isotype of the immunoglobulin (IgG, etc.). The heavy chain is the chain of the molecule that has more amino acids and thus, higher molecular weight. It consists of three or four constant region domains and one variable region domain.

Heat shock proteins – Proteins produced in stressed cells that are responsible for correct folding of proteins.

Hematopoiesis – Development of blood cells. Hematopoiesis occurs in the yolk sack, then liver, and eventually the bone marrow before childbirth. In normal adults it occurs in marrow and lymphatic tissues.

Hereditary angioedema (HAE) – A clinical condition caused by a C1INH deficiency. The condition is characterized by swelling of the mucosa of the gastrointestinal tract and the skin.

Heterodimer – Protein consisting of two peptide chains.

Heterozygous – Having two different alleles of a particular gene.

Highly active retroviral therapy (HART) – Combination chemotherapy for HIV consisting of inhibitors of reverse transcriptase and viral proteases.

Histocompatibility – The sharing of antigens that determine whether a graft will be rejected.

Histogram – A graphical representation of data that shows the frequency of events versus their signal intensity (light scatter or fluorescence). It is used to graphically display the frequency of cells exhibiting a single intrinsic or extrinsic characteristic.

HLA – Acronym for human leukocyte antigen. Analogous to the major histocompatibility complex (MHC) system. A highly polymorphic system of cell surface antigens that is responsible for presenting antigens to T lymphocytes and eliciting antigraft immune responses.

Home-brew test – A procedure developed in-house that uses commercially available or in-house prepared reagents, or any procedure that incorporates modifications of the manufacturer's package insert instructions.

Homolog – One of the members of a chromosome pair in diploid organisms.

Homologous chromosome – The two members of a chromosome pair that have corresponding gene loci, each derived from one parent.

Homozygous – Having two identical alleles of a particular gene.

Horror autotoxicus – Early theory explaining why the immune system did not attack the host.

Humoral immunity – The immunity provided by the production of antibodies (immunoglobulins); type of immune response that involves circulating antibodies; a subset of adaptive immunity mediated primarily by B lymphocytes that produce antibodies.

Hybridization – The binding of two complementary segments of DNA or RNA to DNA to form a double stranded molecule; reannealing of two single strands of DNA to form the original DNA molecule.

Hybridize – Process in which DNA strands that have been denatured (separated) reattach (anneal).

Hydrodynamic focusing – The process of focusing a stream of cells into a narrow column so that they pass single file in a precise fashion through the laser beam. This is necessary so that uniform illumination of the cells takes place.

Hyperplasia – An abnormality resulting from an increase in the number of cells comprising a specific tissue.

Hypersensitivity – Exaggerated or inappropriate immune response that results in pathology to the host.

 I

Idiotype – The variation within the variable domain of the immunoglobulin molecule. The idiotype determines the antigen specificity of the antibody.

IgA – The isotype of antibody defined by the alpha heavy chain. This can be found in the body as monomeric, dimeric, or trimeric forms. This is the isotype of immunoglobulin found in secretions and is associated with innate immunity.

IgD – The isotype of antibody defined by the delta heavy chain. Most IgD is found embedded in mature B cell membranes and, along with membrane IgM, serves as the B cell receptor to recognize antigens.

IgE – The isotype of antibody defined by the epsilon heavy chain. IgE is primarily attached to mast cells and serves as the antigen recognition for Type I hypersensitivity reactions to allergens and immunity to parasites.

IgG – The isotype of antibody defined by the gamma heavy chain. This is the primary immunoglobulin found in human serum.

IgM – The isotype of antibody defined by the μ heavy chain. Found in human serum as a pentamer, but monomers are embedded into mature B cell membranes.

Image analysis – A method used to capture and store images. Image analysis may be used to analyze parameters such as molecular weight, size of nucleic acid fragments, relative abundance, the optical density of objects in the image, and so on.

Immediate hypersensitivity – Antibody-mediated hypersensitivity reaction that occurs within a few minutes to several hours after contact with an antigen; includes Type I, Type II, and Type III hypersensitivity.

Immune adherence – A characteristic of phagocytic cells that allows them to bind to microbial organisms coated with complement fragments.

Immune complex – A circulating complex of soluble antigen and corresponding antibody. Small-sized complexes may initiate an inflammatory process when deposited in tissue.

Immune response – The resultant action of the immune system such as antibody production to an antigen; response of the immune system to an antigen.

Immune surveillance – A normal homeostatic process by which the host immune system recognizes and destroys invading pathogens and perhaps spontaneously arising tumors.

Immune system – System of cells and chemicals that interact to create an immune response to an antigen.

Immune tolerance – Immunologic nonresponsiveness to self antigens.

Immunocompetent – The ability to mount a normal immune response.

Immunodiffusion – Technique employing diffusion of test substance through agar; for identification or quantitation of antibodies.

Immunofluorescence – An antigen identification method using specific antibodies labeled with a fluorescent tag. Antibodies will bind to a desired antigen target and fluoresce when exposed to UV light.

Immunogen – A substance that can elicit an immune response. *See* Antigen.

Immunogenicity – The ability of an antigen to elicit an immune response.

Immunoglobulin – A complex group of serum proteins that are produced by B cells in response to foreign antigens. In humans there are five isotypes: IgG, IgM, IgA, IgD, and IgE. *See also* Antibody.

Immunoglobulin superfamily – Molecules sharing a 100 amino acid long immunoglobulin-like domain with a centrally placed disulfide bridge stabilizing a series of antiparallel B strands organized into an immunoglobulin-like fold. Members include Class I and Class II MHC, T lymphocyte cell receptors, and other molecules not associated with the immune system.

Immunologic deficiency theory – Relates to the balance between T suppressor lymphocytes, T helper lymphocytes, and B lymphocytes. Increased production of autoantibodies and increased immune system deficiency occurs due to age. It suggested that, as an individual ages, suppressor T lymphocytes decline in number and can no longer control the interaction between T helper and B lymphocytes.

Immunologic ignorance – When immunologic response does not occur because the antigen is anatomically sequestered, preventing interaction with the lymphocyte. Cells do not encounter the antigen and therefore remain "ignorant" of it.

Immunoselection – The appearance of antigen loss tumor cell variants, resulting from the immune destruction of antigen expressing tumor cells.

Immunotherapy – Utilization of immune system components to treat select types of human neoplasms.

Imprinting – A modification of DNA during meiosis which prevents or alters transcription during the lifetime of the individual. Both males and females remove the previous imprint and add a new imprint to the appropriate sequences. Mutation or deletions of imprinted regions result in disease specific to the origin of the damaged imprint.

In situ amplification (ISA) – A means to amplify nucleic acid directly from tissues, whole cells, or chromosomes.

In situ hybridization – The use of DNA or RNA probes to detect a complementary sequence in intact cells.

Indirect labeling – Method of attaching a label to a probe in which an intermediary molecule is between the base and the label.

Inflammation – Physiologic reaction to injury involving physical symptoms of pain, redness, swelling, and tenderness due to accumulation of plasma and white blood cells.

Informative locus – One for which at the recipient allele has a different number of repeats than the donor allele; used to determine engraftment after bone marrow/progenitor cell transplants.

Inherit – The receipt of genetic material from a parent.

Innate immunity – Natural form of host protection; nonspecific and is not stimulated by specific antigenic stimuli; immune response that is not directed specifically to an antigen and that is not characterized by specificity and memory.

Insertion – The movement of a segment of DNA between two breaks into a position between a third break before the segments are rejoined. The third break can be on the same chromosome or on a different chromosome. Genes may be disrupted if one of the breaks occurs inside the coding region.

Interferon – A class of mediators that increase the resistance of cells to viral infection by inhibiting viral replication and the growth of some neoplastic cells.

Interleukin (IL) – A type of cytokine originally thought to both be produced by and act upon leukocytes. However, it has since been discovered that other types of cells can elaborate some interleukins and that ILs also have effects on cells other than leukocytes.

Interphase – All collective stages of the cell cycle excluding metaphase. DNA is replicated during interphase.

Intravascular hemolysis – When hemolysis of red blood cells (RBCs) occurs in the circulation releasing hemoglobin into the plasma producing fragmented RBCs called schistocytes. Mechanical trauma, complement fixation, and other toxic damage to the RBC are associated causes of intravascular hemolysis.

Intron – Intervening sequence of DNA between coding sequences (exons); segment of a gene that does not code for a protein.

Isochromosome – A chromosome consisting of two identical arms.

Isotype – Antigenic variation in immunoglobulin molecules that occurs from species to species. It is defined by the domains in the constant region of both heavy and light chains. All members of a species will have the same isotypes.

Inversion – An orientation reversal of a DNA sequence that results from two breaks with the segment between the two breaks rotated 180 degrees before being rejoined.

 J

J chain – Also called the "joining chain." It is a 15 kDa glycoprotein that enables polymerization of IgM and IgA molecules into dimers, trimers, or pentamers.

Job's syndrome – Autosomal dominant multisystem primary immunodeficiency; also known as hyper-IgE syndrome.

K

Karyotype – An organized arrangement of the images of the chromosomes from a single cell arranged according to size, centromere position, and banding pattern.

Kilobase (kb) – A unit of length of DNA equivalent to 1000 nucleotides.

 L

Label – A molecule attached to a nucleotide or reported molecule which allows detection of a probe after hybridization.

Laser – The light source for standard flow cytometers. It produces the beam of light that interrogates cells passing through the beam. Laser is an acronym for light amplification by stimulated emission of radiation.

Law of independent assortment – The chromosomes containing alleles corresponding to different traits are distributed to the gametes independent of one another.

Law of segregation – Inherited traits are controlled by discrete factors (genes) with each individual inheriting two forms (alleles) of a gene, one from each parent. The alleles are separated into different gametes during meiosis and are passed to different offspring.

Leukocyte – A white blood cell the function of which is to protect the host from infections and tissue injury. There are five types, namely, neutrophils, lymphocytes, monocytes, eosinophils, and basophils.

Leukocyte adhesion deficiency (LAD) – Genetic mutation leading to defects in β 2 integrin and impaired leukocyte extravasation.

Ligase chain reaction – A technique that uses pairs of probes and relies on DNA ligase and DNA polymerase for amplification.

Light chain – The second peptide chain type seen in an antibody molecule. It consists on one constant region domain and one variable region domain. It possesses a lower molecular weight and fewer amino acids than the heavy chains.

Light scatter – The result of cells passing through the laser beam of the flow cytometer. Scattered light is collected in the forward and orthogonal (90 degrees) directions to assess the intrinsic and extrinsic characteristics of cells.

Lineage – A specific type of hematopoietic cell, for example, myeloid cells or lymphoid cells.

Linkage – The inheritance of two genes together because of close proximity on the same chromosome.

Linkage disequilibrium – The occurrence of two alleles on the same haplotype at a rate are higher than would be expected on the basis of chance alone.

Liposomes – Intact vesicles composed of a phospholipids bilayer membrane that can be modified to include antibody or antigen in the membrane. Additionally, the liposomes can be made to contain dyes or labeling molecules that aid in visualization.

Locus – The position of a gene on a chromosome.

Lymphocyte – A type of white blood cell that develops not only in the bone marrow but also in other areas such as the thymus, spleen, and lymph nodes.

Lymphopoiesis – Formation of lymphatic tissue.

 M

Macrophage – A mononuclear phagocytic cell that arises from the monocytic cell line.

Major histocompatibility complex – Also known as HLA or human leukocyte antigen, a complex group of protein that code cell surfaces antigens and determine the tissue type and transplantation compatibility; a set of genetic loci with multiple alleles at each locus which encodes proteins involved in presentation of antigen to T cells.

Malignant – A tumor that is invasive and has the potential to metastasize.

Mannose-binding lectin (MBL) pathway – Complement pathway involving activation by carbohydrates such as mannose located on surface of microorganisms. After recognition this pathway follows the same sequence (C2-9) as the classical pathway.

Maturation – The progression of lymphocyte forms from the initial cell made in the bone marrow to the mature cell that is capable of being stimulated to differentiate.

Mediators of inflammation – Cytokines and other chemical substances released by cells that increase the inflammatory response.

Meiosis – Reduction division resulting from two consecutive cell divisions in germ line cells. Meiosis results in four daughter cells, each with a haploid complement of chromosomes.

Membrane attack complex (MAC) – C5-9 components common to all complement pathways that causes cell lysis. The function of this part of the complement cascade is not enzyme driven.

Memory – Enhanced recognition and response to a previously encountered antigen by B or T cells.

Messenger RNA (mRNA) – Molecule carrying genetic information for genes to be translated into protein from the nucleus into the cytoplasm.

Metaphase – The stage of the cell cycle during which the chromosomes are condensed into the visible chromosome structures that align on the equatorial plane of the cell.

Metastatic – A tumor that readily spreads (metastasizes) from an initiative primary tumor.

MHC proteins – Single-use peptide transporters that carry proteolytic degradation products to the cell surface for presenting them to T cells. These proteins allow T cells to distinguish self from nonself. In every cell in the body, antigens are constantly broken up and presented to passing T cells. Without these, there would be no presentation of internal or external antigens to the T cells and other aspects of the immune response cannot occur.

MHC restriction – The observation that immunologically active cells will only cooperate effectively when they share MHC haplotypes at either the Class I or Class II loci.

Microarray – A computer-assisted method of spotting specific DNA segments onto a slide to detect the presence, absence, or amount of a complementary sequence in the specimen or to determine expression levels.

Microbial antigen – Relating or pertains to a microorganism that produces an immune response; molecules (usually proteins or polysaccharides) produced by or found on the surface of a microbe that are recognized and specifically bound by host-produced antibody.

Mitosis – Nuclear division that produces two daughter cells identical to each other and to the parent cell.

Mixed lymphocyte culture (MLC) test – Based on cellular procedures; lymphocytes from two different persons undergo blast transformation and divide when they are mixed in culture in vitro. Also referred to as MLR or mixed lymphocyte reaction test.

Molecular mimicry – Similarity between foreign antigen and self antigen. As a result of this process, antibodies produced to the foreign antigen can cross-react with self antigen.

Monoclonal – Cells that descend from the same lymphocyte. All these cells are identical and will recognize the same specific epitope.

Monoclonal antibody – Antibody with a single (mono) defined specificity; antibody produced by a single B cell clone that secretes immunoglobulin specific for a single antigenic determinant.

Monosomy – The presence of only one copy of a chromosome instead of the normal two copies.

Mosaic – The presence in one individual of two or more cell lines each containing distinctly different genetic material.

Multiple sclerosis – Chronic inflammatory disease characterized by lymphocytic infiltration and demyelination of the white matter in the central nervous system.

Mutation – Any change to the DNA that can be passed from parent cell to daughter cell.

Multiparous – Having experienced two or more pregnancies

Multiplex PCR – Simultaneous amplification of multiple loci in a single reaction tube.

Myasthenia gravis – A neuromuscular disease characterized by presence of antibodies to acetylcholine receptors. When the receptors are blocked by antibody, the nerve impulses to the muscles are blocked, and muscle weakness ensues.

 N

Narcolepsy – Sleep disorder characterized by excessive daytime sleepiness (hypersomnolence), sleep attacks, cataplexy, sleep paralysis, and hypnogogic hallucinations.

Natural-killer (NK) cell – A group of lymphocytes that have the intrinsic ability to recognize and destroy some virally infected cell and tumor cells.

Negative predictive value – A negative result accurately indicates the absence of an analyte or specific disease.

Negative selection – Elimination of cells in generative lymphoid organs which express receptors reactive with self antigens.

Neoantigens – Epitopes produced by posttranslational modifications such as phosphorylation or proteolysis.

Neoplasm – An uncontrolled growing mass of abnormal cells.

Nested – Inclusion of a block of data or subroutine inside another block of data or subroutine.

Neutrophils – A mature white blood cell characterized by a segmented nucleus and granular cytoplasm; makes up the majority of circulating leukocytes.

Nick translation – A technique used to prepare a radioactively labeled DNA strand.

Nitrogenous base – Adenine, thymine, cytosine, guanine, or uracil.

Noise – *See* Background.

Non-self antigen – Antigens (usually from microorganisms) that will stimulate the immune system to mount an immune response.

Nucleic acid probe – A molecule tagged to bind to and detect a specific sequence of nucleic acids.

Nucleic acid sequence based amplification (NASBA) – A procedure that uses the combined activities of a ribonuclease, a reverse transcriptase, and a DNA dependent RNA polymerase to amplify target nucleic acid. NASBA can be performed at one temperature, and does not require a thermal cycler.

Nucleotide – Building block unit of a nucleic acid; a biomolecule that is the building block of DNA and RNA. Nucleotides consist of a five-carbon sugar (deoxyribose for DNA, ribose for RNA), a nitrogenous base (adenine, cytosine, guanine, and thymine for DNA, or adenine, cytosine, guanine, and uracil for RNA), and a phosphate group.

O

Odds ratio – Calculation of the odds that an individual with a given HLA type will develop a given disease.

Oligonucleotide – A small piece of chemically synthesized nucleic acid used as primers or probes in molecular-based assays; a short section of a DNA strand used as a probe or primer in the polymerase chain reaction; a short series of nucleotides, generally artificially produced.

Oligonucleotide probe – A string of nucleotides used to detect the presence of a complimentary nucleic acid sequence.

Omenn's syndrome – Immunodeficiency resulting from mutations in RAG genes and lack of expression of T cell receptors.

Oncogene – A mutated proto-oncogene. Proto-oncogenes are normal genes that play a role in controlling the cell cycle. Oncogenes allow uncontrolled growth and are associated with cancer.

Operon – Complex of structural and regulatory genes in a chromosome which interact to cause expression of the structural genes.

Opportunist – Refers to microorganisms that usually do not produce disease but are capable of causing disease in an individual whose immune system is compromised.

Opportunistic pathogen – *See* Opportunist.

Opsonin – Complement fragment that enhances phagocytosis.

Opsonization – The process by which microorganisms are changed so that they are more easily and readily engulfed by phagocytes and macrophages.

Organ-specific autoimmune disease – Condition in which the autoantibody is specific to antigens on cells of a single organ.

 P

Paint – *See* Whole chromosome paint.

Parasitism – The relationship between species (host and organism) wherein one of the species (parasite) benefits at the expense of the other (host).

Paroxysmal nocturnal hemoglobinuria – Condition characterized by unusual erythrocyte sensitivity to complement activation resulting in lysis.

Pathogen – A microorganism that causes disease.

Pathogenicity – The ability of a microorganism to cause disease.

PCR product – Amplication product as a result of many cycles of the PCR; also called "amplicon." Powerful and sensitive nucleic acid amplification technique.

Pernicious anemia – Megaloblastic anemia caused by defective DNA synthesis as a result of inadequate vitamin B_{12} uptake. Antibodies to intrinsic factor and to parietal cells are primarily responsible for this disease.

Phagocytosis – The process of engulfing or ingesting and digesting foreign particles.

Phagosome – A vesicle that forms around a foreign particle when a phagocytic cell engulfs it.

Phenotype – Observable characteristics produced by genes.

Photodiode – A detector utilized to detect forward scatter signal.

Photomultiplier tube – An electronic device in a flow cytometry that detects side scatter or fluorescent light and amplifies the signals.

Polyacrylamide gel electrophoresis – A gel-like matrix formed from the polymerization and cross-linking of acrylamide. Polyacrylamide gels form a porous support through which DNA or protein molecules can be separated.

Polyclonal – Cells descended from different lymphocytes. Each clone of cells will recognize different specific epitopes.

Polyclonal antibody – A mixture of antibodies produced by different B cells in response to different epitopes of an antigen. There can be a wide variety of binding affinities and specificities among the immunoglobulins produced in response to a single antigen.

Polymerase chain reaction – A method that results in logarithmic increase (amplification) of a segment of DNA.

Polymorphic – Multiple alleles in the human population; maintaining two or more distinct genotypes at a particular locus in a population; the occurrence of multiple alleles in a population; maintaining two or more distinct alleles at a particular genetic locus.

Polymorphism – The presence of different sequences among individuals of a population. Polymorphisms in coding regions may cause nondetrimental phenotypic differences while those in non-coding regions have no phenotypic effect.

Positive predictive value – A positive result accurately indicates the presence of an analyte or specific disease.

Positive selection – Process by which T cells recognizing self-MHC are rescued from apoptosis, thus ensuring self-MHC restriction of T cells.

Precipitin reaction – The concentration-dependent formation of insoluble precipitating complexes by the binding of antigen and multivalent antibody.

Precision – Quantitative agreement between replicate analysis using identical procedures. Precision in qualitative analysis is often referred to as reproducibility. Both terms imply freedom from inconsistency and random error but do not guarantee accuracy.

$$\frac{\text{Number of repeated results in agreement}}{\text{Total number of results}} \times 100$$

Predictive value – The probability that the result is accurate.

Prevalence – The pretest probability of a particular clinical state in a specified population; the frequency of a disease in the population of interest at a given point in time.

Primary biliary cirrhosis – Autoimmune disease affecting small intraheaptic bile ducts and leading to cirrhosis. Antimitochondrial antibody is the typical antibody involved in the process.

Primary immunodeficiency – Immune deficiency is caused by intrinsic defects in the cells of the immune system and are often due to inherited genetic defects.

Primer – An oligonucleotide that is used in amplification reactions to start or "prime" the synthesis of new strands of DNA. A primer has a free 3'-OH group that is used to attach new nucleotides to; an oligonucleotide that determines the section of a DNA strand that will be amplified by the polymerase chain reaction; segment of DNA used to initiate DNA synthesis.

Primer extension – refers to the addition of individual DNA bases (dNTPs) to the primers by DNA polymerase to synthesize a new strand of DNA.

Private epitopes – Antigenic determinants occurring on a single gene product.

Probe – An oligonucleotide that is usually labeled in some manner for detection in molecular-based assays. An oligonucleotide that binds to and identifies a specific section of DNA. A segment of single stranded DNA or RNA used to localize its complementary sequence by hybridization followed by detection of attached labels

Progenitor cell – Pluripotent hematopoietic stem cells that are capable of self-renewal can be isolated from the bone marrow by aspiration, peripheral blood by apheresis, or cord blood and are used to treat patients with leukemias, lymphomas, and other malignancies and genetics defects.

Proliferation – Division of lymphocytes to form daughter cells many times over.

Properdin – A protein in the alternate complement pathway that is responsible for stabilizing the C3 convertase molecule.

Pseudogene – Genes that have structure homologous to other genes but are not expressed.

Public epitopes – Antigenic determinants common to more than one gene product, which may be widely distributed (e.g., Bw4 and Bw6).

Purine – Nitrogenous bases adenine or guanine.

Pyrimidine – Nitrogenous bases cytosine, thymine, or uracil.

 R

RACE – *R*apid *a*mplification of *c*DNA *e*nds. A method employed to determine the sequence of the 5' and/or 3' ends of transcript.

Random primer extension – Synthesis of DNA oligonucleotides from primers generated randomly.

RAST – Radioallergosorbent test; an immunoassay that measures allergen-specific IgE antibodies.

Real-time PCR – A method that usually uses fluorescently labeled probes to detect PCR product. An instrument platform is used to detect fluorescence.

Recognition phase – The stage of an immune response when a carbohydrate or protein of a cell binds to another carbohydrate or protein of another cell; binding of antigen to immunoglobulin on B cells or to the T cell antigen receptor on T cells.

Recognition unit – Complement components (C1qrs) in the classical pathway. These bind to the Fc regions of an antibody molecule to begin the cascade.

Recombination – Process by which genetic material is rearranged during meiosis. Crossing over of genetic material between homologous chromosomes resulting in a complementary exchange. The resulting HLA haplotype is different from that of the original. The frequency of recombination is directly related to the distance between gene loci.

Reporter molecule – A molecule covalently attached to a base at one reaction site and available to react with a fluorochrome molecule at another reaction site.

Resident microbial flora – Microorganisms usually found at a particular body site of healthy individuals and remain at the site for long periods of time or indefinitely.

Resolution – Degree of detail that can be visualized at the microscope, on a physical map of DNA, or by any molecular technique.

Response phase – Effector functions following specific recognition of an antigen.

Restriction enzyme – Enzyme that cuts a DNA molecule at a specific, or restricted, site.

Restriction length-fragment polymorphism (rflp) – DNA segments of varying lengths generated by restriction enzyme digest; function is unknown.

Reticular dysgenesis – A severe form of SCID resulting from a defect in the hematopoietic stem cells and characterized by a lack of both lymphocytes and myeloid cells.

Reverse transcriptase – Enzyme technically known as RNA-dependent DNA polymerase; usually abbreviated "RT." This is an enzyme from retroviruses that will synthesize complementary DNA (cDNA) from an RNA template.

Reverse transcriptase PCR – The conversion of RNA template to complementary DNA (cDNA), then amplification of the cDNA by standard PCR.

Rheumatoid arthritis – Autoimmune disease characterized by chronic inflammation, swelling in the joints, and eventual destruction of the articular surfaces of the joints.

Rheumatoid factor – An IgM antibody directed against the Fc fragment of IgG and found most commonly in patients with rheumatoid arthritis.

Ribonuclease – A family of enzymes (abbreviated RNase) that will degrade RNA. These enzymes are resilient to damage, and must be controlled and/or eliminated when manipulating RNA for molecular tests.

Ribonucleic acid (RNA) – Nucleic acids required for protein translation.

Ribosomal RNA (rRNA) – Structural RNA within a ribosome.

Ribosome – Cellular organelle; site of protein synthesis.

RIST – Radioimmunosorbent test; an immunoassay that measures total serum IgE levels.

RNA polymerase – Enzyme that synthesizes RNA through the use of a DNA template.

RNase – Enzyme capable of degrading RNA.

► S

S protein – Regulator molecule that interferes with ability of C5b67 to bind to cell membrane.

Sarcoma – A tumor arising from connective tissue or muscle cells

Satellite – Repetitive sequences of DNA classified by base pair length.

Scleroderma – An autoimmune condition characterized by fibrosis and thickening of the skin.

Secondary immunodeficiency – Immune deficiencies that occur when damage is caused by an environmental factor. Radiation, chemotherapy, burns, and infections are example of conditions that may contribute to the many causes of secondary immune deficiencies.

Secretory piece – Also known as a secretory component. It is a glycoprotein that is associated with secretory IgA and secretory IgM. It is thought to provide the entire construct with resistance to proteolytic enzymes. These proteins facilitating passage across mucous membranes.

Self-antigen – Antigens of the body to which the immune system normally does not respond because of self-tolerance mechanisms.

Self-tolerance – The state in which an individual's immune system does not respond to its own antigens.

Semiconservative replication – Process responsible for replication of DNA; results in a new DNA molecule containing one newly synthesized strand and one strand from the parent molecule.

Sensitivity – *See* Clinical sensitivity.

Sequestered antigen – Antigens from specific anatomic sites (brain, testes, eye) that may be hidden from recognition by lymphocytes during fetal development.

Serum sickness – Type III (complex-mediated) hypersensitivity reaction caused by exposure to foreign proteins from animal sera.

Severe combined immunodeficiency (SCID) – Class of genetic disorders that affect both B and T lymphocytes.

Sex chromosome – Either the X or Y chromosomes in humans that determine the sex of individuals. Females have two X chromosomes and males have one X and one Y.

Side scatter – Light that has been deflected off of a cell as it passes through the laser beam. It is typically detected at a 90 degree angle to the axis of the laser beam. Side scatter is reflective of the complexity of the cell. Granular cytoplasm or a multilobed nucleus will result in more side scatter light.

Signal transduction – Intracellular process by the binding of a hormone to its receptor at the cell surface is transmitted to the nucleus.

Sjorgen's syndrome – An autoimmune condition characterized by dryness of the mouth and conjunctiva and enlargement of the parotid glands.

Specificity – *See* Clinical specificity.

Spectral karyotype (SKY) – An advanced method of identifying each chromosome by labeling whole chromosome probes for each chromosome a different color.

Split – HLA gene products sharing common epitopes. Defined when a previous (serologically defined) gene product is found to consist of several discrete products as the result of using more discriminating (molecular genetic) test procedures; HLA gene products that share common serologically define epitopes; finding that a previous gene product actually consists of several discrete gene products when using more discriminating molecular genetic procedures.

Spondyloarthropathies – Diseases characterized by inflammation. The site of the inflammation generally determines the disease subset. For example, AS involves the sacroiliac joints and spine, the skin (psoriatic arthritis), ulcerative colitis, Crohn's disease, and Reiter's disease.

Stem cells – Primitive cells that have the capacity of differentiating into functional cells that are committed to specific cell lines; an immature cell that is capable of self-renewal and repopulating a certain lineage(s) of mature cells.

Superantigen – An antigenic molecule capable of binding nonspecifically to both the MHC class II molecule and the T cell receptor.

Symbiosis – The relationship between species (host and organism) wherein both benefit from each other and the relationship.

Syndrome – A group of recognizable characteristics consistent with a particular specific disease.

Systemic autoimmune disease – Disease in which the autoantibody produced reacts to cellular components shared by many cells in the body, resulting damage to multiple organs.

Systemic lupus erythymatosus – autoimmune disease characterized serologically by the presence of antinuclear antibodies (RNA, DNA, and nuclear histone) and by deposits of immune complexes that affect multiple organs.

▶ **T**

Tandem repeats – Multiple copies of an identical DNA sequence repeated throughout a chromosome that is used as a marker in the physical mapping of the genome.

Tandem repeat sequence – Multiple copies of a sequence on a single chromosome usually oriented in the same direction.

Target – The specimen being probed.

Technical accuracy – The nearness of an individual measurement to the true value, as determined by a reference method. Sometimes referred to as test efficiency.

$$\frac{\text{Number of correct results}}{\text{Total number of results}} \times 100$$

T cell receptor (TCR) – antigen receptors on the surface of T cells. T cell receptors enable the cell to bind to and, if additional signals are present, to be activated by and respond to an epitope presented by another cell called the antigen-presenting cell or APC.

Telomere – A specialized structure at the ends of chromosomes that imparts stability to linear DNA, attaches to the nuclear membrane, and plays a role in replication.

Template (as it relates to nucleic acids) – A blueprint for the synthesis of other nucleic acid molecules. Sometimes referred to as the target of molecular-based reactions

T helper (T_H) lymphocytes (CD4+) – T lymphocytes that recognize antigens associated with MHC Class II molecules. The main function of these cells is to modulate the immune response by positively influencing the activity T and B cells and inducing suppressor/cytotoxic functions in CD8+ cells; cells that express CD4 and a T cell receptor on their surfaces and respond to antigen presentation by APCs.

Thermal cycler – An instrument that cycles rapidly to different temperatures; often used for PCR-based assays.

Thymus dependent antigens – Antigens that require mature B cell contact with T helper (T_H) cells for a response to occur.

Thymus independent antigens – Antigens that are able to activate B cells in the absence of T cells.

Titer – The concentration of antibody in serum.

Tm – The melting temperature; the temperature at which 50% of primer has annealed to its target. In order to promote better efficiency of primer annealing (i.e., greater than 50%), the annealing temperature is usually set at a lower temperature than the Tm (often 5° C lower).

Tolerance – A state of specific immunologic unresponsiveness.

Transcription – The synthesis of RNA from a DNA template; process by which mRNA is produced from the DNA template.

Transfer RNA (tRNA) – Group of RNA molecules responsible for conveying amino acids to the mRNA during translation.

Transferrin – A plasma protein that transport iron to the liver, spleen, and bone marrow through the blood.

Transient microbial flora – Microorganisms that reside at body sites for short periods of time, sometimes for days or weeks.

Translation – Process by which polypeptide chains are produced following an mRNA template.

Translocation – The movement of genetic material from one chromosome to another which requires at least two DNA breaks.

Trisomy – The presence of three copies of a particular chromosome instead of the normal two copies.

True pathogen – A microorganism capable of producing disease in both immune competent and immune compromised individuals.

T suppressor lymphocytes (CD8+) – T lymphocytes that recognize antigens associated with MHC Class I molecules. The main function of these cells is to modulate the immune system by decreasing antibody synthesis by B lymphocytes or interfering with the actions of antibody secreting B cells, lymphokine-producing and cytotoxic T cells, null cells, and monocytes.

Tumor-associated antigen (TAA) – An antigen expressed in a native or mutated form by a transformed cell that may also be found in association with normal tissues.

Tumor necrosis factor (TNF) – A cytokine produced by activated macrophages that causes a hemorrhagic necrosis of tumors in vivo while not affecting normal cells.

Tumor-specific antigen (TSA) – An antigen expressed only by a transformed cell and not by any normal tissues.

Tumor-specific transplantation antigen – An antigen that confers resistance to tumor transplantation by virtue of prior immunization.

Tumor suppressor gene – A gene whose product has the property of suppressing the activities of tumor cells. Examples include Rb gene and p53.

Type 1 diabetes mellitus – (insulin-dependent diabetes mellitus) Autoimmune disease in which the combination of lymphocytic infiltration and autoantibodies directed against the islet cells results in destruction of the insulin-producing cells of the pancreas, resulting in insufficient insulin-production.

Type I hypersensitivity – Anaphylactic hypersensitivity; immediate hypersensitivity mechanism involving production

of specific IgE antibodies that sensitize mast cells and basophils, leading to release of histamine and other chemical mediators that produce increased vaso-permeability, smooth muscle contractions, and mucous secretion.

Type IV hypersensitivity – Cell-mediated hypersensitivity; delayed hypersensitivity reaction in which activated T cells release cytokines that stimulate monocytes and polymorphonuclear cells to produce inflammation, granuloma formation, and tissue damage.

Type III hypersensitivity – Complex-mediated hypersensitivity; immediate hypersensitivity mechanism involving production of antigen-antibody complexes that activate complement, leading to chemotaxis of neutrophils, which produce tissue damage and inflammation through their release of lysosomal enzymes.

Type II hypersensitivity – Antibody-dependent cytotoxic hypersensitivity; immediate hypersensitivity reaction in which antibodies directed against a cell surface antigen participate in immunologic mechanisms leading to destruction of the cell or stimulation of the cell's function.

 U

Uniparental disomy – The inheritance of both chromosomes of a pair from the same parent.

Usual or indigenous microbial flora – Microorganisms that are usually found at body sites without causing disease; certain species may produce disease, given the opportunity or when the host's immune system is weakened.

 V

Vaccine – A preparation of killed or attenuated organisms for the purpose of active immunological prophylaxis; dead or attenuated pathogen used to induce an immune response and memory to that pathogen.

Validation – Upon completion of verification, demonstrating that the test is repeatedly giving the expected results over a period of time. This is an ongoing process that generates data to substantiate test algorithms or suggest modifications based on patient population or unique in vitro findings.

Variable region – The region in the immunoglobulin molecule that contains the antigen binding site; the region in an immunoglobulin molecule that shows many sequence differences between antibodies of different specificities.

Variolation – Early form of vaccination with intentional introduction of attenuated smallpox virus or cowpox virus.

Vector – DNA, from a virus, bacteria, yeast or a higher organism, which retains its self replicating ability after integration of a DNA sequence from a foreign source. Vectors infect host cells where they produce large quantities of the inserted DNA. Different size DNA segments can be produced in different vectors. Plasmids, cosmids, and yeast artificial chromosomes (YAC) are frequently used vectors.

Verification – The claims stipulated by the manufacturer in the package insert can be met. Includes performance characteristics such as sensitivity, specificity, positive and negative predictive values, precision, and accuracy. A one-time only process that is achieved before the test is implemented for patient care.

Virulence – The disease-producing ability of a microorganism.

 W

Whole chromosome paints – Fluorescent probe derived from unique and nonshared repetitive sequences that uniquely detect a single chromosome or chromosome arm.

Wiskott-Aldrich syndrome – A rare X-linked recessive immunodeficiency syndrome characterized by thrombocytopenia, eczema, and recurrent infections originally described by Wiskott. The manifestations of bloody diarrhea was added by Aldrich in 1954, with severe immunodeficiency and predisposition to malignancy being recognized subsequently.

 X

X-inactivation – Rearrangement of genes on one chromosome for immunoglobulin or T cell receptor inactivates rearrangement of corresponding genes on the second chromosome.

X-linked – A mutation in a gene occurring on the X-chromosome; affected individuals are predominantly male.

X-linked hyper IgM – Defect in class-switching associated with compensatory increased levels of IgM.

 Z

ZAP-70 – Mutations in the gene encoding this protein are associated with defective TCR-mediated signaling.

Answers to Learning Assessment Questions

CHAPTER 1
1. A
2. C
3. B
4. D
5. C

CHAPTER 2
1. D
2. D
3. E
4. B
5. C

CHAPTER 3
1. D
2. C
3. A
4. A
5. C
6. B
7. B
8. A
9. C
10. D
11. B
12. B

CHAPTER 4
1. C
2. D
3. B

4. C
5. C

CHAPTER 5
1. A
2. D
3. D
4. B
5. B
6. C
7. C
8. A
9. B
10. D
11. C
12. A

CHAPTER 6
1. A
2. C
3. C
4. B
5. C
6. D
7. B
8. D
9. A
10. D

CHAPTER 7
1. B
2. D

3. A
4. D
5. C

CHAPTER 8
1. A
2. B
3. D
4. A
5. C
6. C
7. TRUE
8. B
9. C
10. C

CHAPTER 9
1. C
2. A
3. B
4. D
5. A

CHAPTER 10
1. A
2. C
3. B
4. D
5. C

CHAPTER 11
1. Flow cytometry provides a rapid, precise, and objective method to enumerate cells compared with a microscopic-based method.
2. Monoclonal antibodies are immunoglobulins produce by an immortalized clone of B lymphocytes. They bind to one specific antigen and are thus useful for enumeration of cells that express unique antigens for which a monoclonal antibody is available.
3. A histogram is used to display single intrinsic or extrinsic parameter distribution. A dual parameter dot plot displays the expression of two parameters of interest.
4. The absolute CD4 lymphocyte count is the product of the proportion of CD4+ cells in the lymphocyte population and the absolute lymphocyte count. In this example the absolute CD4 count is 190 cells/ul. The other

cells types in the lymphocyte gate include CD8 positive T lymphocytes, B lymphocytes, and NK cells.

5. The viability of the small should be assessed as a sample this old may have a low cell viability.

CHAPTER 12

1. Refer to the section on transcription, translation, and replication for a description of how mRNA and protein are produced in cells.

2. Refer to the section on differences between prokaryotic and eukaryotic cells and applications of hybridization techniques.

CHAPTER 13
1. B
2. D
3. C
4. B
5. A
6. D
7. B
8. D
9. B
10. A

CHAPTER 14
1. C
2. D
3. C
4. A
5. C
6. B
7. D
8. A
9. D
10. B
11. C
12. B
13. D
14. A
15. A

CHAPTER 15
1. B
2. A
3. B
4. D
5. A

Index